AF147973

MEDICAL RADIOLOGY
Diagnostic Imaging

Editors:
A. L. Baert, Leuven
K. Sartor, Heidelberg

Springer-Verlag Berlin Heidelberg GmbH

G. H. Mostbeck (Ed.)

Duplex and Color Doppler Imaging of the Venous System

With Contributions by

M. Baldt · R. Dorffner · F. Fobbe · S. Grampp · N. Gritzmann · C. B. Henk · A. Hollerweger
F. Karnel · C. Kollmann · R. Kubale · J. Liskutin · P. Macheiner · M. Merz · G. H. Mostbeck
G. Nics · T. Rettenbacher · K.-H. Seitz · G. Strasser · K. Vergesslich · H. P. Weskott
T. Zontsich

Foreword by

A. L. Baert

With 149 Figures in 294 Separate Illustrations, 136 in Color and 27 Tables

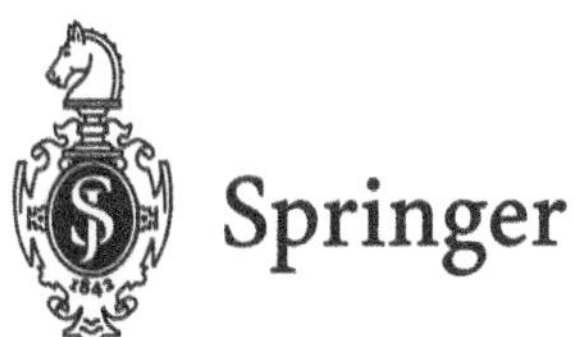

Springer

Gerhard H. Mostbeck, MD
Professor of Radiology
Department of Radiology
Sozialmedizinisches Zentrum Baumgartner Höhe mit Pflegezentrum
Otto Wagner Spital
Sanatoriumstrasse 2
1140 Vienna
Austria

Medical Radiology · Diagnostic Imaging and Radiation Oncology
Series Editors: A. L. Baert · L. W. Brady · H.-P. Heilmann · M. Molls · K. Sartor

Continuation of
Handbuch der medizinischen Radiologie
Encyclopedia of Medical Radiology

ISBN 978-3-540-64168-1

Library of Congress Cataloging-in-Publication Data

Duplex and color doppler imaging of the venous system / G. H. Mostbeck (ed.).
p. cm. -- (Medical radiology)
Includes bibliographical references and index.
ISBN 978-3-540-64168-1 ISBN 978-3-642-18589-2 (eBook)
DOI 10.1007/978-3-642-18589-2
1. Blood-vessels--Ultrasonic imaging. 2. Doppler ultrasonography. 3. Blood-vessels--Diseases--Diagnosis. I. Mostbeck, G. H. (Gerhard H.), 1956- II. Series
RC691.6.U47D87 2003
616.1'307543--dc21 2003042533

http//www.springeronline.com

Originally published by Springer-Verlag Berlin Heidelberg New York in 2004

Cover-Design and Typesetting: Verlagsservice Teichmann, 69256 Mauer

21/3150xq – 5 4 3 2 1 0 – Printed on acid-free paper

Foreword

The human venous system has, in the past, not always attracted the same attention and interest from radiologists as the arterial system. Nevertheless, some of the pathologic conditions of the venous system are either frequently seen in daily practice such as varicosis of the lower extremity, or may relate to more severe and even life-threatening conditions, for instance deep venous thrombosis or liver venous pathology.

However, enormous progress has been achieved during the past decade in the field of duplex and color Doppler imaging necessitating an update in our knowledge of these techniques.

For both reasons, a volume specifically dealing with duplex and color Doppler imaging of the venous system was considered an appropriate addition to the series Medical Radiology – Diagnostic Imaging.

I would like to thank Prof. Mostbeck for his outstanding performance as the editor of this work. I would like to congratulate him and the many contributing authors, all renowned experts in the field, on their comprehensive coverage of the different topics, the up-to-date contents and the superb illustrations.

I strongly believe that this book will encounter the same success as previous volumes published in this series.

Leuven

ALBERT L. BAERT

Preface

Real-time ultrasound has been in clinical use now for more than 30 years. The addition of the pulsed Doppler technique (duplex scanning) and of various color Doppler techniques (color duplex Doppler technique, CDDS) aroused interest in gaining information on normal and disturbed blood flow in arteries and veins. Today, CDDS is a well-established diagnostic tool and is employed not only by radiologists, but by obstetricians, gastroenterologists, surgeons and others in their subspecialties.

However, Prof. Albert Baert's offer to edit a comprehensive textbook on CDDS of the venous system was an challenging opportunity. This book is intended for all who are interested in and confronted by clinical problems regarding various aspects of pathology of the venous system. As reflected by the authors of the chapters, who include radiologists, gastroenterologists and internists, this book is not exclusively intended for the radiologic community.

Nevertheless, it may be easier for those whose background is in the interpretation of images to fully comprehend the dynamic and "functional" significance of Doppler information. In CDDS, probably more than in other ultrasound areas, an appreciation of the physical principles, the examination technique and the hemodynamics and pathophysiology of flow in the venous system is indispensable. This mandatory information is provided in the opening chapters of this book. These are followed by chapters covering CDDS aspects of venous imaging "from neck to toe". Each chapter is primarily intended to answer frequently asked questions, but covers variant anatomy, rare findings and specific problems where necessary. Findings are illustrated by figures obtained with state-of-the-art CDDS machines.

CDDS of the venous system is challenged by various other imaging techniques. Whereas invasive procedures like cavography will soon be outdated for mere diagnostic purposes, modern spiral computed tomography and magnetic resonance venography are excellent diagnostic tools. However, there are superficial veins like those in the neck, the extremities or the scrotum, where the superb contrast and spatial resolution of real-time US and the excellent temporal resolution of Doppler techniques make CDDS the main imaging modality. Regarding abdominal and retroperitoneal veins and their related pathology, CDDS techniques are preferable when examination conditions are excellent, which unfortunately is not always the case. In addition, CDDS of the veins provides unique information on pathologic conditions of other organs, such as the heart. And with regard to radiation protection, the Council Directive 97/43 Euratom of the European Union defines aspects of justification, optimization and responsibilities of medical exposure in favor of techniques without radiation exposure like CDDS.

This book would not have been possible – surprise! – without the work of all authors and co-authors. Many thanks to all of them, but with special emphasis on those who supplied their chapters promptly only to have to update them later. My special gratitude to Prof. Baert for his patience and to Ursula Davis of Springer for her continuous support and belief in this book. Many thanks to the other staff of Springer for their generous help and editorial work; it was an excellent cooperation as seen from my side! I want to extend special thanks to RT Birgit Kloos and RT Maria Markhart for "US modeling" for this book. Last, but not least, I am grateful to my family, Dr. Nicole Grois, Luise and Leonie, for their loving patience with a frequently absent husband and father.

Vienna GERHARD H. MOSTBECK

Contents

1 Basic Principles and Physics of Duplex and Color Doppler Imaging

C. Kollmann

CONTENTS

Introduction

Doppler ultrasound has been used in medicine since the mid-1970s, mainly for the diagnosis of vascular disease like occlusion or stenosis (Keller et al. 1975; Fitzgerald et al. 1977; Weaver et al. 1980; Brown et al. 1982). The first systems developed were based on the continuous-wave (CW) spectral Doppler ultrasound technique with separate transmitter and receiver elements (Brody et al. 1974; Di Pietro et al. 1978). In 1983, pulsed-wave (PW) color Doppler imaging (CDI) systems were introduced clinically for color coding the detected blood flow in real-time (Atkinson et al. 1982). In the past, these early CDI systems were restricted to an evaluation of only a few well-defined medical indications in cardiac disease where the blood velocity is very high. A newer generation of CDI systems has allowed us, since 1986, to detect and display lower blood velocities occurring in peripheral arteries or veins (Kasai et al. 1985; Merritt et al. 1987; Klews 1987; Scoutt et al. 1990). The conventional CDI systems and the newer methods with their different signal processing algorithms (power Doppler, harmonic imaging) evaluate the blood velocity as a consequence of the Doppler effect (Fig. 1.1). Another method that has been clinically available since 1990 is the direct cal-

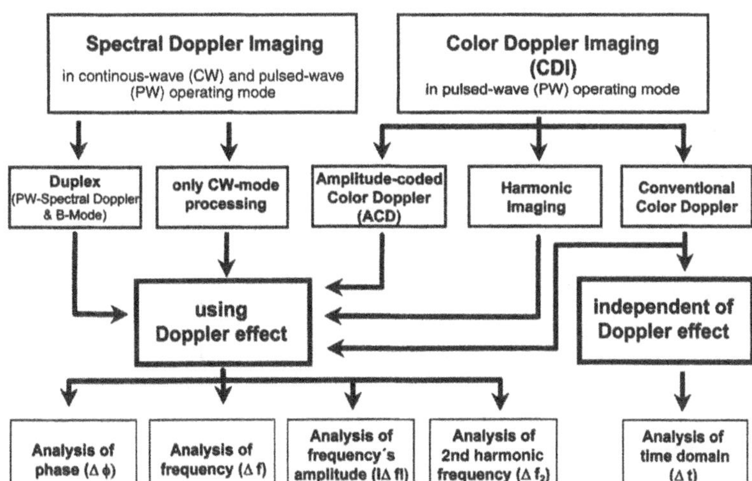

Fig. 1.1. Doppler imaging techniques and the physical principles for detecting blood flow

C. Kollmann, PhD
Department of Biomedical Engineering & Physics, AKH Vienna, Währinger Gürtel 18–20, 1090 Vienna, Austria

culation of the blood velocity using a time domain analysis (Bonnefous et al. 1986; Klews 1991). With this technique, the change of the position of the moving red blood cells between two pulse intervals is detected and used for further signal processing steps (Fig. 1.1).

In contrast to CW Doppler systems, CDI systems were introduced to clinical routine applications rapidly, and the number of systems available in clinics was very large from the beginning (Schneider et al. 1993).

Familiarity with the basic principles of Doppler ultrasound is essential for its proper clinical use and an optimal diagnosis.

CW-Doppler
receiving element
transmitting element
$f_{receive}$
v
depth
α
v
Doppler sample volume
$f_{transmit}$
in both images : $f_{receive} > f_{transmit}$
a

PW-Doppler

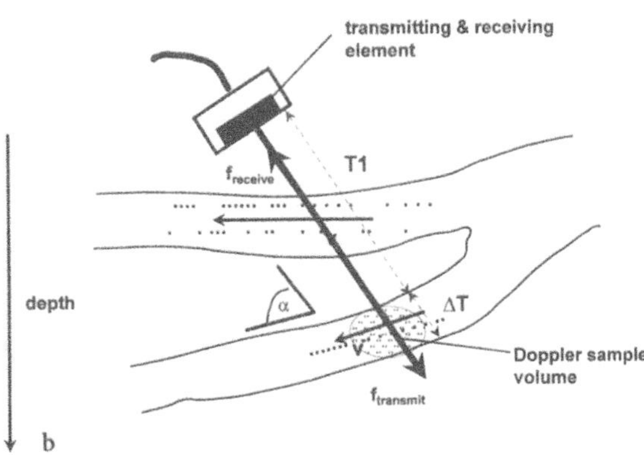

Fig. 1.2a,b. The techniques to acquire flow information from CW and PW Doppler by using the Doppler effect

1.1 Duplex Systems

The simplest technique for detecting blood flow in real-time is a CW Doppler system consisting of two elements for transmitting the frequency signal continuously ($f_{transmit} \approx$ 2–10 MHz) and receiving a frequency signal ($f_{receive}$) modulated by the Doppler effect according to

$$\Delta f = f_{receive} - f_{transmit} = \frac{2f_{transmit}}{c}\cos(\ ) \tag{1}$$

where Δf is the Doppler shift frequency, v the velocity of the erythrocytes, c=1540 m/s, and α the angle between the incident ultrasound beam and the direction of the blood flow (Fig. 1.2a). In the transducer, the two narrow band elements are arranged in a way that both ultrasound beams overlap to provide a small Doppler sample volume. From this volume, the frequency signal of the receiving element is modulated by the moving red blood cells (RBC). This signal is amplified and fed into a demodulator that compares the detected frequency with that from an oscillator to derive a signal difference equal to the Doppler shift frequency Δf. Most demodulators employ a technique called *phase quadrature detection*, which has the capacity to distinguish between blood flow towards or away from the transducer corresponding to a higher or lower received frequency, respectively. This bi-directional demodulation produces two output signals that have a phase relationship determined by the direction of flow. After high-pass filtering, typically in the range 50–250 Hz to reduce low-frequency noise but also low velocities (Fig. 1.3), a stereo audio signal is produced that can be fed to the loudspeakers, headphones, or displayed graphically. The audio signal of each stereo channel varies depending on the selected Doppler angle, transmitted frequency, and RBC velocity and is normally below 20 KHz (Table 1.1).

CW Doppler is a highly sensitive tool for detecting the weak signals preferred for the examinations of smaller vessels like supraorbital arteries and veins or for ophthalmic and transcranial applications. Also, higher velocities than with PW Doppler systems can be monitored, and the effect of aliasing does not occur. The disadvantage with this technique which has led to it being displaced in most clinical diagnostic applications by PW Doppler techniques is the missing depth information of the detected Doppler signal. Because CW Doppler transmits its signal continuously, no run-time information can be used to identify the depth of the origin in the sample volume from which the received signal came (Fig. 1.2a). A CW Doppler

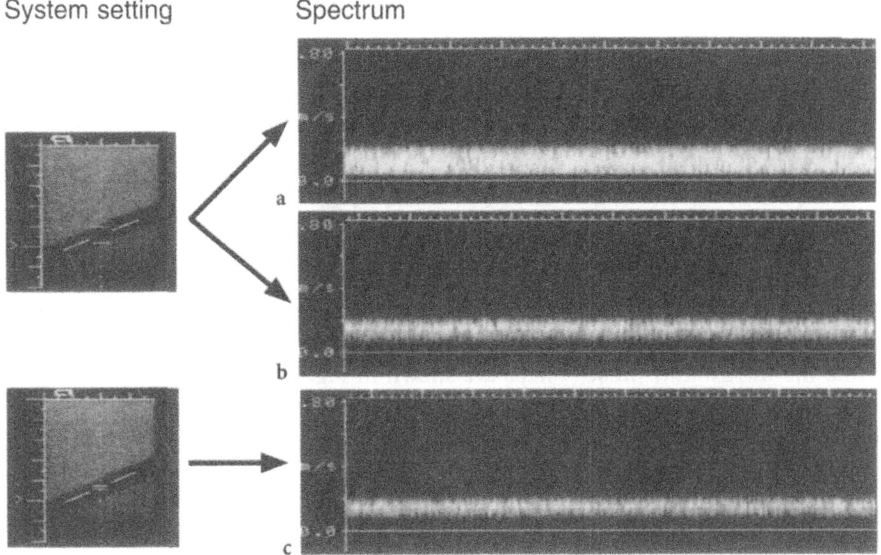

Fig. 1.3a–c. Influence of the sample gate size and the wall-filter settings for PW Doppler spectral analysis measuring small flow velocities. **a** The sample gate is chosen large enough to cover the whole diameter of the vessel, and the wall-filter frequency is minimized (*small black gap* between zero-line and signal). The spectrum appears correct with a broad velocity distribution. **b** The wall-filter frequency is changed to its maximum value. The parts of low velocities are not displayed any more in the spectrum (*black gap*). **c** Additional to **b**, the sample gate size is minimized. This leads to a weaker spectrum. Only the velocities of a special vessel region are detected, i.e., the velocity distribution scanned is not as wide as the whole vessel diameter

Table 1.1. Theoretically derived Doppler shift frequencies in selected arterial and venous vessels (Taylor et al. 1988; Hennerici and Neuerburg-Heusler 1999; Seitz and Kubale 1988; Philips 1989) for an incident 45o ultrasound beam and three different transmit frequencies

	Diameter (cm)	Max $v_{syst.}$ (cm/s)	v_{mean} (cm/s)	RI	PI	Doppler shift frequency f [Hz] for $f_{transmit}$ of		
						3.5 MHz	5.0 MHz	7.5 MHz
Aorta	1.4–1.6	90–140			2–6	2892–4500	4132–6428	6199–9642
A. carotis communis	0.5–0.7	43–150	10–40	0.6–0.7		1382–4821	1974–6887	2962–10331
A. carotis interna		32–100	28–45	0.5–0.6		1028–3214	1469–4592	2204–6887
A. vertebralis		41–70	22–44			1318–2250	1882–3214	2824–4821
A. lienalis								
A. hepatica								
A. femoralis communis	0.6–0.9	116–166	8–24		5–10	3728–5335	5326–7622	7989–11433
A. femoralis superficialis	0.4–0.7	79–107	8–21			2539–3439	3627–4913	5441–7369
A. mesenterica superior	0.6–0.8	120–220		0.7–0.9	2.8–3.5	3857–7071	5510–10102	8265–15152
V. cava	1.0–1.8		7–18			225–579*	321–826*	482–1240*
V. portae	0.7–1.1	18–33	12–18			578–1061	826–1515	1240–2273
V. lienalis	0.4–0.8		6–17			193–546*	275–781*	413–1171*
Vv. hepaticae	0.4–0.8		5–11			161–354*	230–505*	344–758*
V. renalis	0.3–0.6		6–16			193–514*	275–735*	413–1102*

PI: pulsatility index, RI: resistance index, $v_{syst.}$: systolic velocity, v_{mean}: mean velocity
*Data from v_{mean}

technique is therefore not very helpful if many vessels are present in the region of interest. But in the early days of ultrasound Doppler or in low-cost systems where no Duplex technique is available, i.e., to locate the origin of flow within the B-mode image, this CW technique was used to detect blood vessels in a simple and easy way.

1.1.1 PW Doppler (Duplex System)

CW and PW Doppler are equal in the manner of signal post-processing and displaying the spectral results but different in signal generation. In PW Doppler systems, pulsed ultrasound waves are emitted with the same active element that is used for detection (Fig. 1.2b). Therefore, the electronic controller of a PW Doppler system has to switch between transmission and receiving mode. After the first short pulse sequence has been emitted, the system switches to the receiving mode and detects the reflected ultrasound waves after a time T_1 for a certain time interval Δt, then the electronics switches back to transmission mode and emits the next pulse sequence. The time T_1 is assigned to the selected scanning depth (sample volume start position), i.e., twice the time the ultrasound pulse needs to hit the Doppler targets, while during ΔT all the echoes with Doppler information are detected within a specific sample volume size. The maximum possible Doppler pulse repetition frequency (PRF_{max}) of the system is hence dependent on the time period of $T_1 + \Delta T$. According to the Nyquist theorem, the maximum frequency that can be detected without aliasing, that is unambiguously, at this depth is

$$f_{\max} \leq \frac{1}{2} PRF_{\max} \tag{2}$$

If this limit is not exceeded, a PW Doppler system can determine the position of the moving RBCs, and after quadrature signal processing of the echoes, the information about the direction and velocity of the blood flow can be given (Fig. 1.2b).

For all systems that are based on the Doppler effect, this quadrature detector is a key component in the signal processing chain. In this detector, the analog echo signals are mixed with a reference signal from an oscillator (Fig. 1.4) to get information about the flow direction. The final result of this process consists of two different signals, the in-put or cosine component (I-signal) and the quadrature or sine component of the signal (Q-signal) with respect to the reference signal. The I-signal includes the temporal velocity information of the RBC echoes coming towards the transducer, while the Q-signal includes the particle's temporal velocity information flowing away from the transducer. The next signal processing steps are shown in Fig. 1.4. The I- and Q-signals are analog/digitally converted (A/D), and the low-velocity components are removed by a moving target indicator. This can be done in the simplest way by a high-pass filter (wall filter).

Afterwards, the velocity itself of both signal components must be determined. This can be done by phase analysis (Fig. 1.4) or by a discrete Fourier analysis (DFT) of the frequency shift signals (Fig. 1.5). In the first spectral PW Doppler systems, a phase detection algorithm was implemented. In the following, the signal processing of the I-component is considered to describe the function of this detector. The same process is carried out for the Q-component. In the phase detector, the signal ($signal_I$) is compared with a reference signal ($signal_{ref}$). If two waves with the same amplitude but different frequency start with the same phase angle (Φ=0) at a specific time (Fig. 1.4), $signal_{ref}$ with the higher frequency will propagate faster than $signal_I$. The phase angle Φ_{ref} is at a specific moment higher than Φ_I. That means that the wave with the shorter

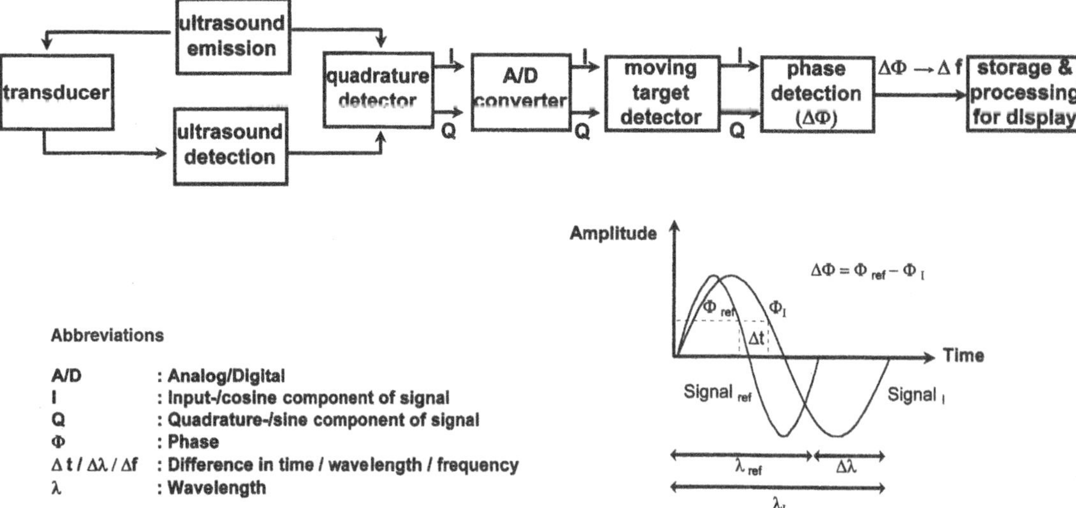

Fig. 1.4. Block diagram showing the modules used for deriving the phase shift information from detected signals in PW spectral Doppler systems

wavelength (λ_{ref}) reaches a particular phase earlier than the wave with the longer wavelength (λ_I). For this reason, it is possible to determine the phase shift ($\Delta\Phi$) and consequently the frequency shift (Δf) or the difference of wavelength ($\Delta\lambda$) by comparing either signal's phases. Now the temporal distribution of the velocity of the RBCs within the sample volume is derived by using Eq. 1 before this information is stored and processed for a spectral display. This flow information in combination with an overlaid B-mode image is known as the spectral Duplex technique. For a rough estimate, the maximum detectable velocities of these systems are proportional to the ratio between PRF_{max} and $f_{transmit}$. The estimated RBC velocities of these systems are only calculated and displayed correctly if the correction of the Doppler angle (α, Fig. 1.2), that can be set with a graphical symbol manually beforehand in the system, takes place in the right way. The errors of the velocity values are relatively low as long as the angle is between 10° and 60°. Other angle settings can lead to severe over- or underestimation of the real velocity and hence, in special cases where an absolute velocity information is needed, to an incorrect diagnosis. For the determination of the pulsatility (PI) or resistance (RI) indices, the Doppler angle is not so critical (Merrit 1991; Haerten and Mück 1992).

1.2 Color Doppler Imaging Based on Doppler Effect

In modern PW Doppler systems, not only the spectral display of the detected flow characteristics is available but also a color presentation. This is known as color Doppler imaging and is often used as a first orientation, whether flow can be detected in the scanned area or not, before a more specialized diagnosis of the flow follows. The presence of flow, its direction, speed, and type (e.g., laminar or turbulent) is indicated in special color schemes with hues, saturations, and brightnesses.

This chapter gives a survey of the basic principles of the favorite methods that are used today in these systems. Not only the frequency shift information (conventional color Doppler) from the echoes can be post-processed for a color representation, but also the strength of the amplitude of this frequency shift (amplitude-coded color Doppler) or the second harmonic of this frequency shift (harmonic imaging, Fig. 1.1). With the last two new methods, Doppler ultrasound has particularly pushed forward in regions that could not be evaluated or displayed with the conventional method before: Low flows in capillaries as well as the vascularity of tumors can be detected now.

1.2.1 Conventional Color Doppler Imaging

In conventional CDI, the signal processing is equal to the spectral Doppler mode (Fig. 1.5). A PW Doppler system emits a relatively long pulse sequence along a scan-line that can be steered by the user. A single gate within the sample volume (Fig. 1.6) is used to acquire the Doppler frequency shift data. In CDI, several gates per scan-line and within the same sample volume are implemented (Fig. 1.6). Each of these gates is capable of detecting Doppler signals at a time. In CDI, many parallel channels are connected to the input of the

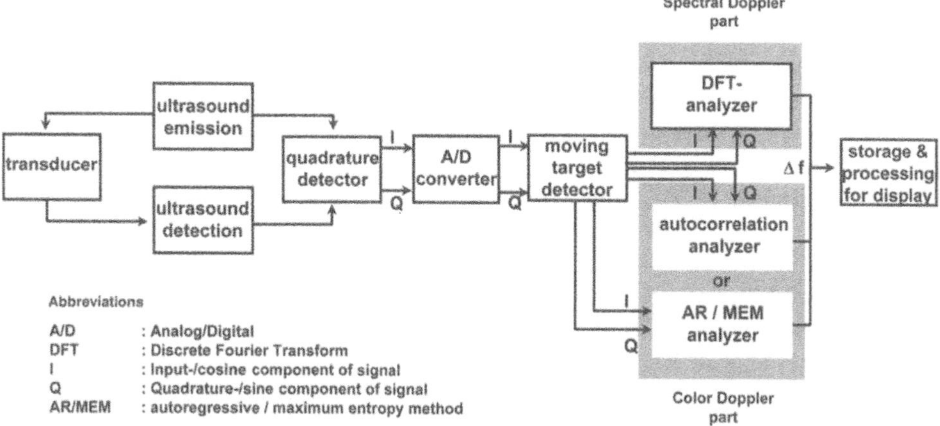

Fig. 1.5. Block diagram showing the technique and the modules used for deriving the frequency shift information from detected signals of real-time blood flow mapping systems

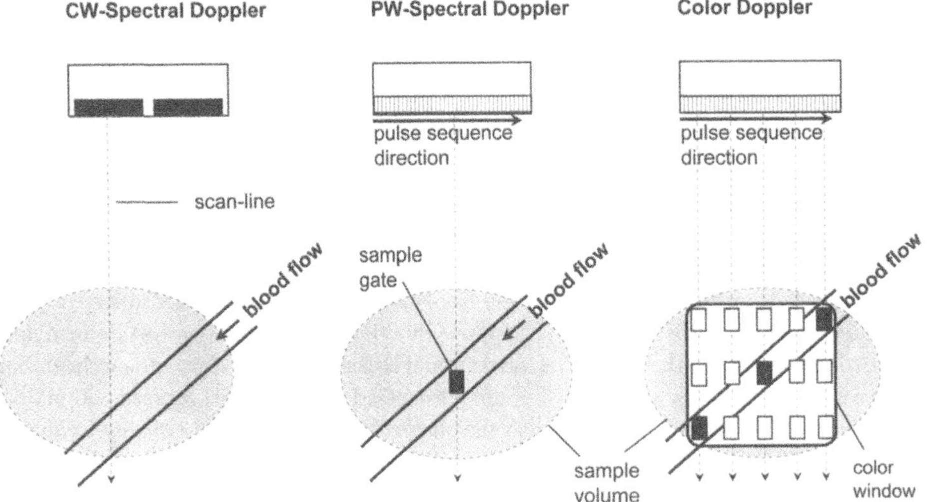

Fig. 1.6. Number and distribution of the sample volume gates for the different Doppler techniques. While the PW spectral Doppler has got only one sample gate, on modern CDI systems there are several gates per scan-line where the velocity is measured for a color-coded representation

quadrature detector, and a large number of Doppler signals have to be processed simultaneously to derive a velocity profile and the spatial velocity distribution across the vessel lumen. Typically, 16–32 gates with approximately 1 mm axial length are available in a modern CDI system (Burns 1987). This causes a timing problem because the ultrasound beam must be stationary for a short time period at each scan-line to collect the Doppler signals. If many parallel channels exist, real-time processing of flow data by discrete Fourier analysis cannot be managed. To obtain the Doppler flow information along a large number of scan-lines and in real time, another method must be used.

The autocorrelation analyzer serves exactly this function (Fig. 1.5). After real-time quadrature detection, the phase information curve of the I- and Q-components from each scan-line is periodical. If the I/Q-components are transferred to an I/Q-diagram (Fig. 1.7), their signal amplitudes can be symbolized by a vector with length L and direction Φ. During different time points (T, 2T, ..), these vectors L are derived. In the autocorrelator, the particular temporal vectors are now multiplied: The I- and Q-components of these signals are multiplied with components from the same line but from a previous pulse (time delay). For a first output of the autocorrelator, 4–16 vector multiplications are used. After this process, there is a resulting vector of length **R** and direction $\overline{\Delta\Phi}$ (Fig. 1.7). From the resulting average phase shift angle $\overline{\Delta\Phi}$, the average Doppler frequency shift $\overline{\Delta f}$. f can be derived easily (as shown for duplex systems earlier). According to Eq. 1, this Doppler frequency shift is proportional to the average flow velocity $\overline{v}$. While the length of the vector **R** is not used for further signal processing, the size and the sign of $\overline{\Delta\Phi}$ are stored and give an estimation in the color image of the average speed and direction of the flow velocity. The standard deviations of particularly DF_i in relation to $\overline{\Delta\Phi}$ are used in the signal processing chain as a unit for flow stability and can be considered an indicator for turbulence.

Because of this way of signal processing, the problem of clutter or motion artifacts is severe in such a CDI system. The echoes of the erythrocytes are 100–1000 times weaker than those of solid targets (e.g., vessel walls) that are stretched by the pulsatility effect and as a result are moving slowly. This effect can inhibit the detection of the weaker Doppler shift echoes. The digital filtering algorithms implemented in the moving target detector or indicator (MTI) of a CDI system to discriminate between blood and tissue are highly sophisticated and averaged over frames to eliminate these clutter artifacts.

In a final step, the color information is overlaid on the B-mode image, creating a real-time color flow mapping system.

The detection of blood flow and its presentation in color can be manually set up using special boxes, the color windows. These windows contain the scan-lines for the color representation process (Fig. 1.6), and their shape can be changed by electronically steering the ultrasound beam coming out of the transducer. Modern transducer technologies with electronic beam steering (phased-array), electronic switching

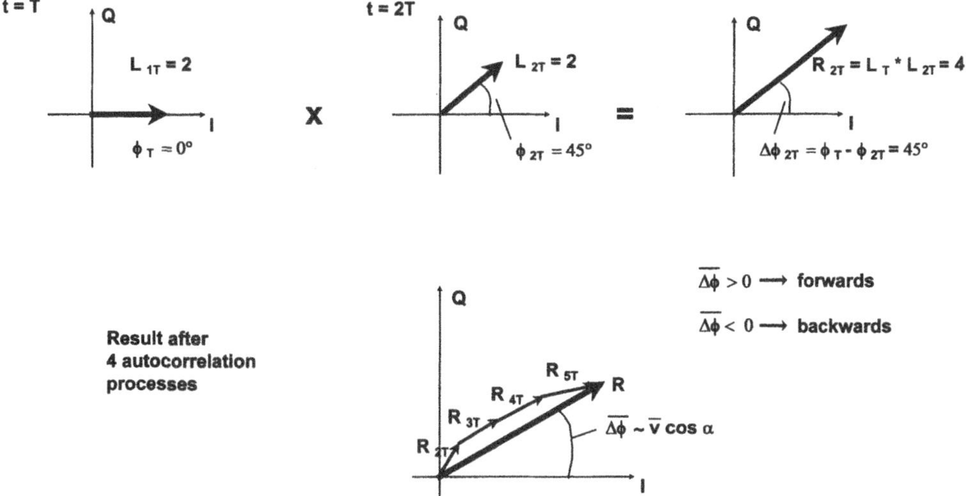

Fig. 1.7. Schematic view of an autocorrelation process. A detailed explanation of the autocorrelation is given in the section on Conventional Color Doppler Imaging

beams (linear-array), or a combination of both techniques can do this well.

Depending on the width, height, and position of this window within the scanned B-mode region, the frame rate (FR), i.e., the number of refreshing cycles of the flow information displayed on the monitor per second, changes. The larger and deeper a color window is set, the lower is the frame rate of the CDI system normally:

$$FR_{CDI} \quad \frac{PRF}{SL \quad N} \tag{3}$$

where PRF is the pulse repetition frequency, *SL* is the number of scan-lines in the color window, and *N* the number of pulses per color line.

If low flows are going to be detected with a CDI system, the PRF is decreased, and as a consequence according to Eq. 3, the frame rate is low (only several Hz). This effect can be sometimes recognized as flickering of the color information update on the monitor.

Another technique that is used for flow signal processing is the maximum entropy method (MEM). It is an autoregressive (AR) technique for spectral density analysis and maximizes the uncertainty, or entropy, of a time series expressed as an autocorrelation sequence. In some newer Doppler systems, this AR processing technique is implemented parallel to the other analyzer modules (Fig. 1.5). Some advantages of the AR technique are its real-time processing method and under certain circumstances its detection of lower flow velocities than with the other CDI techniques (Sohn et al. 1996; Battle et al. 1997).

All CDI methods and their accurate velocity presentation are influenced, of course, by aliasing and the Doppler angle.

The color represents only a single Doppler parameter and does not describe the full Doppler frequency spectrum. However, a spectral analysis (with PW Doppler) has more potential for a diagnosis than the pure color mode and should be preferred.

1.2.2 Amplitude-Coded Color Doppler Imaging (Power Doppler)

In the early 1990s, a new signal processing technique was introduced to internal medical investigations called power Doppler, UltrasoundAngio, color Doppler energy or amplitude-coded CDI (ACD; Rubin et al. 1993/1994; Preidler et al. 1995; Giovagnorio et al. 1995).

This technique encodes the amplitude of the power spectral density of the detected Doppler signal rather than the mean Doppler frequency shift (velocity and direction information) of conventional CDI ultrasound systems. Hence the information of an ACD image and its interpretation are fundamentally different: Neither velocity nor direction information of the blood flow is available, only the strength of the reflected Doppler signal amplitude is color coded, which is sometimes called the 'energy' of the Doppler signal.

However, this technique has opened new areas of clinical applications: Detecting slow blood flows or perfusion in renal blood vessels or kidneys represents only a few examples of many important clinical uses (TURETSCHEK et al. 1998).

Modern CDI systems already have the potential for an upgrade to an ACD system if they contain an autocorrelation analyzer (Fig. 1.5).

The Doppler frequency shift signals are complex functions in a mathematical sense (the I-component corresponds to the real part, the Q-component to the imaginary part of the signal). This simplifies and shortens the signal processing in the complex autocorrelation module to get an average value for the Doppler frequency shift $\overline{\Delta f}$ in real-time:

$$\overline{\Delta f} \quad \overline{\Delta \Phi} = \tan^{-1} \frac{ACF_{im}}{ACF_{re}} \tag{4}$$

where ACF_{im} is the imaginary part, ACF_{re} the real part of the complex autocorrelation function.

This is the information displayed by conventional CDI systems.

In an ACD system, the complex autocorrelation function ACF (t) and the results of Eq. 4 are needed for certain time points t to calculate the power spectral density $P(\Delta f)$ using the Wiener-Khintchine theorem:

$$P(f) = \int_{-\bullet}^{\bullet} ACF(t)\, e^{2\, i f t}\, dt \tag{5}$$

This means that the Fourier transformation of the autocorrelation function is equal to the power spectral density function. Equation 5 is the mathematical description of this relationship, but in ACD systems, an integration from minus infinity to infinity cannot be performed in real-time. The solution to this problem is to replace the integration by a summation of the echo signals that are detected from all transmitted scan-lines. This can be done in real-time regardless of the large number of calculations necessary for creating only one image frame.

Figure 1.8 shows a plot of the power spectral density vs frequency. The integral over the slanted-fill curve (area) is the information that is finally displayed with ACD. The power spectral density measured at the ordinate is the squared amplitude of the signal. In ACD systems, noise has a different representation over the frequency range. After performing the autocorrelation and calculating the power spectral density, noise signals have an uniform distribution, which is quite different from CDI. It can be seen from the figure that this integral is smaller than that from the signal curve and has an uniform distribution over frequency. Therefore, noise detection can be achieved easily in ACD.

Another difference in ACD is that it does not distinguish between positive and negative frequency or phase shifts like conventional CDI does (information of flow direction). All echoes from positive and negative shift components are summarized and displayed as if coming from only one flow direction. This sum-

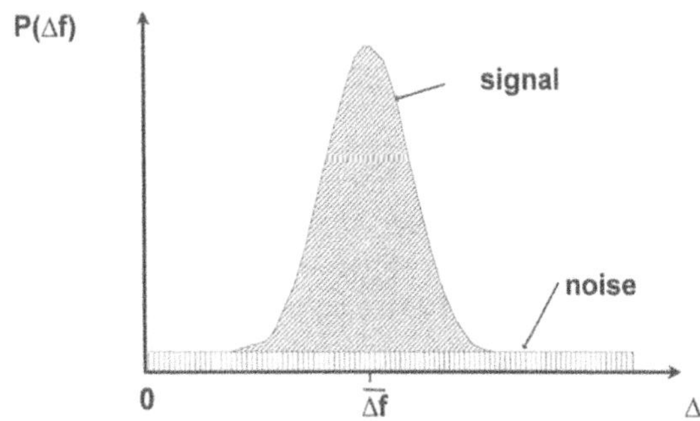

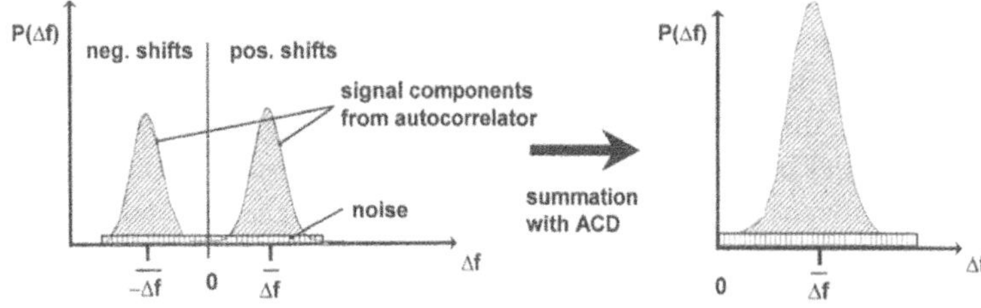

Fig. 1.8. The power spectral density function and its use in ACD systems (from Kollmann et al. 1998, with permission)

mation increases the amplitude of the final signal, as shown schematically in Fig. 1.8b.

The ACD as well as the CDI technique color codes only the flow information because this is the only information available from the moving target detector after eliminating all static echo information.

After the autocorrelation process, the level of noise is lower and totally uniform over the frequency scale compared with the flow signal. Hence, it is easy to separate these two signals and perform a different color coding. While the real flow information is coded in yellow or red colors depending on the signal amplitude, the noise signal gets an uniform color. The signal returning from a region of interest is attenuated by the adjacent tissue on its way back to the transducer, and the height of the signal amplitude decreases with increasing depth of the areas of interest. Less attenuated signals measured with ACD systems have brighter colors than more highly attenuated signals if the system settings are equal and if the same fractional blood volume is moving through the sample volume. The displayed power spectral density distribution is a measure of the amount of the blood volume moving within the considered region.

This color information is mixed with the gray-scale information of the scanned region from the B-mode part of the system before it is displayed.

The influence of the Doppler angle is much less than with conventional CDI. If the incidence beam coming from the transducers changes, the mean Doppler frequency shift will change, but not the power spectral density of the signal. The shape of the frequency distribution (Fig. 1.8) varies, but not the value of the integral (area) of this distribution. However, basically, the ACD technique is not independent of the Doppler angle. Flow signals with a mean Doppler frequency shift around zero (Doppler angle $\approx 90°$) are interpreted as stationary signals coming from soft tissue. The algorithms of the moving target detector suppress these signal components, and no color can be coded to these flow signals. Due to the fact that spectral broadening caused by aperture effects is always present, this effect is eliminated, and a flow can be displayed (NEWHOUSE and REID 1991).

Another effect known as aliasing or 'wrap-around' artifact does not occur, although the flow velocity detected exceeds the Nyquist limit (Eq. 2). The ACD technique evaluates the integral of the power spectrum and not the mean Doppler frequency shift itself, which is influenced by the system's PRF. The value of the integral remains unaffected whether or not the signal wraps around.

Apart from the above properties, ACD should be more sensitive to slow flow velocities than CDI, for the following reasons:

- Amplitude estimations are inherently less noisy than estimations of the mean Doppler frequency shift, particularly if wide-band transducers are used.
- The amplitude of the signal from pulsatile blood flow changes less from image frame to image frame compared with the frequency of the signal from blood because the amplitude does not depend on the velocity of the blood and is therefore not dependent on pulsatility.
- However, the main reason for the enhanced sensitivity is that the ACD technique treats noise differently than flow signals. The noise is displayed in such a way that it is possible to increase the usable dynamic range of the flow signal by extending the range down to the system's electronic noise floor. This increase can, in total, increase the sensitivity to blood flow. In the literature, a three- to five-fold increase of the sensitivity has been reported (BABCOCK et al. 1996; YAMADA et al. 1995). A wider dynamic range obtained with this technique means that slower flow velocities can be detected. Some clinical and in vitro investigations document that increased sensitivity is achieved only under special circumstances but cannot be achieved in all clinical applications (YAMADA et al. 1995; TURETSCHEK et al. 1995; KOLLMANN et al. 1995; SOHN et al. 1996).

In combination with other techniques (3D imaging) and special tools (contrast agents), ACD imaging seems to be a very powerful method for displaying perfusion in very small vessels with very slow flow velocities (see previous section).

1.2.3 Harmonic Imaging

A problem of Doppler imaging during scan processes is the presence of motion artifacts from vessel walls by pulsatility that cannot be suppressed with the moving target detector. One result is that slow flows in small vessel lumens have a mean Doppler frequency shift that is comparable to that from slowly moving tissues. The moving target detector does not distinguish between blood and tissue signal and eliminates these low-frequency shifts. Hence, under a special velocity limit, slow flows cannot be detected at all.

A technique in combination with injection of an ultrasound contrast agent will overcome this problem. This technique, called harmonic imaging, uses the same transducers as conventional imaging (Doppler and B-mode) and involves only software changes inside the imaging system.

Ultrasound contrast agents consist of small uncoated or encapsulated gas microbubbles that are stable and small enough (mean diameter <5 μm) to transverse the pulmonary and capillary circulation after injection into a peripheral vein (Goldberg 1994; Harvey et al. 2001).

If an ultrasound beam is transmitted to the region where contrast agents are present, the microbubbles undergo a nonlinear oscillation caused by pressure changes of the ultrasound field (Fig. 1.9). Depending on their mean bubble radius r and special fluid and bubble parameters, encapsulated microbubbles absorb and scatter ultrasound with high efficiency and oscillate radially with a resonance frequency (Leighton 1994) according to:

$$f_{\mathrm{resonance}} \quad \frac{1}{2\,r}\sqrt{\frac{3}{\rho_{\mathrm{fluid}}}\left(P_{\mathrm{fluid}} + \frac{2\ {}_{\mathrm{st}}}{r}\right)} \tag{6}$$

$3\gamma\,\rho_{\mathrm{fluid}} \ldots P_{\mathrm{fluid}}$ = part for pure hollow shells (uncoated bubbles)

where ρ_{fluid} and P_{fluid} are the fluid density and pressure, σ_{st} the surface tension of the microbubble, and γ the adiabatic ideal gas constant.

For blood, the parameters of Eq. 6 are suitable, as contrast agents with a mean size smaller than 5 μm have resonance frequencies in the range 1–10 MHz. This is the frequency range where broadband transducers of Doppler imaging systems normally operate.

A Doppler imaging system is modified by software so that the transducer emits the signal with a low frequency (e.g., 2.5–4 MHz) and receives at the second harmonic (e.g., 5–8 MHz). Equation 1 for the detected Doppler shift frequency changes in harmonic imaging for the receiving part to:

$$f_{\mathrm{n}} = \frac{2n\,f_{\mathrm{transmit}}}{c}\cos(\ ) \tag{7}$$

where n is the harmonic number.

RBCs for instance do not undergo nonlinear oscillations. Thus, if they are insonated with the fundamental frequency, they do not produce second harmonic echoes, and neither does soft tissue. Only the echoes from the microbubbles within the blood are received. The echoes from RBCs and solid soft tissues are suppressed with this method (Fig. 1.9).

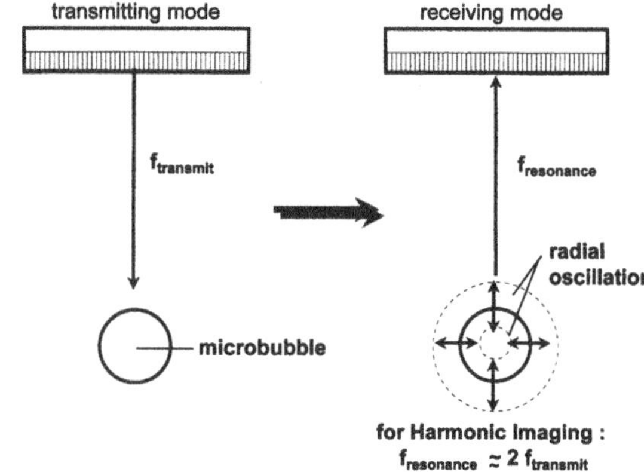

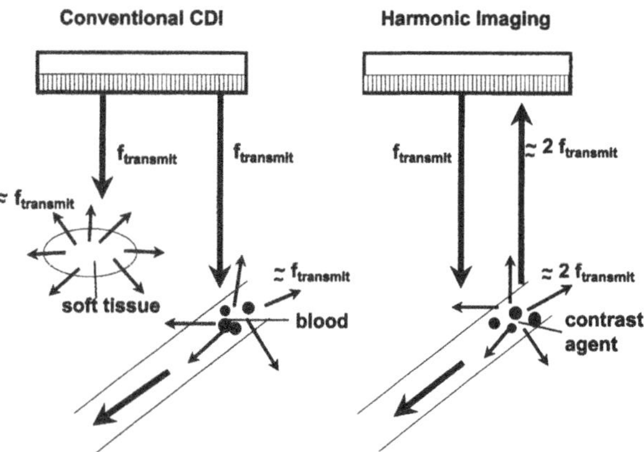

Fig. 1.9. The technique of harmonic imaging: A frequency f_{transmit} is emitted into the tissue, and its second harmonic frequency $2f_{\mathrm{transmit}}$ is detected. With this method, echoes caused by tissue or blood flow can be reduced, while the resonant bubbles of the contrast agent are scanned. The result is an increase of the signal-to-noise ratio

An enhancement of 10–25 dB from the back-scattered blood echoes can be achieved (Chang et al. 1996; Burns 1996). Two effects are responsible for this signal enhancement: First, the large number of microbubbles in the agent acting as scatterers for the ultrasound waves, and second, the increasing scattering cross-section to a magnitude of three in regard to their geometric cross-section caused by the bubble resonance. For some contrast agents, there is more energy in the second harmonic frequency response than in their fundamental one.

Using the harmonic imaging technique for radiological investigations leads to more reproducible spectral waveforms, improves the differentiation and vascularization of lesions, improves the detection of slow blood flows (microcirculation), and can help to reduce the examination time (Missouris et al. 1996;

MADJAR et al. 1996; COSGROVE 1996). On the other hand, there are some drawbacks: The back-scattering of the contrast agent is dependent on the power gain used, and a large ultrasound power output can destroy the agent itself (cavitation), which can lead to harmful biological effects.

Finally, it should be noted that good teamwork between the ultrasound system and contrast agent developers is necessary for optimizing the harmonic imaging technique. The resonance frequency distribution of the contrast agent, for instance, must be harmonized to the receiving frequency of the transducers. For special clinical investigations, it is necessary to develop targeted contrast agents that can enhance vascular or tissue contrast selectively.

1.3 Color Doppler Imaging Independent of Doppler Effect

Another method to determine the intensity-weighted average flow velocity is the 'time-domain processing' that is implemented, e.g., in color velocity imaging (CVI) systems. The technique was developed by BONNEFOUS and PASQUÉ and was published in 1986. There are several benefits of this method over the conventional methods evaluating the Doppler effect. For instance, aliasing as caused by the Nyquist limit does not occur, and the aim to obtain an optimal B-mode image quality simultaneously with the detection of high velocities seems to be reachable.

1.3.1 Time-Domain Analysis

A processing technique that can reduce some limitations of conventional CDI is the time-domain analysis (TDA) of the echo signals back-scattered by RBCs. In Fig. 1.10, two echo signals from two consecutive pulse-echo cycles detected within the same scan-line and scan direction are shown. Both echoes have more or less the same signal signature but are time shifted a little bit, because the special RBC cluster tracked has moved (w_{12}) during the time interval Δt. This time delay between the two echoes is proportional to the RBC's velocity within the scanned sample volume. At this point, it must be noted that this method can only detect axial changes d_{ax} in position and not lateral differences of the cluster movements.

Instead of measuring the Doppler frequency or phase shift information of the echoes in reference to the transmitted signal (as done by the conventional methods), TDA measures the flow velocity directly by evaluating these signal patterns of the two consecutive echoes (signal recognition).

For this special recognition, TDA uses a cross-correlation analysis of the two time-shifted signals, similar to the autocorrelation process.

After A/D conversion of the two echoes and after passing the moving target detector (Fig. 1.11), the digital signals are processed in the cross-correlator. The purpose of this analyzer is to find the position of maximum correlation within both signals. The mathematical way of doing this is to multiply the consecutive signals delayed by time t for a special section (window); later on, this product is integrated from

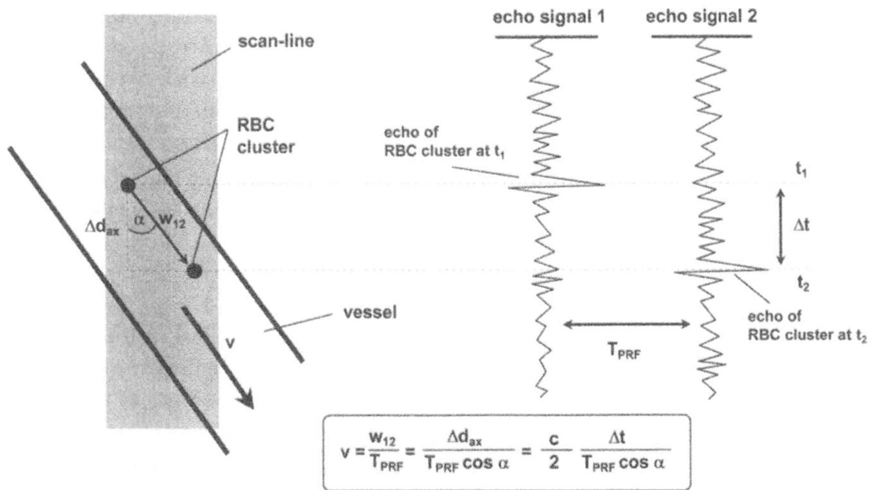

Fig. 1.10. Schematic view of the time-domain processing technique

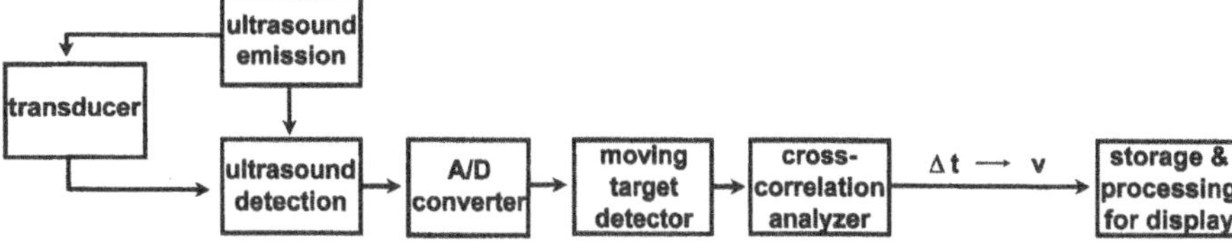

Abbreviations
A/D : Analog/Digital
Δt : Time shift
v : Velocity

Fig. 1.11. Block diagram showing the implementation of the time-domain processing technique. A cross-correlation module is used for deriving the run-time shift information (*ft*) between two detected signals of a real-time blood flow mapping system

minus infinity to infinity. The result is the value of the cross-correlation at time *t*. Finally, the maximum of the cross-correlation function for all time shifts is sought. This is at the certain time $t=\Delta t$. Knowing the pulse repetition period T_{PRF} between two pulses transmitted from the same transducer element, the speed of sound *c*, and the angle α caused by the changes of the scatterer's position within the time shift Δt, the velocity of the RBCs can be calculated with the output value Δt of the cross-correlation analysis:

$$_{RBC} = \frac{c}{2}\,\frac{t}{T_{PRF}\cos(\;)} \tag{8}$$

In a Doppler imaging system using this processing technique, the cross-correlation function is calculated for discrete echo segments to save time and to perform a calculation and display in real time. The length of these segments is a compromise between the accuracy of the calculated flow velocity and the axial resolution. An optimized sampling rate in the A/D converter is essential for correctly corresponding digital values of the signal echoes.

For a high accuracy of the calculated mean velocity, it is necessary to compare several pulse-echo cycles of the same scan-line: The more pulse-echo cycles (higher PRF) that are used, the more accurate is the calculated velocity. Also, the method depends on a good signal-to-noise ratio (>6 dB): If the difference between the echo signal level and the noise signal level is too low, a signal recognition cannot be performed because the algorithm cannot differentiate between peaks coming from noise and real flow echoes. This limits the penetration depth of the technique.

Although this TDA method uses the Doppler angle for its calculation, it is not essential for this process, only a technological limitation that will be overcome (Klews 1991). For TDA, it is not necessary to transmit the same scan-line several times consecutively. Theoretically, it is possible to choose adjacent scan-lines and to detect and evaluate movements parallel to the transducer.

This could have a valuable input for scanning peripheral vessels, because the blood's movement component parallel to the transducer is here generally larger than the vertical one. Detection of both components is also imaginable.

With conventional CDI, 9–17 pulse cycles are needed before an image is displayed; for TDA processing, only 5 cycles are necessary – a higher frame rate is possible (Klews 1991). Another advantage of this technique is that TDA uses the same signal information (A-mode lines) as needed for gray-scale (B-mode) representation. This provides a spatial resolution for the color information as high as the resolution of the B-mode image. Hence, the same output data of the ultrasound pulse should be sufficient for the detection of movements. This is an important point for safety reasons.

1.4 Doppler Artifacts

Artifacts in CDI can be confusing and sometimes lead to misinterpretation of the Doppler information (Fig. 1.12). By using Doppler systems in different clinical fields, the detection and description of many Doppler-related artifacts have ensued. A comprehensive survey of different Doppler artifacts is given in Fig. 1.13. Most detected artifacts fall into three groups:

- those caused by the Doppler technique or system itself
- those generated by inappropriate (subjective) Doppler system settings or
- anatomically related ones.

Knowledge of basic ultrasound physics and the Doppler technique used will help to reduce or to eliminate the artifact which occurred effectively and fast within the image during the investigation. In most cases, it is sufficient to change one or more system settings (e.g., power, PRF, sample gate size) to get an artifact-free Doppler image.

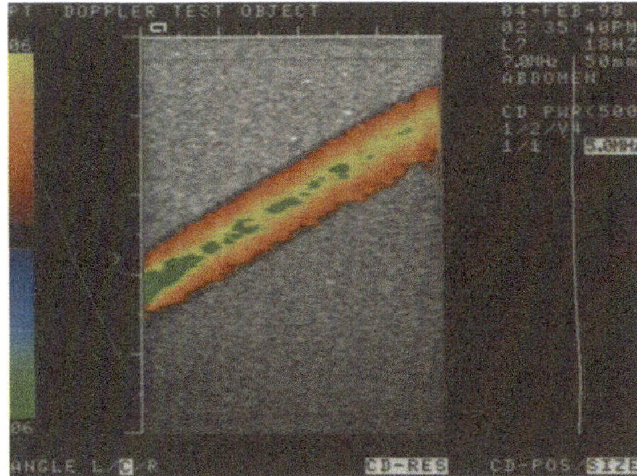

Fig. 1.12. A CDI artifact occurred in a vessel. The flow profile within this vessel is parabolic, with the highest velocity values present in the middle (*yellow*). The artifact appears in the middle of the vessel as a false color coding effect of the highest velocity components (*green* instead of yellow) and wraps the velocities around to the other scale. In this image, the velocity scale chosen was not correct for the detected flow velocity, and aliasing occurred

1.5 Safety and Risks

Almost all CDI systems in hospitals are operating in ultrasonic PW mode; only a limited number of systems with CW mode are used, and in special application fields. This means that the emitted ultrasound energy is concentrated in a small temporal pulse, that can be characterized e.g. by the acoustical exposure parameters power *W* and pressure amplitude *p*. Both parameters are related to the biophysical mechanisms of tissue heating and cavitation.

Published trends of the exposure parameters of modern diagnostic systems show a steady increase towards the use of higher pressure amplitudes, higher powers, or higher time-averaged intensities (Duck and Martin 1991; Henderson et al. 1995). The highest intensities are used in pulsed Doppler systems, while the exposure parameters of CDI systems are comparable to those of M-mode applications.

For an estimation of whether the Doppler mode and the individual front panel settings used are still related to a safe application, two special types of indices have been developed: the thermal (TI) and mechanical (MI) index. All US system developers are required to display these indices on modern systems on-line (AIUM/NEMA 1992) to give valuable information about the way in which changes of system settings during an investigation can alter the acoustic power (and therefore TI) or the pressure amplitude (MI). Different assumptions of 'worst-case' conditions are implemented with these indices.

Displaying of these indices is essential for Doppler techniques because higher exposure values can be generated by using different pulse sequences, e.g., resulting in very focused beams with a high scan-line density (high pressure amplitudes and therefore a high overall acoustic power). The risk is great that a small portion of tissue has to absorb a high amount of ultrasound energy in a short time, which can lead to different biologically induced effects.

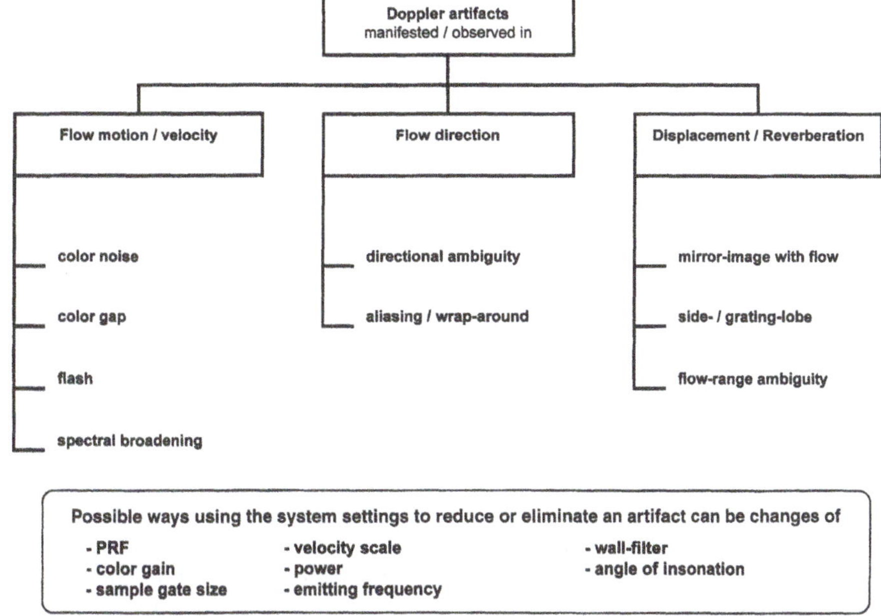

Fig. 1.13. Doppler artifacts and their manifestation in CDI systems

1.5.1 Mechanical Index

MI is calculated from the measured peak negative pressure amplitude p_- [MPa] and the center frequency f_c in MHz:

$$MI = \frac{p_-}{\sqrt{f_c}} \tag{9}$$

MI is quoted without units and shall be an estimation for a threshold where cavitational effects can occur in tissue (no risk: MI <1; potential risk: MI >1). Before this ratio is displayed on the system's screen, the MI value in vivo is derived for a simple tissue model, i.e., the p_- value is calculated by reducing the acoustic pressure (measured in water) with an attenuation coefficient of 0.3 dB cm^{-1} MHz^{-1}. The simple tissue model makes three assumptions: One is that the acoustic pressure in tissue is reduced; the second is that cavitation increases with frequency, although evidence of this dependency in tissue is still sparse (ECURS 1996; Abbot 1999); and last, that no additional cavitation nuclei are present.

When using a Doppler technique in combination with ultrasound contrast agents, it has to be kept in mind that additional nuclei are introduced into the vessels or tissue, and the MI index is not valid any longer, i.e., the risk of causing cavitation is higher with a lower emitted pressure amplitude because more initial microbubbles are present in the scanned region than without contrast agent and can lead to inertial cavitational effects (Miller and Thomas 1995; Dalecki et al. 1997). Also, special harmonic imaging scanning techniques can generate acoustic cavitation nuclei (Brayman and Miller 1997). These investigations should therefore be done under the lowest possible and medically usable exposure parameters to avoid unintentional biological effects.

1.5.2 Thermal Index

A second index, TI, is supposed to warn the user about the potential for tissue heating during Doppler exposure at the system settings used. Three different tissue models (TIS, TIB, TIC) and a differentiation between the scanned and unscanned mode of the Doppler system provide an estimation of the 'worst-case' condition. The temperature rise can be predicted in soft tissue (TIS), in the case where bone is at the focus (TIB), and in a third prediction, where the bone is close to the transducer (TIC, for transcranial applications):

$$TIB = W \quad k_2 \tag{10}$$

$$TIC = W \quad k_3 \tag{11}$$

$$TIS = W \quad f_c \quad k_1 \tag{12}$$

In all three cases, the index depends on the acoustic power W emitted by the Doppler system and special factors k_i, resulting from all the constant values which emerge from the modeling. Only for the soft-tissue heating does the index depend also on the transducer center frequency used (NCRP 1992; AIUM/NEMA 1992; ECURS 1996; Abbott 1999).

Knowing the values of the TI means having an idea of which system settings can produce a temperature increase of more than 1°C, the critical limit, which may, under 'worst-case' conditions, be harmful for the affected tissue.

Various 'watchdog' groups of the ultrasound (WFUMB, EFSUMB) and other societies (WHO, NCRP) keep a special eye on the exposure parameters and the induced biological effects and publish their updated statements about the safety of diagnostic ultrasound periodically in different journals (Barnett et al. 1997, 1998, 2000; Docker and Duck 1992; WFUMB 1997).

In conclusion, the first safety information given to the user is already available with the TI and MI indices or the older p_- and intensity values on the display.

It is very important to recognize that there are difficulties in obtaining a complete representation of heating and cavitation on-line. Hence, the displayed MI and TI values should be taken as a general indicator of possible safety concern, and not as validated measurements of the true heating or cavitation risk in tissue.

1.6 Quality Assurance of Doppler Systems

For a Doppler or CDI system, a quality assurance (QA) concept should be worked out to guarantee its optimal functioning as long as the system is used. Not only the regular service checks or eventually software upgrades belong to this QA, but also quality control tests that are performed periodically and give information about the long-time constancy of special Doppler parameters. These parameters are, e.g., the maximum Doppler penetration depth, the sample volume position error, or system sensitivity.

A second point that can be managed with such a check is specifying the measurement errors produced by the Doppler system.

A Doppler system should measure flow velocities (mean and peak) or volume flow data as accurately as possible. Knowledge of the individual system tolerances is therefore a crucial point.

For this kind of quality control, special Doppler test objects are suitable. Such a test object should mimic the ultrasound properties of the human body as closely as possible and should be standardized. The latter aspect is very important since long-term constancy checks are carried out, and the properties of the test object are not allowed to vary, which would lead to irreproducible measurements.

The international standard for Doppler test objects (IEC 61685) is the basis for these quality control checks.

A model of a Doppler test object that fulfills the requirements of this standard is shown in Fig. 1.14 (Kollmann et al. 1999; Teirlinck et al. 1998). A blood-mimicking fluid is pumped through two vessel-mimicking materials with different diameters that are inside the test object body (Fig. 1.14 middle). A wide laminar flow velocity range can be used that enables, e.g., measurement of the minimum and maximum detectable velocity limits of a Doppler system.

Other Doppler parameters can be measured with this test object, too, to characterize the checked system and to create an individual system profile (Kollmann et al. 1999).

Quality controlling by using a test object should follow after a regular service check or software change to document the present system status, to obtain data for the long-term constancy properties of the measured Doppler parameters, and last but not least, to verify the success of the service.

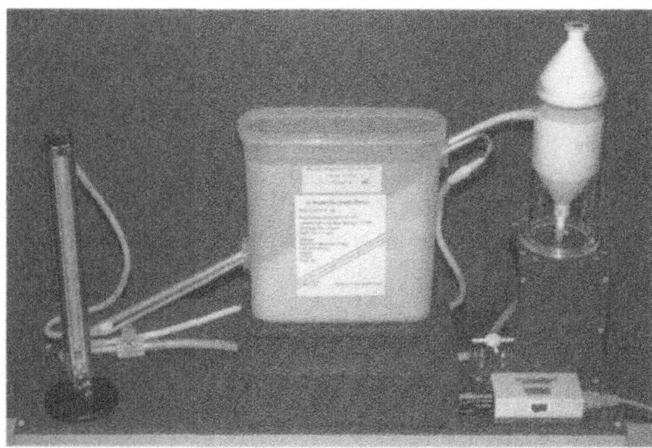

Fig. 1.14. Prototype of a Doppler test object that can be used for quality assurance checks of Doppler systems

1.7 Ongoing Developments and Future Aspects in Color Doppler Imaging

As shown in the previous sections, the potential of CDI systems is limited by the hardware and software used. New developments of Doppler systems must try to accommodate and overcome these technical factors.

Meanwhile, modern CDI systems have a signal generation and processing that are completely digital. In combination with new transducer concepts that contain 2D-array elements (matrix transducer) with more than 1024 single channels, it is possible to focus the ultrasound beam not only axially but also laterally (Rizzatto 1998; Stetten 2001; Hoskins 2002). A marginal increase of the image and flow resolution by reduced processing time can be expected in combination with faster signal-processing algorithms.

The classic CDI techniques are currently being developed and improved: To overcome the dependency on the Doppler frequency shift and hence the estimated 'true' flow velocity in combination with the measured Doppler angle, echo information from 2–3 or more independent beam directions is used to obtain calculations of 2–3 or more velocity components and to reduce refraction errors. These *vector Doppler systems* combine the different velocity data to get an angle-independent 'true' velocity estimation or to measure changes in velocity directions that represent the 3D nature of hemodynamics (Dumire et al. 1995; Hoskins 1997, 1999; Steel 2002).

Detecting and displaying the 2D and 3D blood flow geometry are important aspects for diagnosis. A 3D visualization of organ and vessel perfusion and vascularization, e.g., allows us to detect and measure the volume of arterial plaques as well as the velocity distribution behind a stenosis or to calculate the shear stress for the endothelial layer of an artery. More and more investigations are reporting clinical applications by using 3D or real-time 3D (4D) CDI or ACD techniques (Downey et al. 1995; Hashimoto et al. 1995; Ritchie et al. 1996; Guo et al. 1996; Adam and Burstein 1997; Barry et al. 1997; Carson et al. 1997; Lyden et al. 1997; Berg 2000; Li 2002; Mehwald 2002; Sitges 2003).

Another aspect of the ACD technique is that it is a powerful tool for visualizing perfusion with a very sharp definition and in regions with very low velocities and hence a small moving blood volume. Because of the different method of signal processing, the ACD information can be used for a quantitative estimation of fractional moving blood volume within the observed sample volume (Carson et al.

1993; Rubin et al. 1995; Adler et al. 1995; Kollmann et al. 1996a,b). This estimation can be derived only for special cases because several factors and parameters from the Doppler system (e.g., beam geometry, gain) and the moving medium (e.g., packing factor, viscosity) have an important influence on the echo signal and must be considered for evaluation (Jain et al. 1991). Future investigations will show if there are practicable solutions and implementations for clinical applications in general.

Further very promising projects for detecting blood flow in the microcirculation are the developments of high-frequency Doppler imaging systems (>40 MHz for CW and PW). Initial investigations with a PW Doppler system with emitting frequencies of 40 and 50 MHz reveal that they are very suitable for measuring low blood flow velocities (<5 mm/s) in capillaries and arterioles with very high spatial, temporal, and velocity resolution (Christopher 1997; Phoon 2000). The diameters that can be detected with this system are around 20–35 µm. One drawback for a wide application field of this transducer is the limited penetration depth of 2 mm, but further miniaturization could overcome this problem by developing an intravascular transducer.

A second technique that permits the detection of the microcirculation is harmonic imaging. Although the interactions of the ultrasound beam with the microbubble contrast agents that are responsible for this effect are yet not fully understood, the method alone or in combination with the ACD techniques has already shown its important impact on small vessel imaging (Burns et al. 1994, 1995). Similar to the conventional CDI technique, there are two different signal (echo) processing techniques of the harmonic imaging method: The conventional 'normal' harmonic imaging technique uses the non-linear reflective characteristics of the microbubbles to increase the contrast (signal-to-noise ratio) for signal processing, while a second technique, called transient response or intermittent imaging, uses another interaction effect of the contrast agent with ultrasound: A high negative ultrasound peak amplitude can destroy gas-filled microbubbles (cavitation). This inertial cavitation is the basic effect for intermittent imaging and was first observed in cardiology. It requires waiting for some period after imaging (usually within a few cardiac cycles for the contrast to reperfuse the observed region), then imaging again, which leads to a brief but dramatic increase in myocardial contrast (Porter et al. 1996, 1997a,b). The technique and the image information have to be validated carefully, and its usefulness is still to be proven before this special method has a chance of being adopted into other clinical application fields.

Miniaturization of systems and data (information) merging of different imaging modalities are the key words for the next decade: There are already some mobile hand-held or portable Doppler imaging systems available for a quick bedside diagnosis and emergency applications with implemented CDI and ACD modes. These systems have been evaluated by physicians and seem to be very comfortable to use, light-weight, ready-to-operate in seconds, and equal in flow representation to conventional systems.

However, once an easy-to-use concept has been found that combines the dynamic ultrasound Doppler flow information from these systems with the exact anatomical information of other imaging modalities, this so-called 'fusion' of 2D or 3D images will revolutionize flow diagnosis again. The first steps towards this development are already being taken (Langer 2001; Kollmann 2001).

References

Abbott JG (1999) Rational and derivation of MI and TI–a review. Ultrasound Med Biol 25:431–441

Adam DR, Burstein P (1997) Vascular imaging by ultrasound: 3D reconstruction of flow velocity fields for endothelial shear stress calculation. Adv Exp Med Biol 430:177–185

Adler RS, Rubin JM et al (1995) Ultrasonic estimation of tissue perfusion: a stochastic approach. Ultrasound Med Biol 21: 493–500

American Institute of Ultrasound in Medicine, National Electrical Manufacturers Association (eds) (1992) Standard for real-time display of thermal and mechanical acoustic output indices on diagnostic ultrasound equipment. AIUM/NEMA, Rockville

Atkinson P, Woodcock JP (1982) Doppler ultrasound and its use in clinical measurement. Academic, London

Babcock DS, Patriquin H et al (1996) Power Doppler sonography: basic principles and clinical applications in children. Pediatr Radiol 26:109–115

Barnett SB (1998) Update on thermal bioeffects issues. Ultrasound Med Biol 24 [Suppl 1]:S1–S10

Barnett SB, Rott H-D, Ter Haar G, Ziskin MC, Maeda K (1997) The sensitivity of biological tissue to ultrasound. Ultrasound Med Biol 23:805–812

Barnett SB, Ter Haar GR, Ziskin MC, Rott H-D, Maeda K (2000) International recommendations and guidelines for the safe use of diagnostic ultrasound in medicine. Ultrasound Med Biol 26:805–812

Barry CD, Allott CP, John NW, Mellor PM, Arundel PA, Thomson DS, Waterton JC (1997) Three-dimensional freehand ultrasound: image reconstruction and volume analysis. Ultrasound Med Biol 23:1209–1224

Battle DJ, Harrison RP, Hedley M (1997) Maximum entropy image reconstruction from sparsely sampled coherent field data. IEEE Trans Image Process 6:1139–1147

Berg S, Torp H, Haugen BO, Samsted S (2000) Volumetric blood flow measurements with the use of dynamic 3-dimensional ultrasound color flow imaging. J Am Soc Echocardiogr 13: 393–402

Bonnefous O, Pasqué P (1986) Time Domain formulation of pulse-Doppler ultrasound and blood velocity estimation by cross correlation. Ultrasonic Imaging 8:73–85

Brayman AA, Miller MW (1997) Acoustic cavitation nuclei survive the apparent ultrasonic destruction of Albunex7 microspheres. Ultrasound Med Biol 23:793–796

Brody WR, Meindl JD (1974) Theoretical analysis of the CW doppler ultrasonic flowmeter. IEEE Trans Biomed Eng 21: 183–192

Brown PM, Johnston KW, Kassam M, Cobbold RS (1982) A critical study of ultrasound Doppler spectral analysis for detecting carotid disease. Ultrasound Med Biol 8:515–523

Burns PN (1987) The physical principles of Doppler and spectral analysis. J Clin Ultrasound 15:567–590

Burns PN (1996) Harmonic imaging with ultrasound contrast agents. Clin Radiol 51:50–55

Burns PN, Powers JE et al (1994) Power Doppler imaging combined with contrast-enhancing harmonic Doppler: new method for small-vessel imaging. Radiology 193:366

Burns PN, Powers JE, Hope-Simpson D et al (1995) Harmonic power mode Doppler using microbubble contrast agents. An improved method for small vessel flow imaging. J Echogr Med Ultrason 16:132–142

Carson PL, Li X, Pallister J et al (1993) Approximate quantification of detected fractional blood volume in the breast by 3D color flow and Doppler signal amplitude imaging. In: Levy M, McAvoy BR (eds) 1993 Ultrasonics Symposium Proceedings, IEEE Catalog No. 93CH33001-9. Institute of Electrical and Electronic Engineers, Piscataway, pp 1023–1026

Carson PL, Moskalik AP, Govil A, Roubidoux MA et al (1997) The 3D and 2D color flow display of breast masses. Ultrasound Med Biol 23:837–849

Chang PH, Shung KK, Levene HB (1996) Quantitative measurements of second harmonic Doppler using ultrasound contrast agents. Ultrasound Med Biol 22: 1205–1214

Christopher DA, Burns PN, Starkokoski BG, Foster FS (1997) A high-frequency pulsed-wave Doppler ultrasound system for the detection and imaging of blood flow in the microcirculation. Ultrasound Med Biol 23:997–1015

Cosgrove D (1996) Why do we need contrast agents for ultrasound? Clin Radiol 51:1–4

Dalecki D, Raeman CH, Child SZ, Penney DP, Carstensen EL (1997) Remnants of Albunex7 nuclate acoustic cavitation. Ultrasound Med Biol 23:1405–1412

Di Pietro DM, Meindl JD (1978) Optimal system design for an implantable CW Doppler ultrasonic flowmeter. IEEE Trans Biomed Eng 25:255–264

Docker MF, Duck FA ed. (1992) The safe use of diagnostic ultrasound. British Institute of Radiology, London

Downey DB, Fenster A (1995) Vascular imaging with a three-dimensional power Doppler system. Am J Roentgenol 165: 665–668

Duck FA, Martin K (1991) Trends in diagnostic ultrasound exposure. Phys Med Biol 36:1423–1432

Dumire BL, Beach KW, Labs KH, Detmer PR, Standness DE (1995) A vector Doppler ultrasound instrument. IEEE Ultrason Symp Proc 2:1477–1480

European Committee for Ultrasound Radiation Safety (1996) Tutorial paper: thermal and mechanical indices. Eur J Ultrasound 4:145–150

Fitzgerald DE, Drumm DE (1977) Non invasive measurement of human fetal circulation using ultrasound: a new method. Br J Obstet Gynaecol 2:1450–1451

Giovagnorio F, Quaranta L (1995) Power Doppler sonography enhances visualization of orbital vessels. J Ultrasound Med 14:837–842

Goldberg BB, Liu J-B, Forsberg F (1994) Ultrasound contrast agents: a review. Ultrasound Med Biol 20:319–333

Guo Z, Fenster A (1996) Three-dimensional power Doppler imaging: a phantom study to quantify vessel stenosis. Ultrasound Med Biol 22:1059–1069

Haerten R, Mück M (1992) Doppler- und Farbdoppler-Sonographie: Eine Einführung in die Grundlagen. Siemens Bereich Medizinische Technik

Harvey CJ, Blomley MJK, Eckersley RJ, Cosgrove DO (2001) Developments in ultrasound contrast media. Eur Radiol 11:675–689

Hashimoto H, Shen Y, Takeuchi Y, Yoshitome E (1995) Ultrasound 3-dimensional image processing using power Doppler image. IEEE Ultrason Symp Proc 2:1423–1426

Henderson J, Willson K, Jago JR, Whittingham TA (1995) A survey of the acoustic outputs of diagnostic ultrasound equipment in current clinical use. Ultrasound Med Biol 21:699–705

Hennerici M, Neuerburg-Heusler D (1999) Gefäßdiagnostik mit Ultraschall. Thieme, Stuttgart

Hoskins PR (1997) Vector Doppler. Eur J Ultrasound 6 [Suppl 2]:S7

Hoskins PR (1999) A review of the measurement of blood velocity and related quantities using Doppler ultrasound. Proc Inst Mech Eng 213:391–400

Hoskins PR (2002) Ultrasound techniques for measurement of blood flow and tissue motion. Biorheology 39:451–459

International Electrotechnical Commission (2001) Ultrasonics-flow measurement systems-flow test object. IEC 61685 Standard. IEC Technical Committee 87, Geneva

Jain SP, Fan PH, Philpot EF et al (1991) Influence of various instrument settings on the flow information derived from power mode. Ultrasound Med Biol 17:49–54

Kasai C, Namekawa K, Koyano A, Omoto R (1985) Real-time two-dimensional blood flow imaging using autocorrelation technique. IEEE Trans Son Ultrason 32:458–464

Keller H, Muller A, Meier W, Schonbeck M (1975) Transorale Doppler-Sonographie unter Schleimhautanasthesie zur Beur-teilung der Strömungsverhältnisse in den Aa. vertebrales (Vertebralis-Doppler). Dtsch Med Wochenschr 100:937–938; 943–946

Klews PM (1987) The Philips quantum angiodynograph: an ultrasound system for vascular diagnostics. Medicamundi 32:77–79

Klews PM (1991) Color velocity imaging – ein Vergleich der Verfahren zur farbkodierten Sonographie. Röntgenstrahlen 65:1–8

Kollmann C, Turetschek K, Backfrieder W et al (1995) Untersuchungen zur Detektion von low flow mit neuen Ultraschall-Farbdoppler-Techniken. Ultraschall Med 16:S81

Kollmann C, Turetschek K et al (1996a) Quantitative Untersuchungen mit dem amplitudenkodierten Farb-dopplergerät. Ultraschall Med 17:S5

Kollmann C, Turetschek K, Backfrieder W et al (1996b) Quantitative Untersuchungen mit dem amplitudenkodierten

Farbdopplergerät (in-vitro Studien). Gemeins. Jahrestagung DGMP, ÖGMP & SGSMP, Graz 1996. In: Medizinische Physik 1996, Tagungsband. DGMP, ÖGMP & SGSMP, Graz, pp 181–182

Kollmann C, Turetschek K, Mostbeck G (1998) Amplitude coded color Doppler sonography. Eur Radiol 8:649–656

Kollmann C, Bezemer RA, Fish P, Fredfeldt KE et al (1999) Ein Testobjekt für die apparative Qualitätssicherung bei Ultraschall-Doppler-(Duplex) Geräten, ausgehend vom Normenentwurf IEC 61685. Ultraschall Med 20:248–257

Kollmann C, Greiffenberg B, Schlachetzki F et al (2001) 2-dimensional fusion of cerebral cross-modality images employing a mutual information algorithm. Phys Med 17: 267–270

Langer SG, Carter SJ, Haynor DR et al (2001) Image acquisition: ultrasound, computed tomography, and magnetic resonance imaging. World J Surg 25:1428–1437

Leighton TG (1994) The acoustic bubble. Academic, San Diego

Li X, Wanitkun S, Li XN et al (2002) Quantification of instantaneous flow rate and dynamically changing effective orifice area using a geometry independent three-dimensional digital color Doppler method: an in vitro study mimicking mitral regurgitation. J Am Soc Echocardiogr 15:1189–1196

Lyden PD, Nelson TR (1997) Visualization of the cerebral circulation using three dimensional transcranial power Doppler ultrasound imaging. J Neuroimaging 7:35–39

Madjar H, Pfleiderer A et al. (1996) Diagnosis by color Doppler and contrast agents. In: Figueira AS et al (eds) Mastology—breast diseases. Elsevier Science, Amsterdam, pp 69–75

Mehwald PS, Rusk RA, Mori Y et al (2002) A validation study of aortic stroke volume using dynamic 4-dimensional color Doppler: an in vivo study. J Am Soc Echocardiogr 15: 1045–1050

Merritt CRB (1987) Doppler color flow imaging. J Clin Ultrasound 15:591–597

Merritt CRB (1991) Doppler US: The Basics. Radiographics 11:109–119

Miller DL, Thomas RM (1995) Ultrasound contrast agents nucleate inertial cavitation in vitro. Ultrasound Med Biol 21:1059–1065

Missouris CG, Allen CM et al (1996) Non-invasive screening for renal artery stenosis with ultrasound contrast enhancement. J Hypertens 14:519–524

National Council on Radiation Protection and Measurements (1992) Exposure criteria for medical diagnostic ultrasound. I. Criteria based on thermal mechanisms. NCRP Report No. 113. NCRP, Bethesda

Newhouse V, Reid J (1991) Invariance of the Doppler bandwidth with flow displacement in the illuminating field. J Acoust Soc Am 90:2595–2601

Philips Medizin Systeme (1989) Duplexsonografische Referenzwerte. Produktinformation 794

Phoon CK, Aristizabal O, Turnbull DH (2000) 40 MHz Doppler characterization of umbilical and dorsal aortic blood flow in the early mouse embryo. Ultrasound Med Biol 26:1275–1283

Porter TR (1997) Transient response during contrast echocardiography. Adv Card Echo Contrast 5:47–55

Porter TR, Xie F, Li S et al (1996) Increased ultrasound contrast and decreased microbubble destruction rate using triggered ultrasound imaging. J Am Soc Echocardiogr 9:599–605

Porter TR, Li S, Kilzer K, Deligonul U (1997) Effect of significant two-vessel versus one-vessel coronary artery stenosis on myocardial contrast defects observed with intermittent harmonic imaging after intravenous contrast injection during dobutamine stress echocardiography. J Am Coll Cardiol 30:1399–1406

Preidler KW, Szolar DM et al (1995) Comparison of colour Doppler energy sonography with conventional colour Doppler sonography in detection of flow signals in peripheral renal transplant vessels. Br J Radiol 68:1103–1105

Ritchie CJ, Edwards WS, Mack LA, Cyr DR, Kim Y (1996) Three-dimensional ultrasonic angiography using power-mode Doppler. Ultrasound Med Biol 22:277–286

Rizzatto G (1998) Ultrasound transducers. Eur J Radiol 27 [Suppl 2]:S188–195

Rubin JM, Adler RS (1993) Power Doppler expands standard color capability. Diagn Imaging 15:66–69

Rubin JM, Bude RO, Carson PL et al (1994) Power Doppler US: a potentially useful alternative to mean frequency-based color Doppler US. Radiology 190:853–856

Rubin JM, Adler RS et al (1995) Fractional moving blood volume: estimation with power Doppler US. Radiology 197: 183–190

Schneider KTM, Dumler EA, Lippert A (1993) Umfrage zur Verbreitung und Anwendung der Dopplersonographie im deutschsprachigen Raum. Geburtshilfe Frauenheilkd 53:56–60

Scoutt LM, Zawin ML, Taylor KJW (1990) Doppler US. II. Clinical applications. Radiology 174:309–319

Seitz K, Kubale R (1988) Duplexsonographie der abdominellen und retroperitonealen Gefäße. VCH, Weinheim

Sitges M, Jones M, Shiota T et al (2003) Real-time three-dimensional color Doppler evaluation of the flow convergence zone for quantification of mitral regurgitation: validation experimental animal study and initial clinical experience. J Am Soc Echocardiogr 16:38–45

Sohn C, Weskott HP, Schiesser M (1996) Sensitivity of new color systems: "Maximum entropy method" and angio-color. Comparative in vitro flow measurements. Ultraschall Med 17:138–142/Surg Endosc (1997) 11:1040–1046

Steel R, Fish PJ (2002) Error propagation bounds in dual and triple beam vector Doppler ultrasound. IEEE Trans Ultrason Ferroelectr Freq Control 49:1222–1230

Stetten G, Tamburo R (2001) Real-time three-dimensional ultrasound methods for shape analysis and visualization. Methods 25:221–230

Taylor KJW, Burns PN, Wells PNT (1988) Clinical applications of Doppler ultrasound. Raven, New York

Teirlinck CPJM et al (1998) Development of an example flow test object and comparison of five of these test objects, constructed in various laboratories. Ultrasonics 36:653–660

Turetschek K, Kollmann C, Hittmair K et al (1995) Power Doppler versus color Doppler US in the detection of low flow: in vitro results. Radiology 197:338

Turetschek K, Kollmann C, Mostbeck G (1998) Amplitude coded Doppler sonography: clinical applications. Eur Radiol 9:115–121

Weaver RG Jr, Howard G, McKinney WM, Ball MR, Jones AM, Toole JF (1980) Comparison of Doppler ultrasonography with arteriography of the carotid artery bifurcation. Stroke 11:402–404

World Federation for Ultrasound in Medicine and Biology (1997) Secretary's report: WFUMB administrative council meeting, San Diego, March 26–27, 1997. In: WFUMB News. WFUMB, San Diego, pp 2–3

Yamada R, Hirai T et al (1995) Evaluation of power Doppler imaging for renal diseases. Jpn J Med Ultrason 22:15–20

2 Venous Duplex Doppler and Color Doppler Imaging Techniques

J. Liskutin, R. Dorffner, G. H. Mostbeck

CONTENTS

Both the patient's position and the US equipment, especially the scan head, change according to the region and vein being examined and the clinical objectives. To a certain extent, there is individual variability of these parameters, and some of the recommendations presented in this chapter are based on subjective experience. However, the basic recommendations will enhance the understanding of "how to do" a venous color duplex Doppler imaging (CDDS) study.

J. Liskutin, MD
CT und MR Institut Hernalser Spitz, Jörgerstrasse 52, 1170 Vienna, Austria
R. Dorffner, MD
Associate Professor of Radiology, Department of Radiology, Hospital of the Brothers of St. John, Esterhazystrasse 26, 7000 Eisenstadt, Austria
G. H. Mostbeck, MD
Professor of Radiology, Sozialmedizinisches Zentrum, Baumgartner Höhe mit Pflegezentrum, Otto Wagner Spital, Sanatoriumstrasse 2, 1140 Vienna, Austria

2.1 Upper and Lower Extremity Veins

2.1.1 Veins of the Lower Extremity

2.1.1.1 Technical Equipment

When investigating the deep veins of the lower extremities, in most cases a 5.0 to 12.0 MHz linear probe is used for the inguinal region and the proximal thigh, while lower MHz curved array probes may be optimal for the mid- and distal thigh, in which the femoral vessels are located in a deeper intermuscular plane. Obese patients frequently require lower frequencies. For the inferior vena cava (IVC) and the iliac veins, abdominal probes, preferably curved array, provide more effective penetration. High-resolution, low-penetration 5.0 to 12.0 MHz linear probes may be used to examine the popliteal vein (POPV) as well as the calf veins.

When frequency-encoded color Doppler is used, venous flow should be coded blue, and an appropriate color scale should be selected to detect slow flow velocities (slow flow technique). Greater sensitivity to slower flow can be achieved by reducing the sampling rate for the returning Doppler signal, thus reducing the dynamic range. The color gain of the US unit should be adjusted so that the recorded flow occupies the full diameter or cross-sectional area of the vessel during the phase of maximum venous flow. Color noise should be avoided.

2.1.1.2
Anatomy

When studying the veins of the extremities, it is useful to divide the venous system into the deep and the superficial systems. The deep venous system lies subfascially and follows a course within a vascular sheath parallel to the arteries. The superficial veins are generally epifascial, with the exception of the proximal portion of the small saphenous vein, and have no accompanying arteries along their course. Both systems are connected by perforating veins (Fig. 2.1) (ROUVIERE and DELMAS 1985; WILLIAMS et al 1989).

2.1.1.2.1
Superficial Venous System

The great saphenous vein (GSV) originates at the medial margin of the dorsum of the foot and continues to the lower leg in front of the medial malleolus. Thereafter, it moves along the medial side of the calf, crossing the medial condyle of the femur dorsolaterally, until it joins the common femoral vein (CFV) or superficial femoral vein (SFV) approximately 2–3 cm below the inguinal ligament. In the calf, the GSV courses between the posterior arcuate and the anterior arcuate vein, which all unite, as a rule, around the

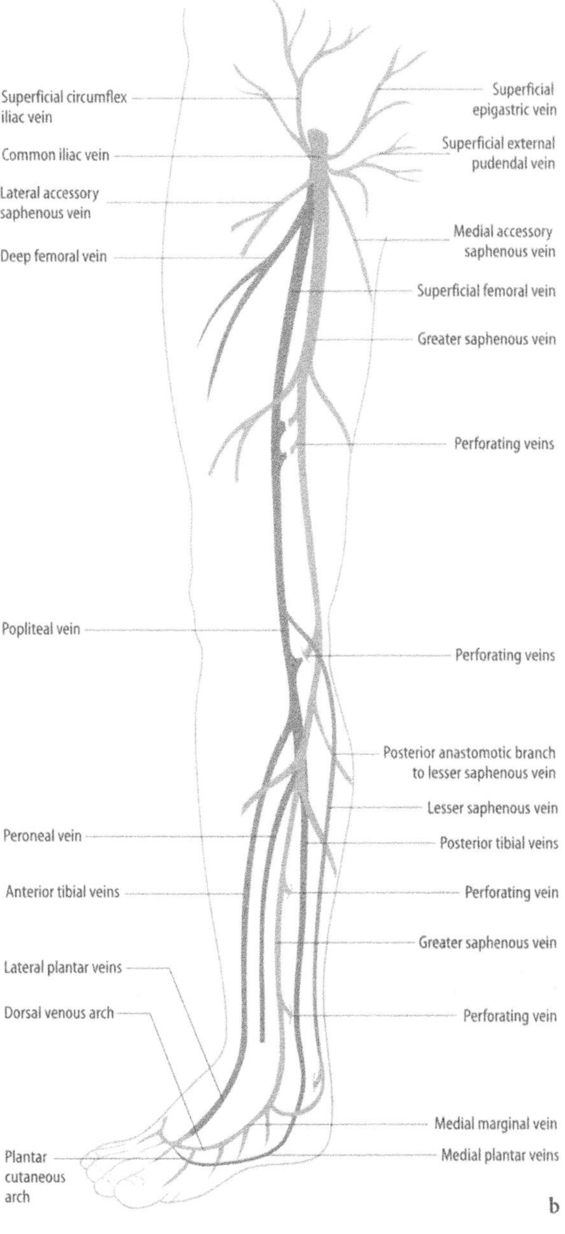

Fig. 2.1a,b. Anatomy of the pelvic and lower extremity veins. **a** Pelvic veins. **b** Lower extremity veins

level of the knee to one vessel. In 73% of cases, a single, unpaired GSV is found, while in the remaining 27%, it is paired. There are between 8 and 10 valves.

The small saphenous vein (SSV) originates from the lateral margin of the dorsum of the foot and proceeds dorsally to the lateral malleolus towards the lower leg. In the distal portion of the calf, it moves epifascially. More proximally, it runs between the two heads of the gastrocnemius muscle in a subfascial course until it joins the POPV, usually around the level of the knee. However, the level of the junction is very variable. In about 79% of cases, the junction lies 3–5 cm above, in 20% about, and in 1% below the level of the interarticular space. Furthermore, in up to 50%, the SSV is paired (Hennerici and Neuerburg-Heusler 1998, p. 202). There are between 6 and 12 valves.

2.1.1.2.2 Deep Venous System

The deep subfascial venous system of the lower leg consists of at least six veins, which accompany the three corresponding arteries in pairs. The posterior tibial veins (PTV) arise dorsal to the medial malleolus from the medial plantar veins, while the fibular veins (FV) collect the blood of the dorsal foot and join the PTV in the proximal portion of the lower leg. The anterior tibial veins (ATV) originate from the lateral plantar veins. In the proximal portion of the calf, they reach the interosseal membrane and, after crossing it, join the PTV to form the POPV. Each of the deep lower leg veins has at least 10 valves.

A special group which also belongs to the deep veins is termed muscle veins. They are located in the calf muscles and consist of the gastrocnemius and soleus veins. They flow into the PTV and ATV and are quite variable.

The POPV proceeds upwards between the heads of the gastrocnemius muscle and is also closely related to the biceps femoris muscle laterally and the semitendinous muscle medially. In the lower portion of the popliteal fossa, the vein lies medial to the artery. In the proximal portion, after having crossed the artery dorsally, it flows posterolaterally into the adductor canal, where it becomes the SFV. On its upward course, it runs mainly dorsal to the artery; only in the proximal portion is it found medially. After having joined the deep femoral vein (DFV) approximately 2–12 cm below the inguinal ligament, it becomes the CFV. The CFV always lies medial to the artery. Very constantly just below the femoral vein junction, a valve is found. The SFV is a single vessel in 62% (Weber and May 1990), while in 21% there are paired vessels in the distal segment, in 13% multiple veins are found, and in only 3% is the vein completely paired.

Usually, the SFV has 3–5 valves. Above the inguinal ligament, it becomes the external iliac vein (EIV), which first runs medially and then posteriorly to the external iliac artery and, after joining the internal iliac vein (IIV), continues as the common iliac vein (CIV) into the IVC. The junction of the CIVs with the IVC is to the right of the spine (May 1974). The right CIV is located dorsal to the corresponding artery, while the left CIV lies medial to the artery. Shortly before its junction, it is crossed by the right common iliac artery and pressed against the body of the 5th lumbar vertebra. At this point, the left CIV may be obstructed by a venous spur, a membrane that projects into the venous lumen. In addition, there is a higher rate of left-sided CIV thrombosis (67% on the left vs 33% on the right side) due to this arterial compression, which may cause a reactive intima proliferation. EIV and CIV usually have no valves.

2.1.1.2.3 Perforating Veins

The blood vessels termed the perforating veins (PVs) connect the superficial, epifascial, and deep subfascial veins. Physiologically, they transport blood from the superficial venous system into the subfascial veins. Reverse blood flow is prevented by valves. Of the approximately 150 PVs throughout the lower extremity, only a few, the majority of which are located in the lower leg, are of clinical significance. For the calf, the Cockett perforating veins I–III, the Sherman and the Boyd group are of importance, while in the thigh the Dodd PVs are of clinical interest in case of PV insufficiency.

2.1.1.3 Examination Technique

For US examination of the iliac, CFV, and SFV, the patient should be positioned supine with the leg slightly abducted and externally rotated. Elevation of the body can be offered to highly dyspneic patients. The POPV is examined with the patient decubitus or prone. The knee should be flexed approximately 20–30°. This prevents stretching and compression of the POPV by the gastrocnemius tendons and facilitates its compression by the transducer during the investigation. The POPV can also be examined with the patient in a supine, lateral, or sitting position. If a supine position is necessary, e.g., in bedridden patients, the foot should be held a little upward by a second person.

The lower leg veins can be examined with the patient seated with dangling lower legs. In more incapacitated patients, the calf may also be examined in the supine position, with the leg abducted and externally rotated. Physiologic changes (gravity) to venous morphology in different patient positions have to be considered. As a general rule, gravity (sitting or standing patient position) increases the venous cross-sectional area and decreases flow velocity in the lower extremity.

The US investigation consists of B-mode imaging using compression of the veins and CDDS in combination with several maneuvers including increased respiration, Valsalva's maneuver, and manual signal amplification as described in Chapter 3.

When using the B-mode, veins are displayed as round or oval-shaped structures in a transverse section; the venous lumen is usually anechoic. The venous lumen can be compressed completely by applying pressure via the scan head (Fig. 2.2). When CDDS is used, the vessel should be investigated in the longitudinal and transverse planes. The lumen should be entirely occupied by the color flow signal. Care should be taken to place the duplex Doppler sample volume in the center of the vein, usually in longitudinal scans of the vein.

The examination starts with a transverse scan of the proximal thigh (Foley 1991, pp. 128–151). The transducer should be positioned just below the inguinal ligament, where the CFV is easily found medial to the femoral artery (Fig. 2.3). The course of the vein is now followed distally to the SFV (Fig. 2.4), and soft pressure is applied with the transducer. In contrast to the accompanying arteries, the patent vein can be totally compressed. Under compression, the transducer is moved a few centimeters caudally, then pressure is briefly reduced until the vein shortly opens, followed by another compression. Proceeding from a dorsal direction, the POPV is examined in the popliteal fossa, where it is close to the transducer. As in the thigh, a sequential change of compression and release is applied (Fig. 2.5).

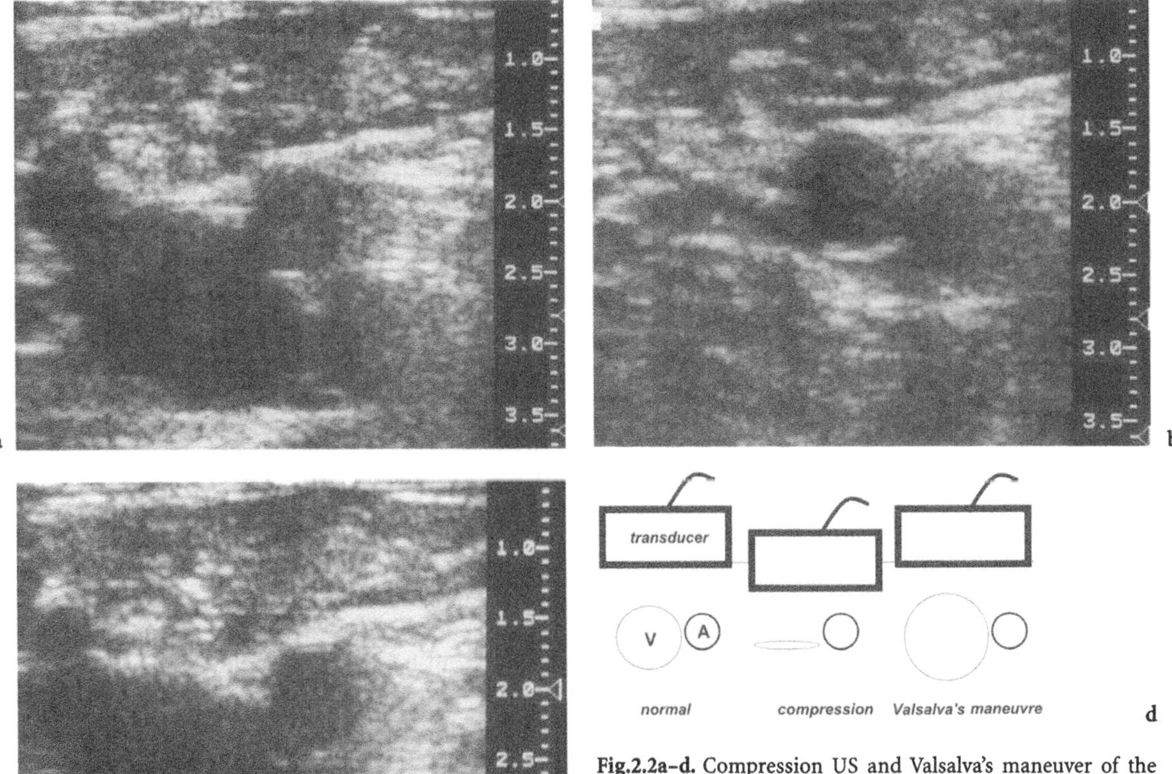

Fig. 2.2a–d. Compression US and Valsalva's maneuver of the left common femoral vein (CFV, *V*). **a** Normal, quiet respiration and gentle compression of the transducer. Manual compression (**b**) and Valsalva's maneuver (**c**). Note complete compression of the normal CFV lumen in **b** and increase in diameter in **c** while the diameter of the common femoral artery (CFA, *A*) remains constant. Corresponding graph demonstrated in **d**

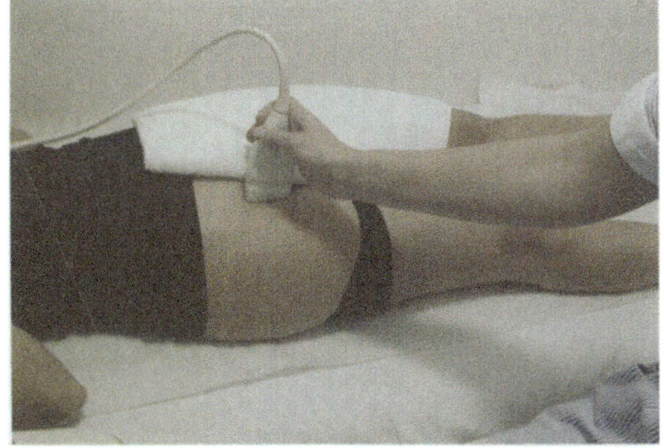

a

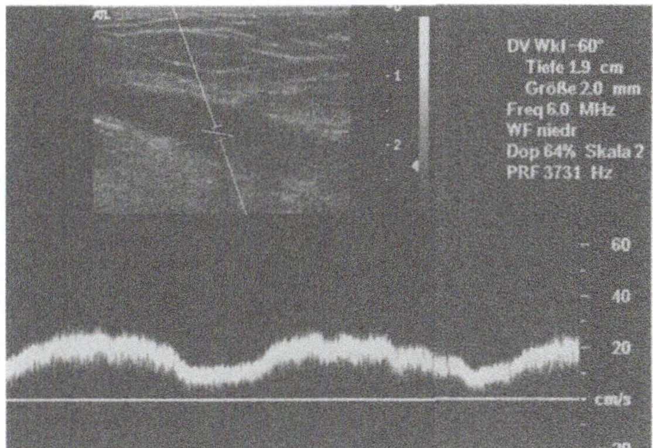

b

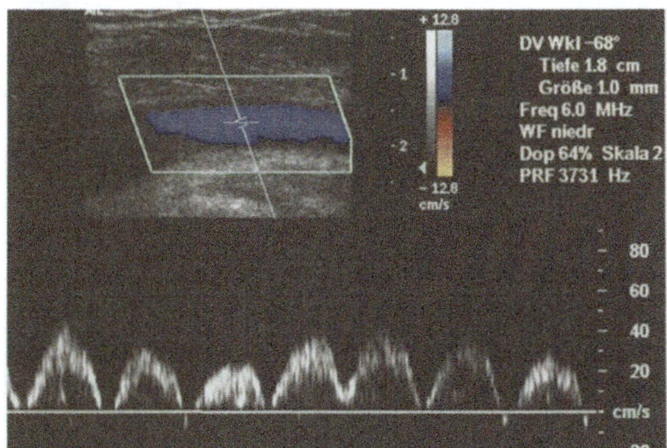

c

Fig. 2.3a–c. Longitudinal CDDS imaging of the CFV. **a** Position of the scan head. CDDS demonstrating normal respiratory variability in a volunteer (**b**) and marked cardiac variability in another volunteer (**c**)

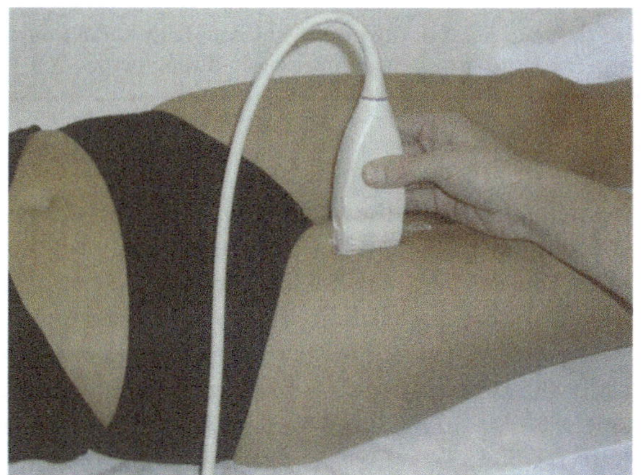

a

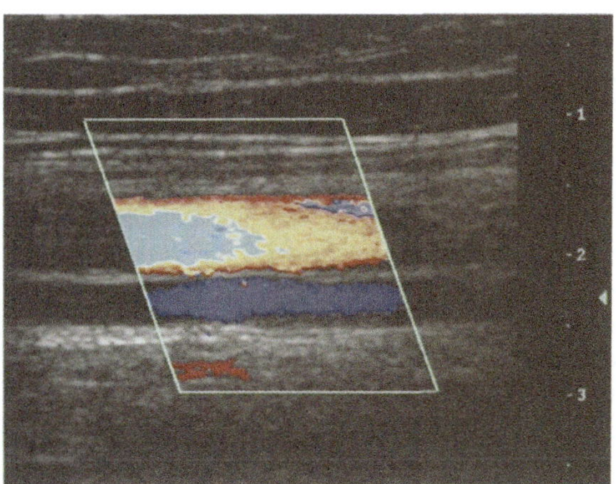

b

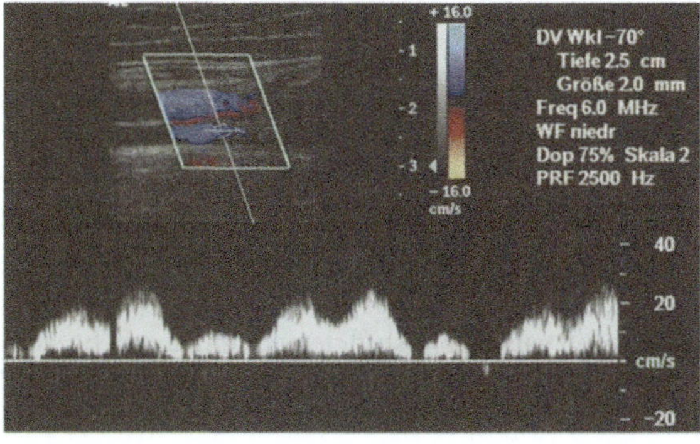

c

Fig. 2.4a–c. Longitudinal CDDS imaging of the superficial femoral vein (SFV). **a** Position of the scan head. CDDS demonstrating color flow both in the SFA and SFV (vein encoded in blue, below artery) (**b**) and Doppler curve with respiratory and cardiac variability (**c**)

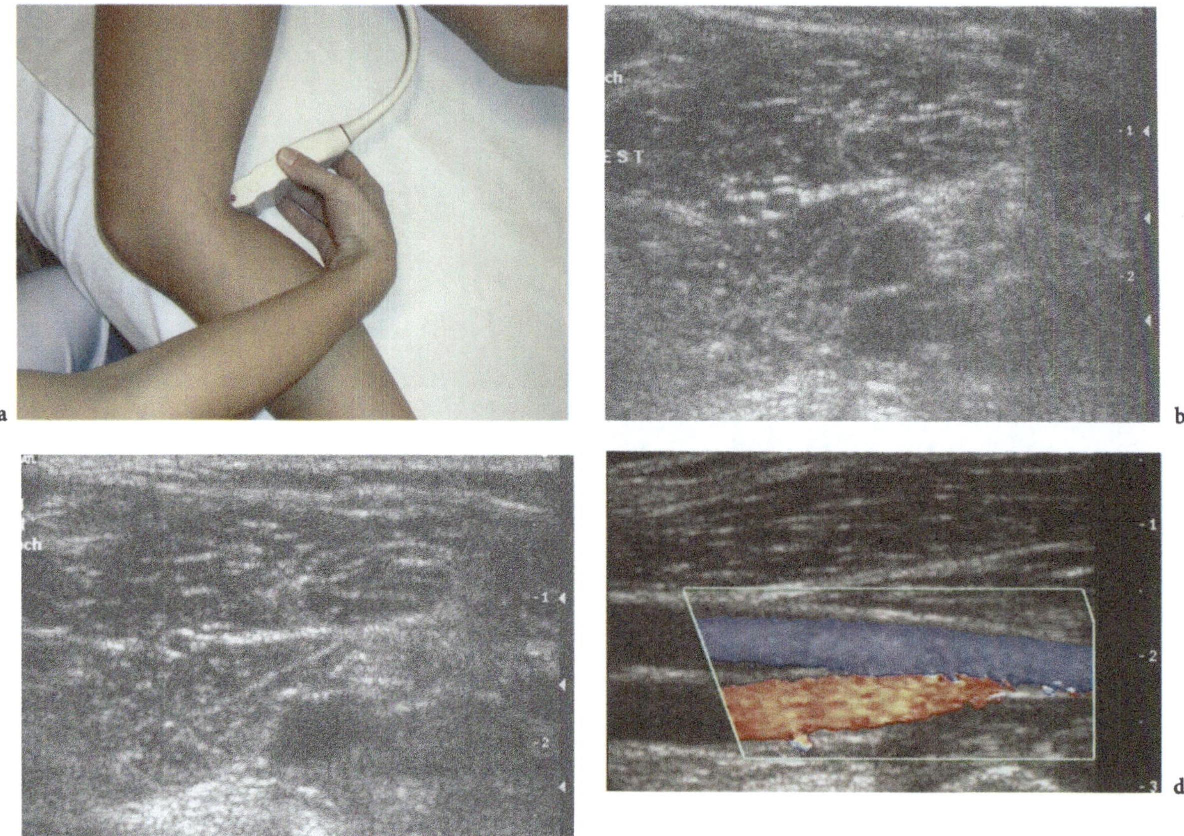

Fig. 2.5a–d. Imaging of the popliteal vein (POPV). **a** Position of the scan head in the popliteal fossa. Transverse image of POPV and popliteal artery without (**b**) and with compression (**c**). Note complete compression of the normal POPV in **c**. **d** Longitudinal CDDS image of the POPV encoded blue

The PTV, ATV, and FV can be visualized in the majority of patients. However, the vessels' slower venous flow and smaller diameter (only a few millimeters) make this task more difficult. The vessels can be imaged longitudinally using a coronal approach, with the transducer placed on the medial posterior calf. It is usually not possible to image each of the paired venae comitantes simultaneously with a coronal longitudinal imaging plane. Therefore, the same vessels should be re-evaluated in a transverse plane. In very obese legs, it may be difficult to examine the ATV; the latter can be found by a ventrolateral access between the tibia and the fibula (Fig. 2.6).

Pelvic veins can only be compressed in thin patients. In order to evaluate their patency, several maneuvers using B-mode and CDDS are helpful as described in Chapter 3 in detail. Distal manual compression increases the vessel diameter and flow velocity. Valsalva's maneuver increases the vessel diameter and stops the blood flow. However, demonstrating normal blood flow and patency of the iliac veins and the IVC may be difficult in obese patients or in cases of poor visibility due to bowel gas.

Indications to examine the superficial veins, especially the GSV and SSV, include varicosis, phlebitis, and valvular and chronic venous insufficiency. The best results are achieved with the patient standing. Linear scanners with transmission frequencies between 5.0 and 12 MHz are recommended. The GSV is examined in longitudinal scans starting in the groin. The normal response to Valsalva's maneuver is an increase in venous diameter to the first proximal valve and a stop of the blood flow (Fig. 2.7). Valvular insufficiency is demonstrated by CDDS in Valsalva's maneuver as a long reflux. Assessing the SSV may be difficult if the vein is normal and of small diameter. In case of valvular insufficiency, reflux can be augmented by manually compressing the POPV or SFV just above the inflow of the SSV. To examine the PVs,

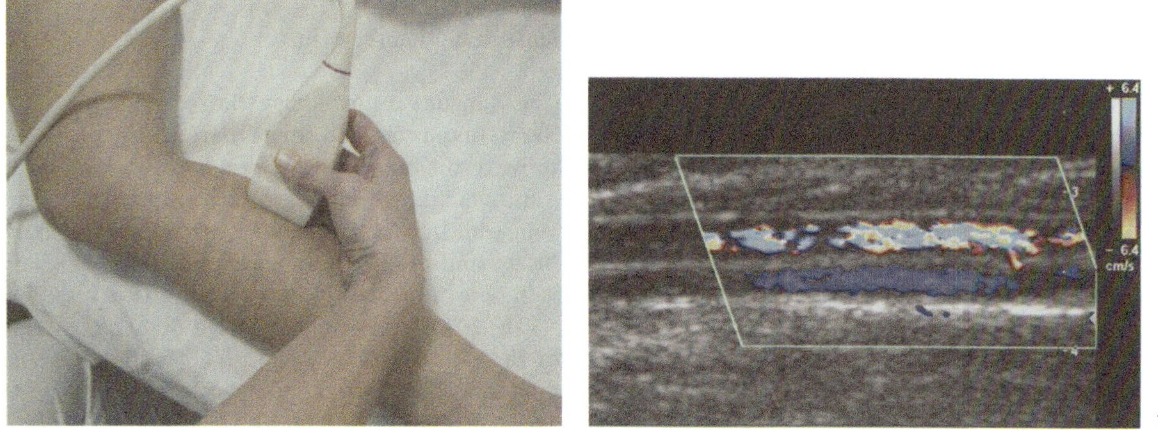

Fig. 2.6a,b. Longitudinal CDDS imaging of the posterior tibial vein (PTV). Position of the scan head (**a**) and CDDS image with PTV encoded in blue (**b**)

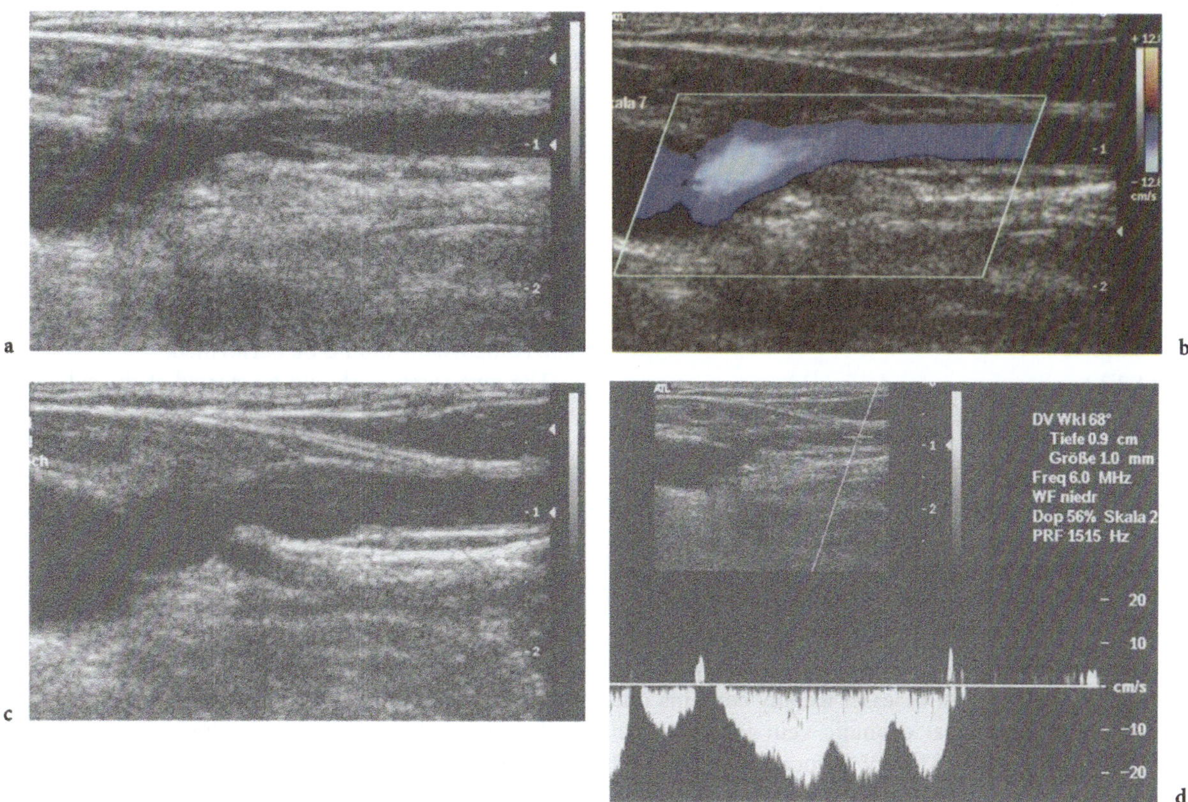

Fig. 2.7a–d. CDDS imaging of the great saphenous vein (GSV) using longitudinal US scans. **a** GSV at rest with the patient supine. Diameter (between crosses) 0.3cm. Note normal proximal valve leaflets near the crosses (**a**). **b** CDDS demonstrating laminar flow at rest towards the heart. **c,d** Normal response toValsalva's maneuver. Note increase in diameter in B-mode US (**c**) and cessation of flow in CDDS indicating a competent valve (**d**)

the patient should be made to sit with legs dangling. Proximal and distal to the PV, a tourniquet should be placed in order to compress the superficial vein, and the soft tissue manually compressed. In cases of insufficient PVs, flow from the deep veins towards the transducer will be observed in the PV.

2.1.2 Veins of the Upper Extremity

2.1.2.1 *Technical Equipment*

As with the lower extremities, linear array probes with frequencies from 5.0 to 12.0 MHz are preferred. Small sector probes with frequencies from 5.0 to 10.0 MHz may be helpful to examine the veins of the thoracic outlet and the brachiocephalic veins via a jugular approach. Again, in CDDS, flow sensitivity should be set so that the color flow is demonstrated through the full diameter or cross-section of the vein during the phase of maximum venous flow.

2.1.2.2 *Anatomy*

As in the lower extremities, the venous system can be divided into a superficial and a deep part (Fig. 2.8).

2.1.2.2.1 Deep Venous System

The ulnar and radial veins, collecting blood from the deep palmar arch, follow the course of the corresponding arteries in pairs. They flow slightly above the elbow joint into the brachial veins (BV), which are normally also paired, and unite at the lower margin of the pectoral muscle to form the axillary vein (AV) together with the basilic vein, which is only paired in 1% of cases. It usually contains one valve. The superficial cephalic vein joins 2–3 cm distal to this point. The AV is located ventral and caudal to the corresponding artery and becomes the subclavian vein (SV) after passing below the clavicle. The SV flows cephalad to the first rib and unites ventral to the anterior scalene muscle with the internal jugular vein (IJV) to form the brachiocephalic vein (BCV); the last valve is located in this so-called venous angle. The BCVs join in the upper anterior mediastinum to form the superior vena cava (SVC).

2.1.2.2.2 Superficial Venous System

The cephalic vein arises from the radial margin of the dorsal venous rete and crosses the forearm diagonally to reach the cubital fossa. From here, a side branch – the cubital medial vein – flows towards the basilic vein, while the main stem flows medially between the biceps and the brachioradial muscle to the axillary vein. The cephalic vein contains 6 to 10 valves.

The basilic vein proceeds from the ulnar margin of the dorsal venous plexus, follows the ulna, and crosses at the proximal region of the antebrachii to the volar side. At the elbow, it is joined by the cubital medial vein and continues into the medial bicipital sulcus to the middle section of the upper arm, where it perforates the deep fascia and flows into the medial brachial vein. The basilic vein contains 4 to 8 valves and may be paired, especially in the forearm.

2.1.2.3 *Examination Technique*

The upper extremity veins are examined with the patient positioned supine. The patient's arm should be placed at his or her side in a neutral or slightly abducted position, with the hands supine. It is a matter of personal preference whether the sonographer sits at the left side or behind the patient. As is recommended for the lower extremities, a side-to-side comparison should be performed.

The investigation should be started at the subclavian jugular junction, although imaging of the proximal infraclavicular SV may be difficult, depending on the patient's body. When turning the transducer parallel to the longitudinal axis and moving it laterally, the infraclavicular portion of the subclavian vein can be visualized and evaluated. To examine the AV and BVs, the arm is abducted and externally rotated. The proximal portion of the AV often has to be investigated in the same way as the SV, while the distal portion as well as the BVs and the veins of the forearm are evaluated in the same fashion as is done for the lower extremity veins (Fig. 2.9). In other words, the most important criteria in B-mode US is compressibility. Analogously to the leg veins, the transducer is slowly guided distally, while applying a continuous alternation of compression and release in the transverse plane. Care has to be taken when the epifascial veins are being investigated. In this setting, the transducer should be guided with no more than a light touch.

With the exception of patients with a mediastinal mass, lymphadenopathy, or lipomatosis, it is not pos-

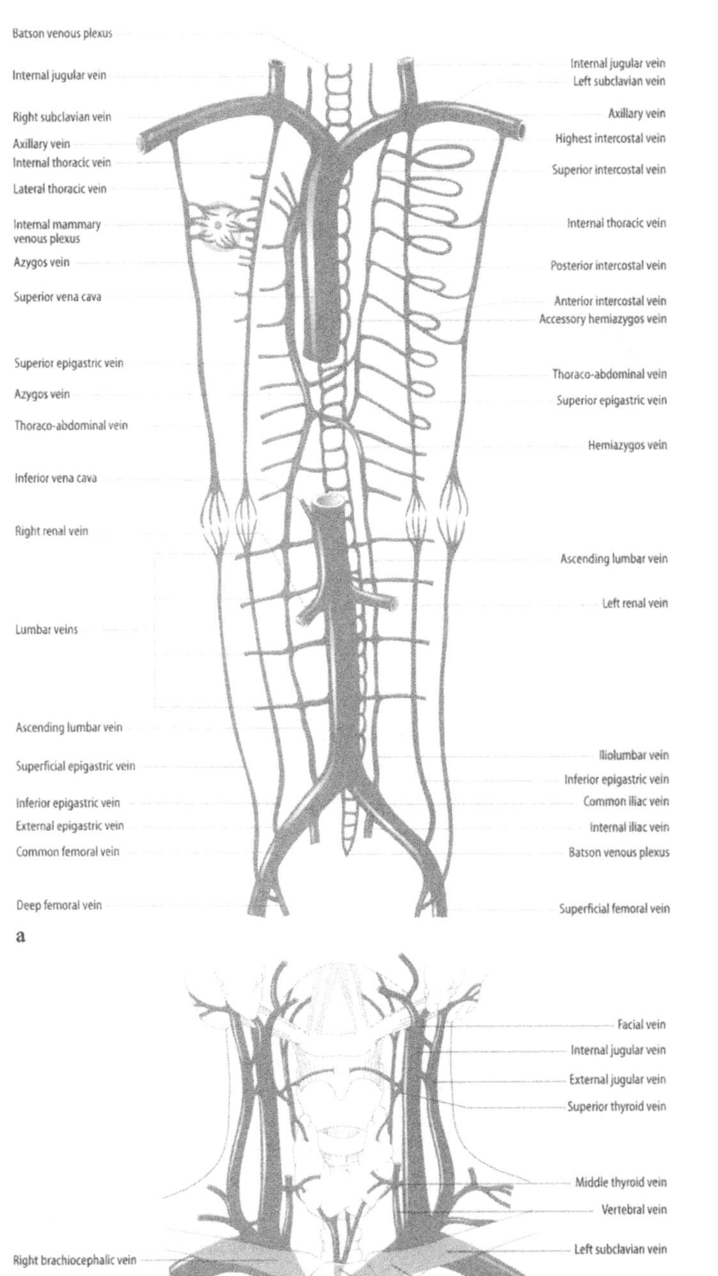

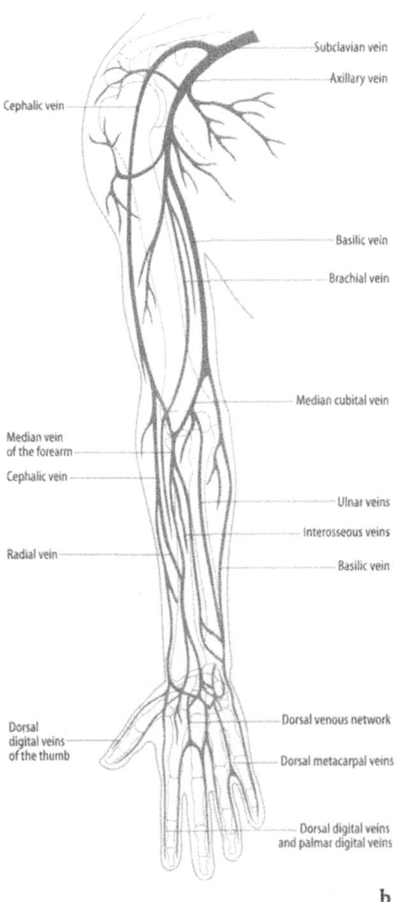

Fig.2.8a–c. Anatomy of the veins of the neck, arms, chest, abdominal wall, and retroperitoneum

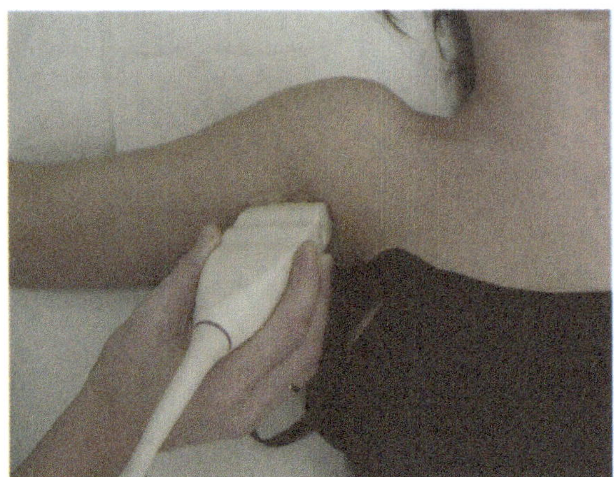

a

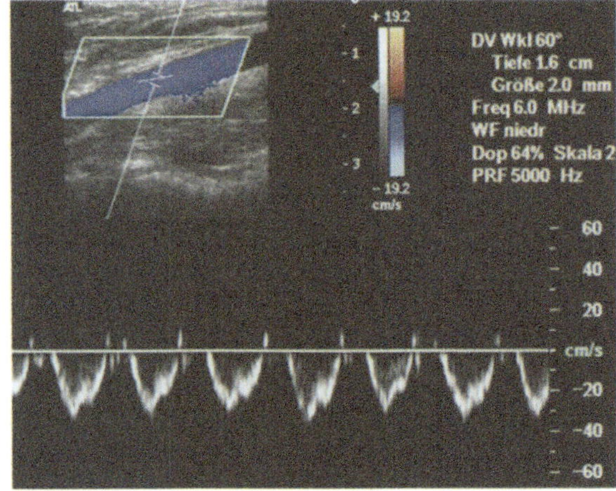

b

Fig. 2.9a,b. CDDS imaging of the axillary vein (AV) in the right axilla. Position of the scan head for a longitudinal scan (**a**) and corresponding CDDS image with AV encoded in blue and some cardiac variability in AV flow (**b**)

sible to image the entire BV and the SVC sufficiently by US. However, normal cardiac and respiratory variability of blood flow obtained by CDDS and normal response to augmented flow maneuvers in the SV or IJV are indicators of normal venous blood flow up to the right atrium.

2.2 Extracranial Veins – Internal Jugular and Vertebral Vein

2.2.1 Anatomy

The IJV is located lateral to the common and the internal carotid artery. It can be followed caudally up to the vascular angle where it forms the BCV together with the SV. The vertebral vein can be examined discontinuously above C6, as the vein is in part obscured by the transverse processes of the vertebral bodies. It can be found ventral to the vertebral artery (Rouveire and Delmas 1985).

2.2.2 Examination Technique

To investigate the vessels of the neck, 5.0 to 12.0 MHz linear array transducers are recommended. The patient is positioned supine with the head turned to the opposite side. For the IJV, a posterolateral and/or anterolateral approach is used, often employing the sternocleidomastoid muscle as an acoustic window. The vertebral vein may also be examined with a posterolaterally positioned probe in longitudinal section. The IJV should be examined both in longitudinal and transverse scans (Fig. 2.10). Using CDDS, flow sensitivity should be adjusted so that the recorded flow occupies the full diameter of the vessel. Various maneuvers are useful to demonstrate venous patency and normal venous flow (see Chapter 3).

2.3 Abdominal Veins

US and CDDS are powerful tools in assessing the abdominal venous anatomy, pathology, and blood flow (Foley 1991, p. 67). In general, standard curved array abdominal transducers operating from 2.0 to 5.0 MHz are required. For CDDS, the use of a "windows" function in order to increase the Doppler frame rate is standard. Low-velocity scales (pulse repetition frequency), low wall filter adjustment, and adequate gain settings just below the disappearance of color noise are mandatory for good results.

Patients are usually positioned supine, additionally in the left or right anterior oblique position, depending on the vessel being examined. Care should be taken to place the patient in a relaxed position, since any tension in the abdominal muscles will increase the intra-abdominal pressure and affect the venous flow relationships. For examination of the deep intra-abdominal veins like POV or IVC, putting the patient in the standing position sometimes dramatically improves US visibility, as overlying gas-filled bowel loops drop down and give free access to

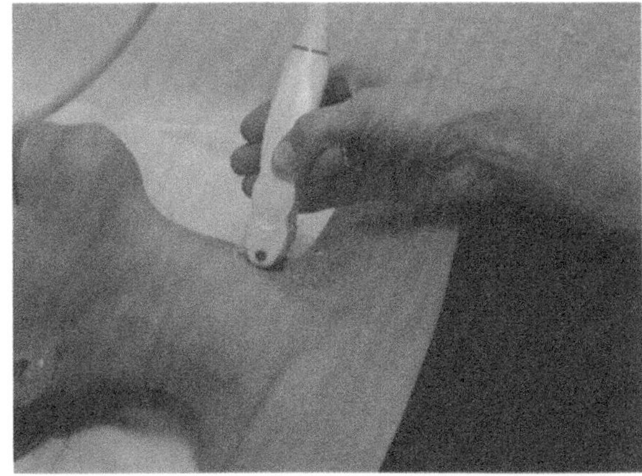
a

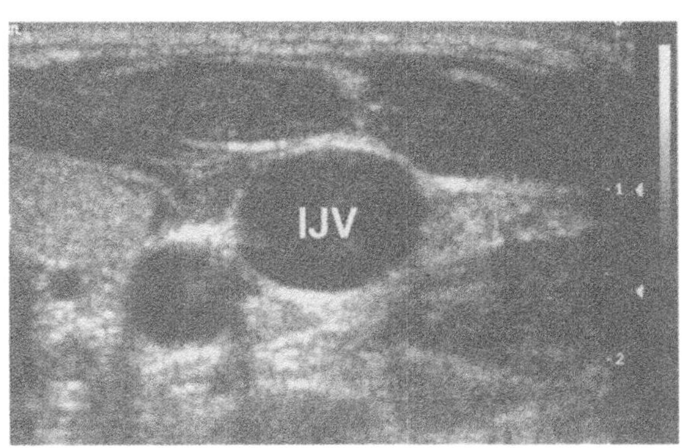

b

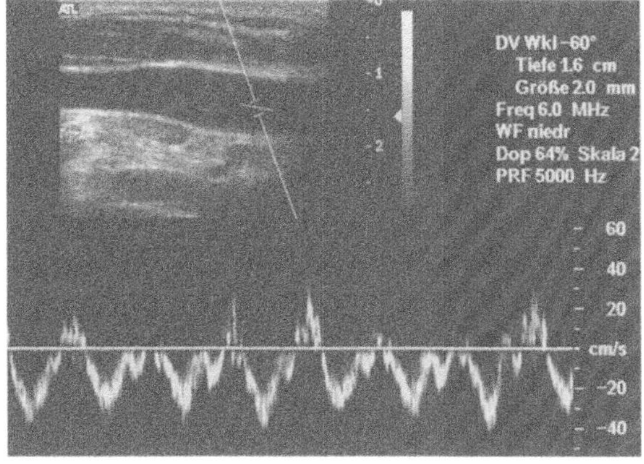

c

Fig. 2.10a–c. Imaging of the internal jugular vein (IJV). Position of the scan head for a transverse scan of the left IJV (**a**), corresponding B-mode US image with left IJV lateral to the common carotid artery (**b**), and CDDS demonstrating marked cardiac variability in IJV flow (**c**)

these vessels – sometimes using the left lobe of the liver as an acoustic window.

2.3.1
Anatomy and Examination Technique

2.3.1.1
Inferior Vena Cava

The CIVs join at the level of the 4rth and 5th lumbar vertebra to form the IVC (Fig. 2.11). It runs right to the abdominal aorta and passes through the vena caval foramen into the thorax. The IVC is joined by the right ovarian (testicular), the renal, the right suprarenal, the lumbar, and the phrenic veins. Finally, 2–5 hepatic veins (usually 3) join the IVC below the diaphragm. The diameter varies with respiration. The maximum diameter is achieved during Valsalva's maneuver. The diameter of the IVC is modulated by the heart, as well as by the flow dynamics. These dynamics are seen on B-mode US as marked caliber changes of the IVC, referred as the "double beat" of the IVC (Fig. 2.12).

Variant anatomy of the IVC is not rare and may be found in up to 7% of patients. Due to the rather complex embryological development, the more common variants are a left-sided or paired IVC (Bürggemann et al. 1993; Kubale et al. 1992; Pierro et al. 1990). Agenesis of the infrarenal or hepatic segment of the IVC leads to azygos or hemiazygos continuation of blood flow of the lower body to the SVC.

Using B-mode imaging and CDDS, the IVC is investigated in longitudinal and transverse scans from ventral and right lateral. Under good sonographic conditions, it is possible to image the IVC from the junction of the hepatic veins to the confluence of the CIVs (Hennerici and Neuerburg-Heusler 1998, p. 283; Kubale 1993). Normal B-mode findings are a lumen free of reflections, a delicate wall, and a "double beat". Normal CDDS findings are demonstrated in Chapter 3.

2.3.1.2
Renal Veins

Numerous arcuate and interlobar veins form a single renal vein (RV). On the right side, the RV is about 2.5 cm in length and reaches the IVC almost at an right angle. On the left side, the RV measures approximately 8 cm, crosses the aorta ventrally, courses dorsal to the superior mesenteric artery, joins with the left testicular (or ovaric) and the suprarenal veins,

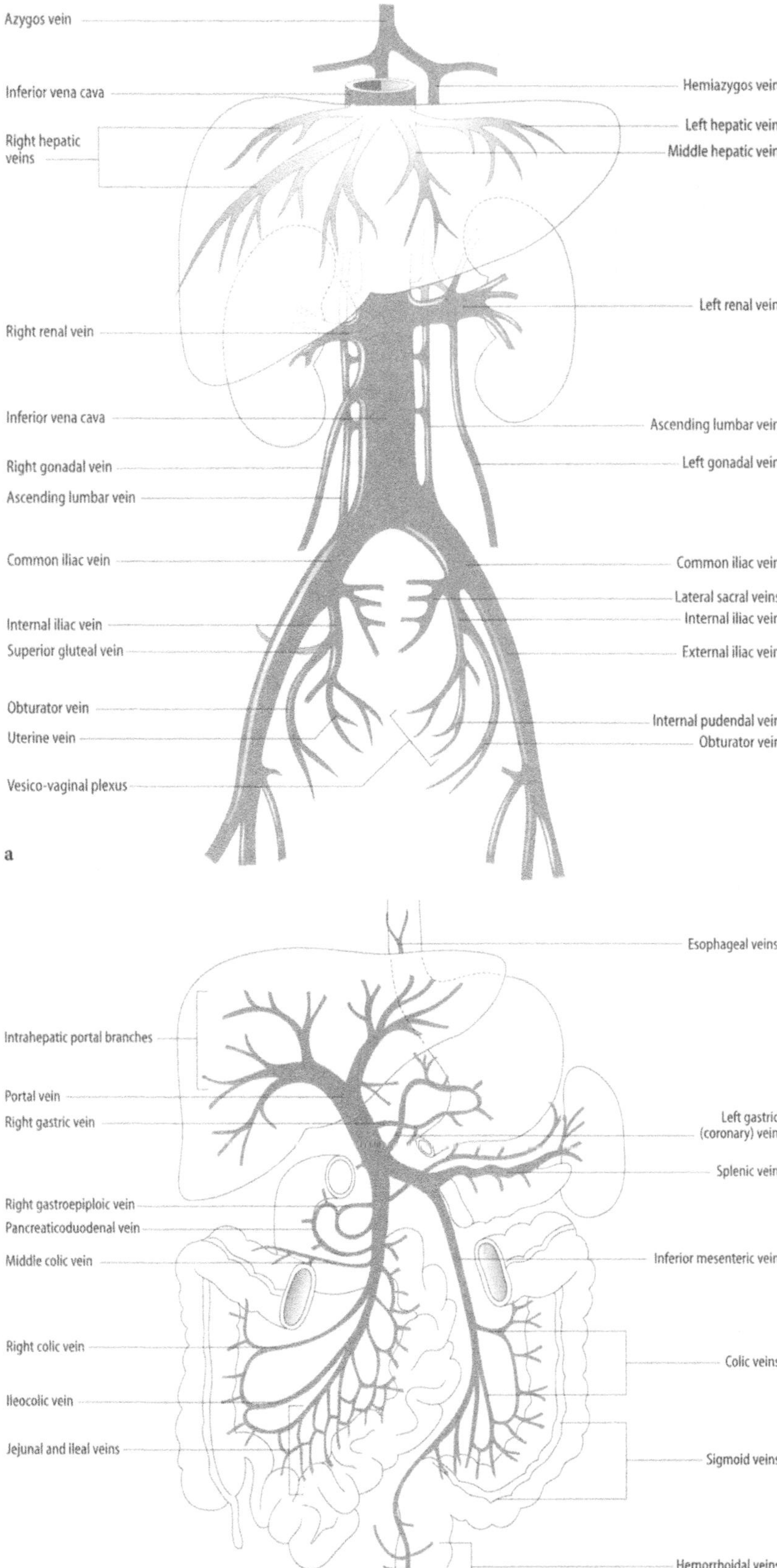

Fig.2.11a,b. Anatomy of the intra-abdominal and retroperitoneal veins

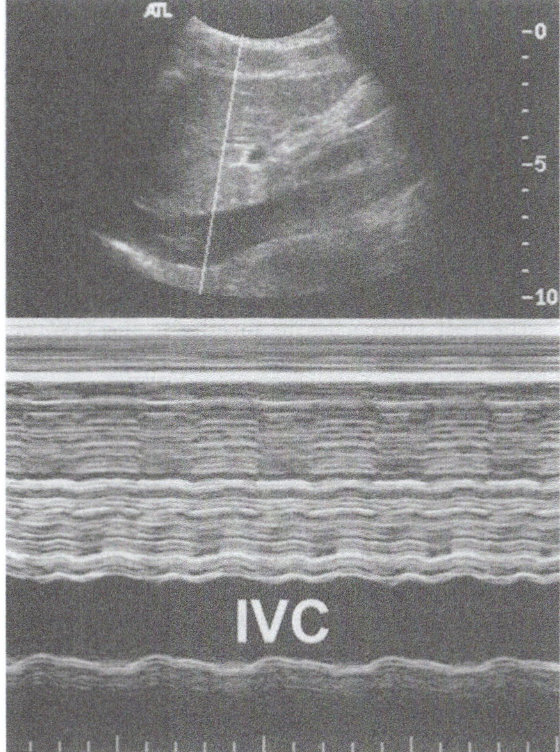

Fig.2.12. B-mode longitudinal scan (*top*) and M-mode (*bottom*, along the *white line* in the B-mode image) of the inferior vena cava (*IVC*). Note cardiac modulation changing the IVC diameter ("double beat")

and reaches the IVC also at the level of the first or second lumbar vertebra. The most common variant in this region is a retroaortic course of the left RV.

RVs can be examined in the transverse plane or by oblique dorsolumbar sections (Fig. 2.13). The examination is started at the level of the superior mesenteric artery by drawing the transducer slowly in a caudad direction, until the left RV is found between the superior mesenteric artery and the aorta. Tilting the transducer slightly to the right and caudad, the right RV becomes visible. Normal CDDS findings are demonstrated in Chapter 3.

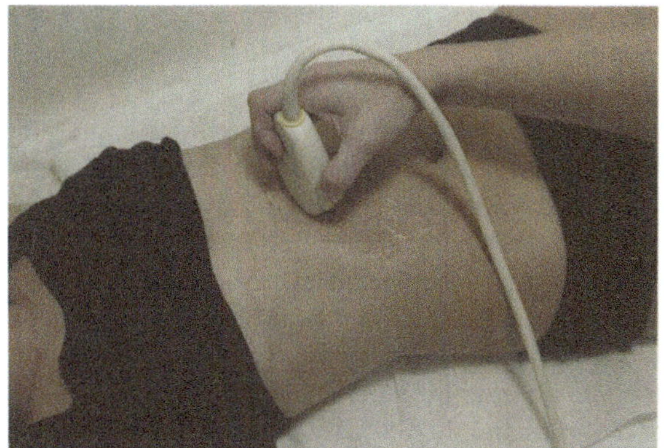
a

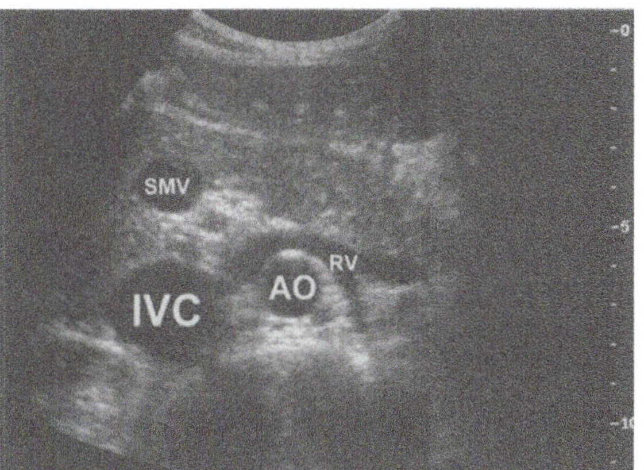

b

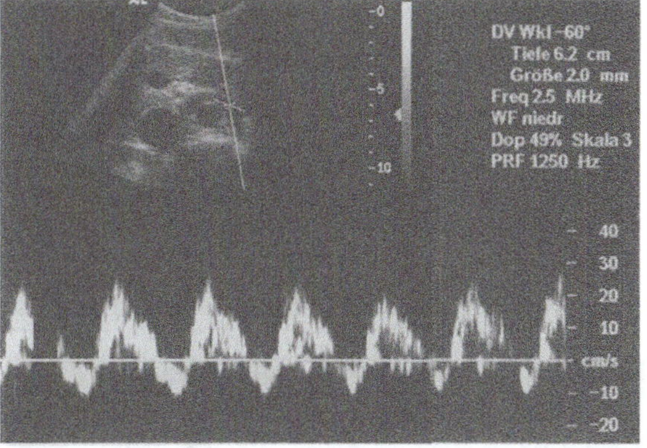

c

Fig.2.13a–c. Imaging of the left renal vein (*RV*). **a** Position of the scan head. **b** Corresponding B-mode US image demonstrating left RV crossing from left to right to the IVC between abdominal aorta (*AO*) and mesenteric root (*SMV* superior mesenteric vein). **c** Note cardiac variability of left RV flow in the Doppler curve

2.3.1.3 Hepatic Veins

Usually three hepatic veins (HVs; right, middle, and left) lead blood from the liver to the IVC. However, there is marked anatomic variability regarding the number and course of these veins. They can be followed in B-mode US from the periphery to their confluence with the IVC through a right sub- or intercostal oblique approach. In B-mode imaging, the HVs, in contrast to the POV, demonstrate no walls except in situations when the course of the veins and the US beam reach an angle of about 90°. Using CDDS, there is marked cardiac modulation of the flow velocity as in the IVC (Fig. 2.14).

2.3.1.4 Portal Venous System

Anatomically, the portal venous system consists of the portal vein (POV) and its sources, the superior mesenteric vein (SMV), the splenic vein (SPV), the coronary vein of the stomach (right and left gastric veins, prepyloric vein), and directly or indirectly the inferior mesenteric vein (IMV). The portal vein originates behind the isthmus of the pancreas at the confluence of the SMV and SPV and proceeds in the hepatoduodenal ligament to the liver, together with the bile duct and the hepatic artery. Intrahepatically, it is divided into a right and left main branch and further into 6–10 smaller branches that supply the corresponding liver segments.

The best approaches to investigate the POV are paramedian, transcostal, and lateral subcostal sections. In B-mode imaging, it has an oval, echo-free lumen and is only minimally affected by respiratory modulation. The flow direction is hepatopetal, and the mean flow velocity varies between 10 and 25 cm/s (Seitz and Kubale 1988; Wermke 1989), although postprandial peak velocities of up to 40 cm/s have been reported.

In CDDS, the POV is usually filled homogeneously, demonstrating the same color as the accompanying

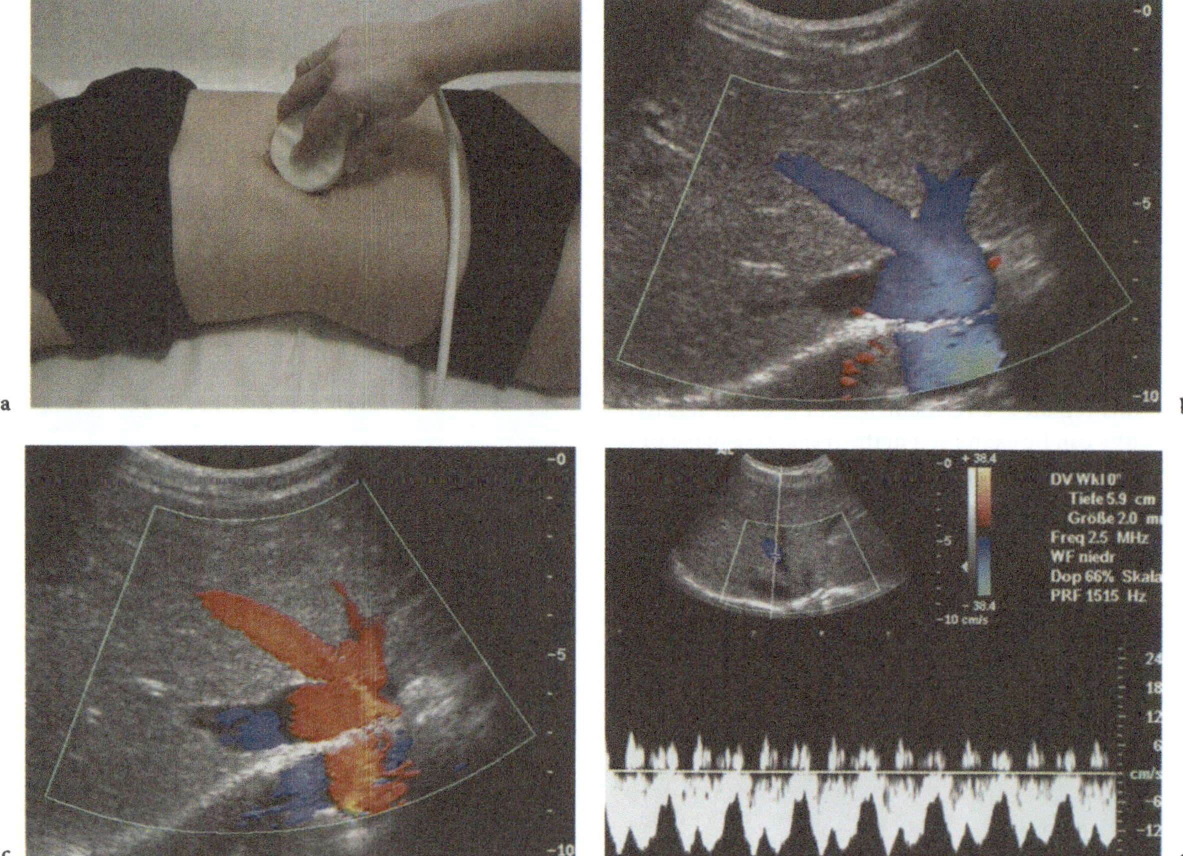

Fig. 2.14a–d. CDDS of the liver veins. **a** Position of the scan head for a subcostal approach. Corresponding CDDS image with liver veins encoded in blue (**b**) and red (**c**) depending on the point in time of the cardiac cycle. **d** Doppler curve demonstrates marked cardiac variability with flow towards and away from the transducer

hepatic arteries. In the majority of cases, there is laminar, monochromatic color flow. Only in a small percentage can one find alternating or parallel red and blue bands, which indicate helical flow in the main POV and should not be mistaken for simultaneous bidirectional portal venous flow. Although helical flow may be an indicator of liver disease, it may be a normal appearance in 2%.

The SPV is formed in the hilum of the spleen. It proceeds dorsal to the pancreas and caudal to the splenic artery over a length of about 15 cm to the confluence with the SMV, and also collects blood from the IMV in 70% of cases. In about 30% of cases, the IMV connects to the SMV directly. Additional venous pathways to the SPV are the short gastric veins, the left gastroepiploic vein, and numerous small veins of the pancreatic tail and the duodenum. The SPV is investigated in transverse sections of the upper abdomen angled along the course of the vessel. In CDDS, hepatopetal flow with a mean velocity of approximately 5–12 cm/s is the normal finding (Fig. 2.15).

The SMV drains blood from the jejunum, ileum, the ascending and transverse colon, as well as the pancreaticoduodenal arcades. It moves adjacent and right to the superior mesenteric artery and joins the SPV dorsal to the pancreas. The diameter is usually larger than that of the accompanying artery, and the mean flow velocity ranges between 9 and 18 cm/s, with significant increases in flow velocity and diameter in the postprandial state. The SMV is best investigated in transverse and longitudinal scans in the same way as the IVC.

The IMV collects blood from the left-sided colon. It joins the SPV or the SMV behind the pancreas. The IMV is rarely seen on US scans due to its small diameter and variable course.

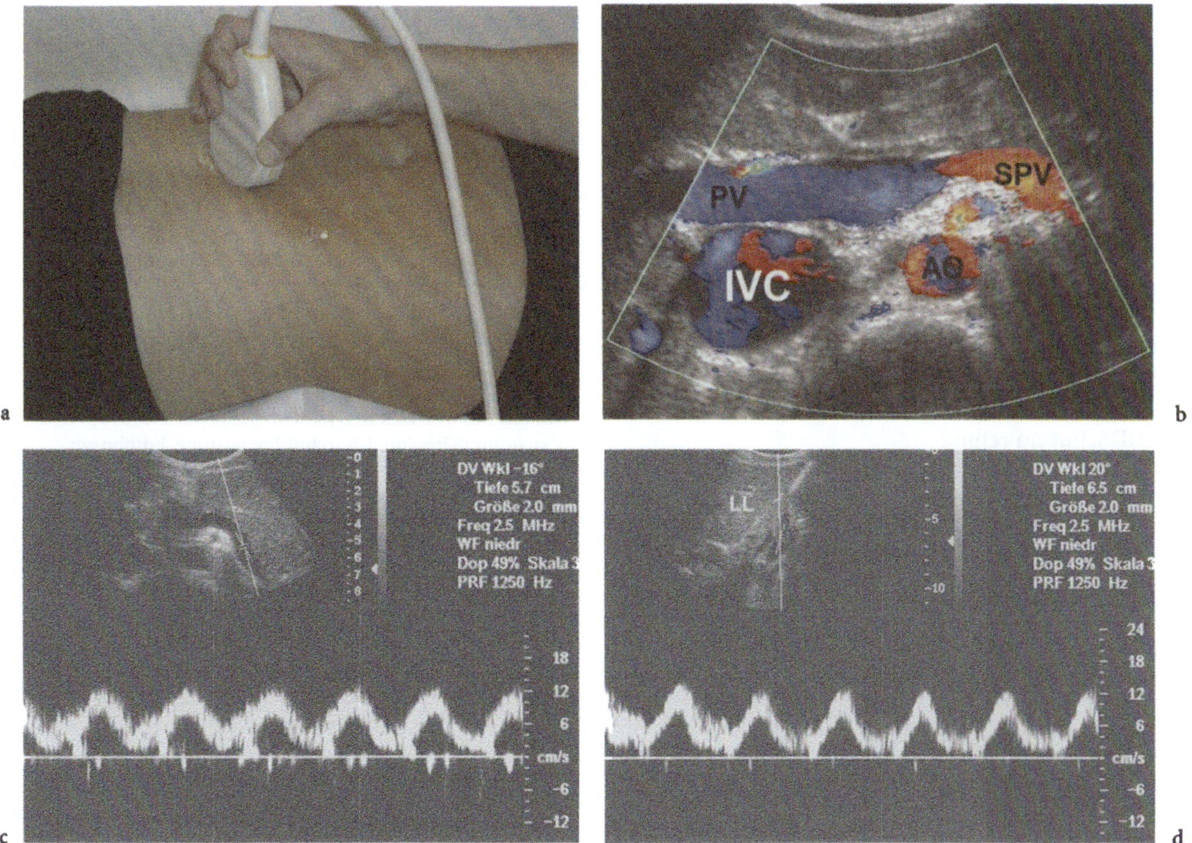

Fig. 2.15a–d. CDDS of the splenoportal axis. **a** Position of the scan head for a longitudinal US scan of the splenoportal axis. **b** Corresponding CDDS image with portal vein (*POV*) and splenic vein (*SPV*) changing color from red (flow towards the transducer in the SPV) to blue (flow away from the transducer in the POV) with normal hepatopetal flow direction. **c** Doppler flow curve obtained in the SPV in the longitudinal direction shows cardiac variability. **d** SPV might be demonstrated behind the pancreas by rotating the scan head 90° and tilting the imaging plane along the direction of the pancreatic tail. *LL* left lobe of the liver

2.4 Scrotal Veins

2.4.1 Anatomy

Numerous veins collect blood from the testicles and gather at the hilum, where they form the pampiniform plexus, a venous network and the main structure of the spermatic cord. The left testicular vein drains into the left RV, while the right testicular vein joins the IVC directly (Gösfay 1959; Hamm 1991; Fobbe 1993).

2.4.2 Examination Technique

Sonography is generally performed with the patient first in the supine and then in the standing position. The patient is asked to keep the penis away from the scrotal area, which can be easily elevated by some paper or towel. The 5.0 to 12.0 MHz transducers should be used, and CDDS parameters should be adjusted to their most flow-sensitive settings. The pampiniform plexus is best seen cephalad and lateral to the head of the epididymis both in the longitudinal and transverse planes (Fobbe 1993). After localizing the spermatic cord, it is first scanned at rest. The patient should then be asked to perform a Valsalva's maneuver. In normal cases, the diameter of the single vessel remains constant, measuring no more than 2 mm. As a normal finding, there should be cessation of venous flow with the Valsalva's maneuver at CDDS, but no reflux.

References

Brüggemann A, Schmid A, Wüstner M, Klinge B, Lepsien G (1993) Sonographische Darstellung einer Dopplung der Vena cava inferior. Ultraschall Klin Prax 8:37–40

Fobbe F (1993) Skrotum. In: Wolff KJ, Fobbe F (eds) Farbkodierte Duplexsonographie. Thieme, Stuttgart, p 197

Foley D (1991) Color Doppler flow imaging. Andover Med, Boston

Gösfay S (1959) Untersuchungen der Vena spermatica interna durch retrograde Phlebographie bei Kranken mit Varikozele. Z Urol 2:105–115

Hamm B (1991) Sonographische Diagnostik des Skrotalinhaltes, Lehrbuch und Atlas. Springer, Berlin Heidelberg New York

Hennerici M, Neuerburg-Heusler D (1998) Vascular diagnosis with ultrasound. Thieme, Stuttgart

Kubale R (1993) Abdominelle Venen, portalvenöses System und Leber. In: Farbkodierte Duplexsonographie. Thieme, Stuttgart, p 163

Kubale R, Grimbach M, Walter F, Girmann M, Güttner B, Boos H, Heger N (1992) Nicht invasive Diagnostik isolierter Thromben der Vena mesenterica superior. Ultraschall Klin Prax 7:238

May R (1974) Chirurgie der Bein- und Beckenvenen. Thieme, Stuttgart, p 168

Pierro JA, Soleimanpour M, Bory JL (1990) Left retrocaval ureter associated with left inferior vena cava. Am J Roentgenol 155:545–546

Rouviere H, Delmas A (1985) Anatomie humaine, tête et cou, tome 1. Masson, Paris, pp 225–243

Seitz K, Kubale R (1988) Duplexsonographie der abdominellen und retroperitonealen Gefäße. Edition Medizin, Weinheim, pp 57–127

Weber L, May R (1990) Funktionelle Phlebographie. Thieme, Stuttgart, p 25

Wermke W (1989) Sonomorphometrische und dopplersonographische Untersuchungen bei chronischen Leberkrankheiten. Habilitationsschrift, Humboldt-Universität, Berlin

Williams PL, Warwick R, Dyson M, Bannister LH (1989) Gray's anatomy, 37th edn. Churchill Livingstone, Edinburgh

3 Venous Hemodynamics and Normal Doppler Findings in the Venous System

G. H. Mostbeck, G. Strasser, and J. Liskutin

CONTENTS

3.1 Introduction

The venous system guides blood back towards the right heart and stores blood not needed for current circulatory requirements. Venous blood is drained from the superficial to the deep veins and from the periphery towards the heart. The splanchnic circulation, where blood is sampled from the gastrointestinal tract and flows through the liver sinusoids towards the heart, has some different flow conditions. In addition, the veins play an important function in the orthostatic circulatory regulation. Compared with the arterial system, which has been investigated extensively by various CCDS techniques, the hemodynamic properties of venous blood flow have been studied to a lesser extent by duplex Doppler and color Doppler ultrasound. This might be due to the fact that the venous system is isolated from the pulsatile pressure in arteries by the capillary bed. Thus, venous pressure gradients and venous flow velocities are much lower, and the flow is more continuous, making disturbed flow conditions rather unusual, even in pathologic conditions. However, veins near the right heart like the superior or inferior vena cava (SVC, IVC) or liver veins demonstrate extreme pulsatility in flow velocity due to heartbeat. In addition, energy to return the blood toward the heart is derived from additional factors. These are the muscle pump, gravity, respiration, and physiologic action of the venous valves.

In order to understand these complex factors and to use some physiologic aspects of venous flow for optimal results in venous CDDS investigations, studying the basic principles of fluid dynamics and of venous hemodynamics will aid us in the application of CDDS techniques.

G. H. Mostbeck, MD; G. Strasser, MD
Sozialmedizinisches Zentrum,Baumgartner Höhe mit Pflegezentrum, Otto Wagner Spital, Sanatoriumstr. 2, 1140 Vienna, Austria
J. Liskutin, MD
CT and MR Institut Hernalser Spitz, Jörgerstrasse 52, 1170 Vienna, Austria

3.2 Hemodynamic Basics

3.2.1 Steady Flow

The ideal properties of continuous, laminar (see below) flow are found only occasionally in human vessels. Whereas arteries are prone to pulsatile flow, there are cardiac and respiratory variations on central venous flow and variations in surrounding pressure affecting the venous diameter more peripherally.

3.2.2
Basic Physics

With continuous flow, the velocity v of flow of an element of fluid does not change over time. Velocity v is simply the distance s between any points in the flow direction divided by the time t taken for the element to traverse it.

$$v = s/t \tag{1}$$

There is only flow if some force is applied to the fluid to overcome its tendency to resist flow. This resistance is the result of fluid-immanent friction or viscosity. This force, returning to the venous system, may be transmitted to the fluid (blood) via contraction of the left ventricle (vis a tergo), as an aspirative force resulting from the right heart movements and contractions and from respiration (vis a fronte), or even by the action of gravity in the standing position. The relationship between the flow (volume over time), viscosity ('inner friction', η), the length of the vascular segment l, the radius of the vessel lumen r, and the pressure difference $P_{2\_}P_1$ is described by the Hagen-Poiseuille law

$$P_2 - P_1 = 8\, l\eta\ \Theta/\pi r^4 \tag{2}$$

In accordance with Ohm's law, which relates a steady electrical current I to the potential difference E and the electrical resistance R,

$$E = RI \tag{3}$$

this equation can be used to calculate the fluid resistance R

$$R = 8\, l\eta\ \Theta/\pi^4 \tag{4}$$

It is easily seen that resistance increases 16-fold if the radius of the vessel cross-sectional area is divided by two and 256-fold if the radius is divided by four. Accordingly, it has been shown that the greatest contribution to overall vascular resistance in the human body occurs at the arteriolar level. Pressure differences in the venous system are low and mainly due to hydrostatic pressure changes (see below).

3.2.3
Laminar Flow

As long as the flow is steady, the fastest flowing fluid elements are in the center of the vessel, with a decreasing velocity towards the edge. This is known as the velocity gradient within a vessel. This velocity gradient is influenced by the inner friction of a fluid, where viscosity and cohesion are important factors. In addition, outer friction or adhesion of the fluid to the vessel wall influences the velocity gradient. If all velocity vectors are parallel (or anti-parallel) to the vessel wall, this flow is called laminar. In laminar flow, the velocity gradient is smooth and continuous, and the velocity vectors are parallel to each other. The resulting velocity profile has the form of a parabola or, to be precise for the case of a cylindrical pipe, a paraboloid of rotation (Fig. 3.1).

Investigating laminar flow within a vessel by CDDS reveals the brightest color saturation within the center of a vessel representing the highest velocity, whereas darker shades of color near the vessel edge indicate lower flow velocities. Under physiologic conditions, the flow in veins is laminar (Fig. 3.2).

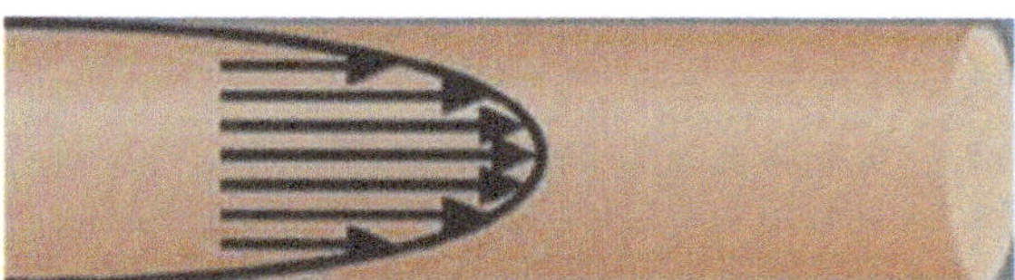

Fig. 3.1. Parabolic velocity profile in a vessel with laminar flow

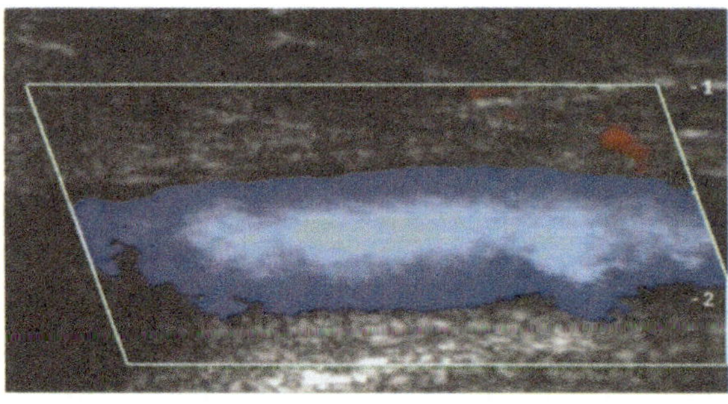

Fig. 3.2. Laminar blood flow in the common femoral vein. Color saturation is bright in the center of the vessel, indicating higher flow velocity compared with the vessel wall. Color saturation 'parallels' the vessel wall, indicating laminar blood flow

3.2.4
Continuity Equation and Hemodynamics of Stenosis

Everybody with some experience of canoeing knows quite well that the flow velocity of fluid (the river flow velocity) speeds up when entering a narrow passage. As rivers are not within a tube, the cross-sectional area usually increases (the water becomes deeper within a narrow passage) as well (Fig. 3.3). When dealing with flow in a tube, the quantity of fluid *p* flowing per time interval is the product of average velocity *v* and the cross-sectional area *A*:

$$\Theta = v_1 A_1 \quad (5)$$

As the flow volume remains constant within the narrow passage,

$$\Theta = v_1 A_1 = v_2 A_2 \quad (6)$$

and

$$v_2/v_1 = A_1/A_2 = d_1^2/d_2^2 \quad (7)$$

Thus, narrowing the diameter of a vessel by 50% (50% stenosis) results in a fourfold increase in average velocity. According to Bernoulli's principle and assuming that there is no energy loss in a stenosis, velocity measurements allow estimation of stenosis in percentage reduction of the normal vessel diameter and estimation of the pressure gradient within the stenosis, as energy is lost in 'real' vessel stenosis (Fig. 3.4). However, whereas velocity measurements by CDDS of the carotid artery are well-established criteria for the estimation of the severity of a stenosis, in the venous system there are no established criteria for the estimation of a stenosis by CDDS velocity measurements. Indeed, the low pressure differences within the venous system under normal and pathologic conditions as well as the rapid development of a venous collateral circulation make such measurements rather meaningless. In clinical settings, quantification of venous stenosis is usually judged by 'best guess', but it is essential to know that the velocity increases in venous stenosis, especially if there is no time to develop venous collaterals or alternative pathways of flow towards the right atrium (Fig. 3.5).

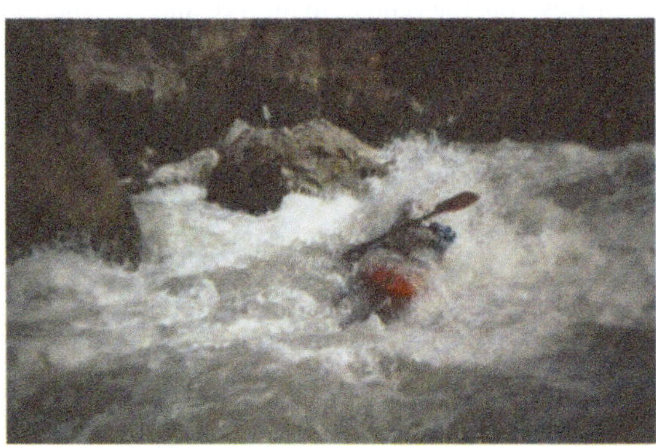

Fig. 3.3. Turbulent flow in white water canoeing

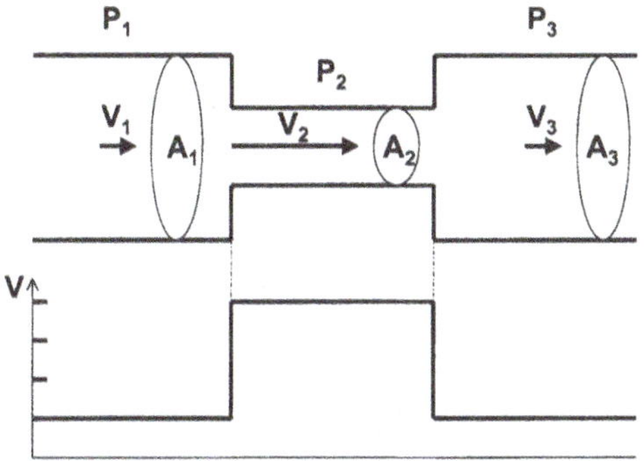

Fig. 3.4. Schematic drawing of a 50% stenosis: *A* cross-sectional area, *V* velocity, *P* pressure

3.2.5 Disturbed Flow and Turbulence

Under physiologic conditions in the human venous system, no vessel is ideal for the conditions of laminar flow. There is physiologic tapering, there are venous valves and entering vessels, as well as bending and curvature, leading to disturbed flow conditions. Whereas in the arterial system this disturbed flow (e.g., the physiologic flow reversal in the carotid artery at the origin of the internal carotid artery) has been studied by CDDS, probably due to the much lower flow velocities in the venous system these conditions are of no clinical importance there. However, turbulent flow might occur in tight venous stenosis. It is defined as a chaotic flow condition, where all velocity vectors face in random directions (Fig. 3.6). However, the sum vector of these velocity vectors points in the direction of flow within the vessel. The occurrence of turbulence is dependent on the vessel diameter (2*r*), the average velocity *v*, the viscosity η, and the density ρ of the fluid and is expressed by the Reynolds number

$$Re = v2r\ / \quad (8)$$

Re is without a dimension. Re>2000 is assumed as the critical value for the occurrence of turbulence in blood vessels. As peak flow velocities within the venous system are much lower than peak systolic velocities in the major arteries, it is questionable whether turbulence occurs under pathologic flow conditions within the venous system.

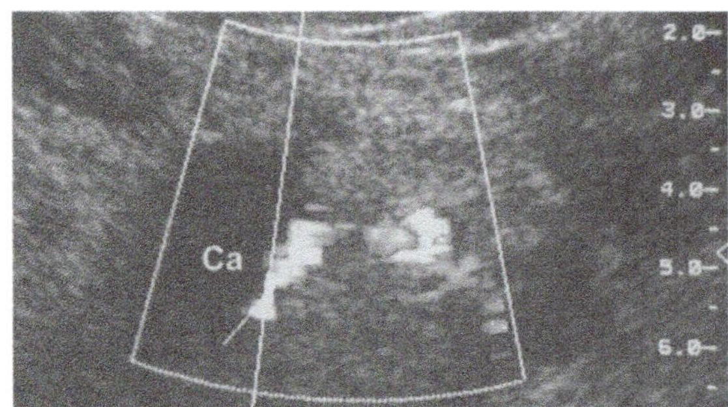

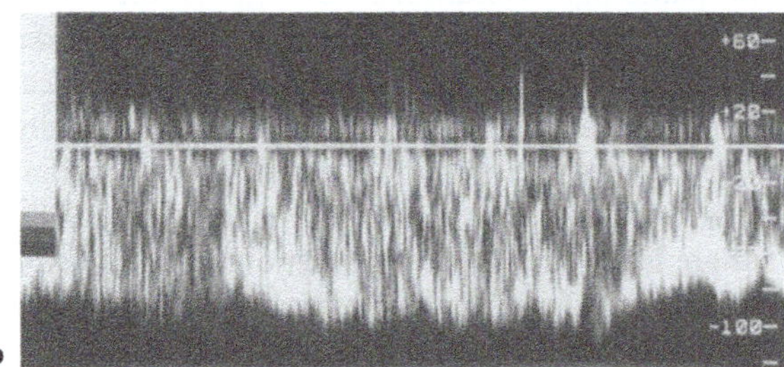

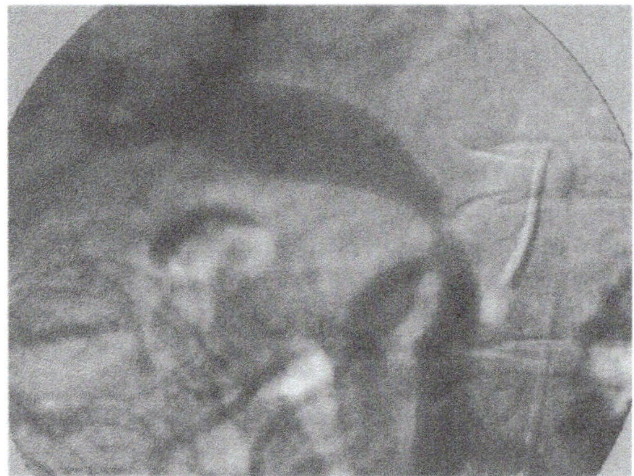

Fig. 3.5a–c. Ductal adenocarcinoma (*Ca*) of the pancreatic head with hemodynamically significant stenosis of the portal vein. Tumor (*Ca*) shown as hypoechoic mass ventral to the portal vein. **a** Duplex Doppler sample volume within the portal vein. **b** Flow velocity profile demonstrating peak velocities of up to 100 cm/s (normal values around 20–40 cm/s). **c** DSA demonstrating stenosis of the portal vein

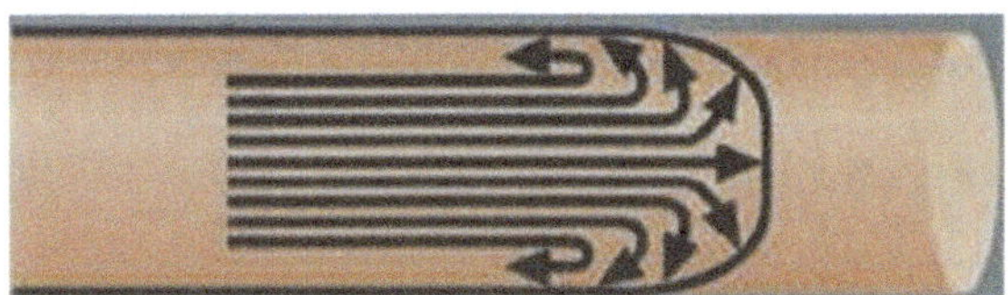

Fig. 3.6. Disturbed blood flow with flat velocity profile

3.3 Hemodynamics of Venous Flow

In the venous circulation, various factors are of influence, in addition to the vis a tergo, the left-sided cardiac output. These factors are predominantly pressure changes within the thoracic and the abdominal cavities, the muscle pump, and gravity.

3.3.1 Pressure and Flow in the Venous System

We have to differentiate between the transmural pressure which influences the cross-sectional area of the veins and the intravascular venous pressure, which is very low compared with the arterial system. When a healthy volunteer assumes a horizontal position, there is a continuous pressure drop from the venoles (15–25 mmHg) to the large extremity veins (8–20 mmHg) to the right atrium, where the central venous pressure is 5–7 mmHg. This pressure gradient is sufficient to guide the blood towards the heart. Consequently, as the overall venous cross-sectional area decreases from the venoles to the SVC and IVC, there is an increase in average flow velocity from the periphery to the central veins. Time-average flow velocities in the large veins are in the range of 10–20 cm/s.

3.3.2 Hydrostatic Pressure

Both arterial and venous pressure are influenced by hydrostatic pressure. Gravity leads to an increase in venous pressure (+0.77 mmHg/cm) below and to a decrease in venous pressure (–0.77 mmHg/cm) above the level of the right atrium. In the standing position, the intravascular pressure becomes negative within the supracardiac veins. Conversely, pressure increases in the lower extremity veins. Thus, veins of the upper extremity have the tendency to collapse in the standing position, whereas the veins of the lower extremity increase in size, and vice versa if a subject is in the Trendelenburg position (Fig. 3.7). In addition, moving from the supine to the sitting or standing position shifts approximately 300–350 ml blood out of the thorax to the peripheral veins of the lower extremity, leading to a dilatation of these capacity vessels (Kappert 1976). With passive dangling of the lower legs, this venous pooling is increased compared with an active standing position. These factors influence the normal aspect of the upper and lower extremity

a 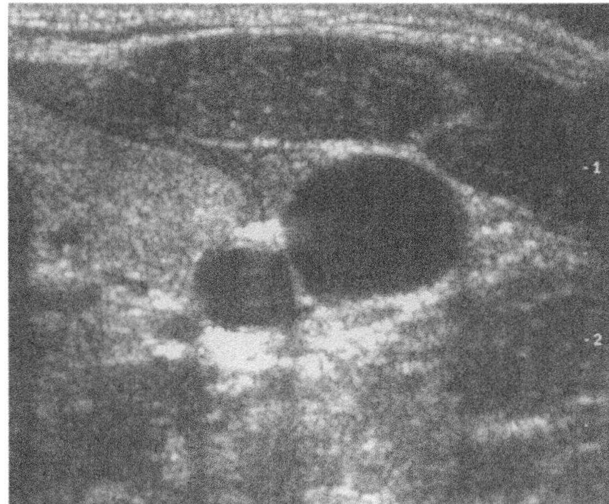

b 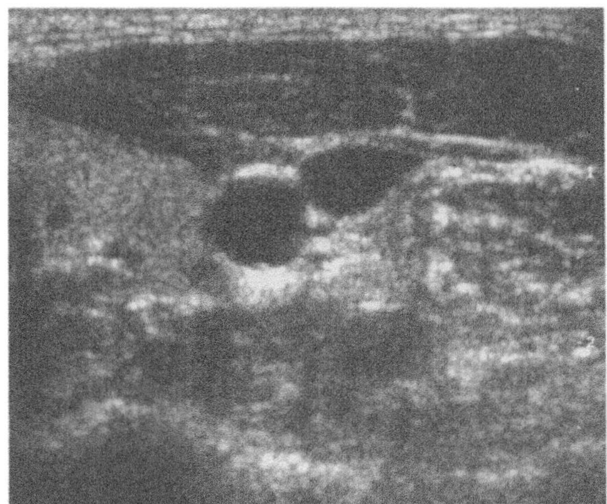

Fig. 3.7a, b. US cross-section through the left internal jugular vein obtained in the prone (**a**) and standing (**b**) position. Note the decrease in cross-sectional area in the upright position

veins in different positions (prone, supine, sitting, standing) during CDDS examinations.

3.3.3 Respiratory Changes in Thoracic and Abdominal Cavity Pressures

During inspiration, the intrapleural pressure falls from -2.5 mmHg to -6 mmHg (GANONG 1991). This negative pressure is transmitted to the great veins so that the central venous pressure fluctuates from about 6 mmHg during expiration to approximately 2 mmHg during quiet inspiration. This pressure drop during inspiration aids venous return from the upper body as the pressure gradient between the right atrium and veins is increased. In addition, the descent of the diaphragm during inspiration increases the intra-abdominal pressure and squeezes blood towards the heart as backflow is prevented by the venous valves (GANONG 1991). However, as the abdominal pressure exceeds the venous pressure in the legs, the venous flow from the lower extremity to the heart stops (BOLLINGER et al 1970). During expiration, the pressure within the abdominal cavity falls, and the blood flows from the lower extremity veins to the abdominal cavity. However, as the pressure gradient between the lower extremity veins and the central venous pressure decreases, flow into the chest from the upper extremity veins decreases. BOLLINGER et al. (1968) termed this process the 'abdominothoracic two-phase pump'. The Valsalva maneuver (a brief period of forced expiration against a closed glottis) increases the intrathoracic and intra-abdominal pressure. High intrathoracic and intra-abdominal pressures compress the intrathoracic and intra-abdominal veins and decrease the venous return from the upper as well as from the lower extremity and consequently cardiac output. Peripheral veins increase dramatically in diameter, as blood flow towards the heart is prohibited but inflow over the capillaries is preserved, and demonstrate stagnant blood flow if the venous valves are intact (MÜLLER-LISSE et al. 1998). However, insufficient venous valves lead to venous reflux during the Valsalva procedure. Immediately after the Valsalva maneuver, an increased flow towards the right atrium is noted (Fig. 3.8).

3.3.4 Effects of Heartbeat

The sucking of the blood into the atria during systole and the rapid ventricular filling in early diastole lead to two peaks of heart-directed flow in the veins near the right atrium and to marked pulsatility of venous flow. As valves within the SVC, IVC, and pelvic veins are absent, this venous pulsatility is detectable by CDDS not only within these central veins but also in the proximal upper and lower extremity veins (Fig. 3.9). For more details, see the chapter by HENK et al. in this book.

3.3.5 Muscle Pump

In the limbs, the veins are surrounded by muscles, and contraction of these muscles during activity compresses the veins (GANONG 1991; HACH and HACH-

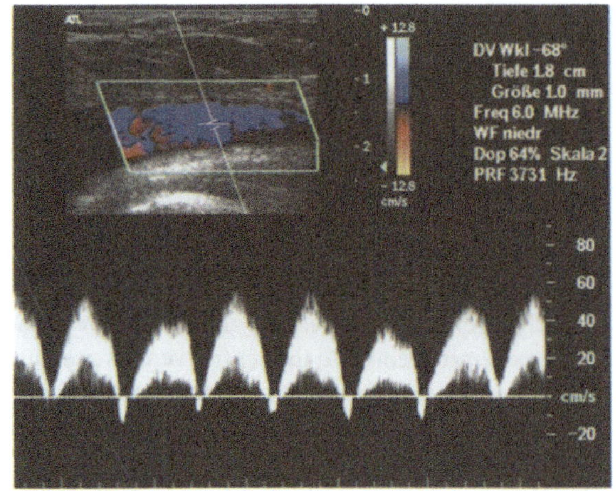

a

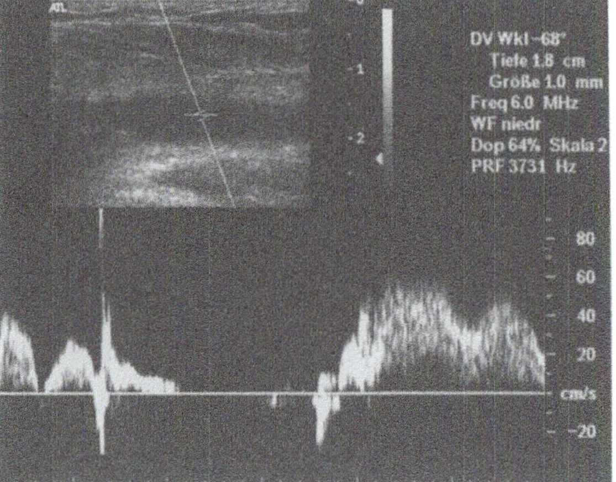

b

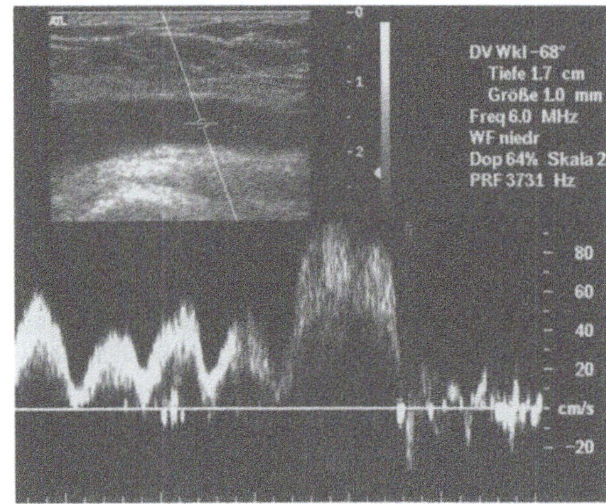

c

Fig. 3.8a–c. Doppler spectra obtained in the common femoral vein in a young female volunteer, supine position. **a** With normal, quiet respiration, there is flow towards the heart with marked cardiac and some respiratory variation. **b** The Valsalva maneuver leads to stasis in the vein without any reflux, but there is an increase in flow velocity after the Valsalva maneuver. **c** With distal compression of the calf, there is increased flow velocity

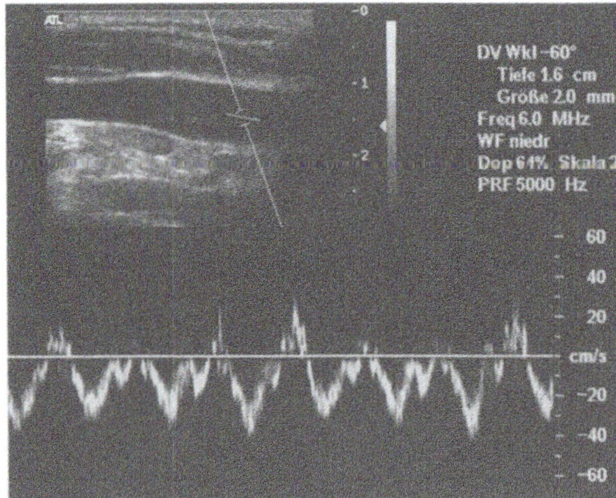

a

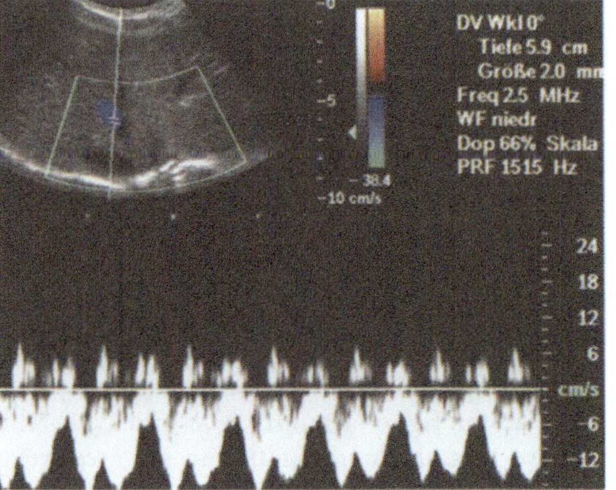

b

Fig. 3.9a, b. Normal cardiac variability of the Doppler spectrum in veins near the right atrium. **a** Left internal jugular vein of a normal volunteer in supine position and quiet respiration. **b** Middle liver vein

Wunderle 1996). It is essential to note that without the muscle pump, the venous valves would not work or, to express it another way, the muscle pump only works if the venous valves are competent. During muscle contraction, the muscular volume increases and compresses the deep veins, as the muscle fascia surrounding both deep veins and muscle cannot be extended. Thus, the venous blood is forced towards the heart due to the action of the venous valves. When the muscles relax, there is decompression of the deep veins; they can increase in diameter, and blood is directed from the superficial to the deep veins via the perforating system (Hach and Hach-Wunderle 1996). In addition, pulsation from nearby arteries may also compress veins (Gardener and Fox 1989) as the perivascular interstitial tissue is not extensible. However, this effect is of minor importance, whereas many different anatomical muscle pumps (the soleus and quadriceps femoris muscles are the most important ones) have been described for the lower extremity (Hach and Hach-Wunderle 1996). In addition, different suction pumps have been proposed at the level of the knee, the thigh, and the inguinal ligament. With contraction of fascia in these specific regions and active or passive movement in the knee and hip joint, the diameter of the deep veins may increase and induce suction of venous blood towards the heart (Gardener and Fox 1989; Staubesand 1980). In addition, with active walking, venous return from the plantar veins is enhanced, thus increasing the flow velocities in the deep venous system.

3.3.6 Autonomic Tone of the Veins

The veins are no longer considered rigid and inert tubes. Mobility is under the control of two different, antagonistic forces: the vasoconstrictive sympathetic and the vasodilative parasympathetic nervous system. Today, this seems to be rather simple. In fact, there are various other factors making this more complicated. (e.g., temperature, circulating vasoactive factors). For CDDS imaging purposes, these autonomic regulations are of minor importance (Hugue 1997).

3.4 Normal CDDS Findings in the Venous System

3.4.1 Lower Extremity Veins

According to the chapter on examination technique, normal Doppler findings and provocatory maneuvers are described for the deep and superficial veins and for the perforating veins. Using continuous wave (CW) Doppler sonography, spontaneous respiration (S-sounds) and augmented sounds (A-sounds) have been differentiated using small CW probes (Hennerici and Neuerburg-Heusler 1998). It is useful to employ similar maneuvers for CCDS examination of the veins of the lower extremity.

3.4.1.1 Deep Venous System

Near the groin and within the pelvic veins, venous blood flow is usually phasic. It increases towards the heart with expiration and decreases during inspiration. These phasic changes can be augmented with deep respiratory excursions. As pointed out in the article by Henk et al. in this book, there may be some cardiac variability within the Doppler spectrum of the pelvic and thigh veins overlying respiratory variations. It is not completely understood whether this reflects cardiac disease, but clinical practice teaches that especially in thin patients, there is some cardiac variation without underlying cardiac disease. This may be due to the fact that venous valves in the IVC and pelvic veins are absent, thus leaving central flow velocity changes dampened, but recognizable by CDDS technique to the groin. This variability in deep venous blood flow may be suggested by color techniques, but duplex Doppler is extremely helpful in the assessment of the normal Doppler spectrum. B-mode and CDDS findings in various maneuvers are summarized in Table 3.1. These maneuvers are extremely helpful in cases where B-mode US findings remain indeterminate for a pathologic process or where only weak duplex or color Doppler signals are recognized. It is noteworthy that when examining the patient in the standing or sitting position with dangling legs, deep calf veins and muscle veins of the calf may become highly echogenic due to low flow velocity and red blood cell and/or platelet aggregation. This phenomenon is completely reversible and also dependent on the US frequency used (Battino 1991, 1992; Sigel et al. 1983; Van der Heiden et al. 1995).

Table 3.1. Normal and normal augmented CDDS findings in the deep lower extremity venous system

Maneuver	B-mode	Duplex Doppler	Color Doppler (frequency encoded)
Normal respiration, supine position	Smooth venous contour, normal valves	Flow towards heart with respiratory phasicity (decrease to stop during inspiration; increase during expiration)	Laminar venous flow with respiratory phasicity
Deep inspiration/expiration, supine position	Smooth venous contour, normal valves	More pronounced respiratory phasicity with stop during inspiration	Pronounced respiratory phasicity, no color flow during inspiration
Valsalva maneuver, supine position	Increase in venous diameter, closure of venous valves	No venous blood flow, augmented flow after Valsalva maneuver	No venous blood flow, augmented flow after Valsalva maneuver
Normal respiration, distal manual compression	Short increase in venous diameter due to augmented flow	Peak flow during compression towards the heart	Peak flow during compression towards the heart
Normal respiration, proximal manual compression	Increase in venous diameter	Flow cessation, short peak flow towards heart after relief of compression	Flow cessation, short peak flow towards heart after relief of compression
Compression via US transducer	Vein collapses, accompanying artery remains unchanged	No flow in compressed, collapsed vein	No flow in compressed, collapsed vein
Normal respiration, supine position, distal muscle contraction ("muscle pump")	Short increase in venous diameter due to augmented flow	Peak flow during muscle compression towards the heart	Peak flow during muscle compression towards the heart
Supine to standing position or loosely hanging calf in the sitting position, normal respiration	Increase in venous diameter, deep veins and muscle veins in the calf may become highly echogenic	Decrease in flow velocity towards heart	Decrease in flow velocity towards heart

3.4.1.2 *Superficial Venous System*

Examination of the great and small saphenous veins is only done when valvular insufficiency or thrombophlebitis are suspected. Normal CDDS findings and normal augmented findings are summarized in Table 3.2.

3.4.1.3 *Perforating Veins*

The perforating veins can be assessed for insufficiency by CDDS. Under normal conditions and without the presence of varicosis, these small vessels are not easily found. Their flow direction should go from the superficial to the deep venous system.

3.4.2 Upper Extremity Veins

As imaging of the superficial and perforating venous system of the upper extremity is of minor clinical importance [with the exception of superficial thrombophlebitis and before and after hemodialysis shunts and fistulae (Robbin et al. 2000)], the focus is on the deep venous system. The most important aspect to note is that the flow behavior is the opposite of what is found in the deep system of the lower extremity (Müller-Lisse et al. 1998). Hence, during inspiration, with low pressure in the thoracic cavity, blood flow towards the right atrium is increased, and it decreases or even ceases during expiration. In addition, there is usually marked cardiac pulsatility overlying this respiratory phasicity, at least in the proximal veins (brachiocephalic, subclavian, and internal jugular veins) (Patel et al. 1999). As for the lower extremity venous system, augmented flow maneuvers are helpful but usually restricted to forced inspiration, Valsalva maneuver, and distal compression (Table 3.3). Interestingly, forced, quick inspiration leads to complete collapse of the proximal veins (Gooding et al. 1986). The Trendelenburg position may be used for anatomic landmark or US-guided central venous catheterization. Using the internal jugular vein, it has to be noted that these veins are asymmetric (more than 50% difference in cross-sectional area) regarding their diameter in 62% of patients, the right being dominant in 68% of cases (Lichtenstein et al. 2001). In addition, anatomical variations (Benter et al. 2001) and the influence of respiration on the venous diameter (Hayashi et al. 2000) have to be taken into consideration when catheterization is going to be performed. In general,

Table 3.2. Normal and normal augmented CDDS findings in the superficial lower extremity venous system (great and small saphenous vein)

Maneuver	B-mode	Duplex Doppler	Color Doppler (frequency encoded)
Normal respiration, supine position	Veins may be collapsed or of small diameter, normal valves visible with high-resolution equipment	Flow towards heart with/without some respiratory phasicity as deep veins	Laminar venous flow with/without some respiratory phasicity
Valsalva maneuver	Increase in diameter near the groin or popliteal fossa, closure of the proximal valve	No blood flow, augmented flow after Valsalva maneuver	No blood flow, augmented flow after Valsalva maneuver
Supine to standing position	Increase in diameter	Decrease in flow velocity towards heart	Decrease in flow velocity towards heart

Table 3.3. Normal and normal augmented CDDS findings in the central deep upper extremity veins (brachiocephalic, subclavian, and internal jugular veins)

Maneuver	B-mode	Duplex Doppler	Color Doppler (frequency encoded)
Normal respiration, supine position	Smooth venous contour, normal valves	Flow towards heart with respiratory phasicity (decrease to stop during expiration; increase during inspiration) and cardiac pulsatility	Laminar venous flow with respiratory phasicity and cardiac pulsatility
Deep, quick inspiration, supine position	Collapse of the veins	Rapid increase in flow velocity towards heart	Rapid increase in flow velocity towards heart
Valsalva maneuver, supine position	Increase in venous diameter, closure of venous valves	No venous blood flow, augmented flow after Valsalva maneuver	No venous blood flow, augmented flow after Valsalva maneuver
Normal respiration, distal manual compression (subclavian and brachiocephalic veins)	Short increase in venous diameter due to augmented flow	Peak flow during compression towards the heart	Peak flow during compression towards the heart
Compression via US transducer (where possible)	Vein collapses, accompanying artery remains unchanged	No flow in compressed, collapsed vein	No flow in compressed, collapsed vein
Trendelenburg position (internal jugular vein)	Increase in venous diameter	Decrease in flow velocity towards heart	Decrease in flow velocity towards heart
Supine to standing position	Decrease or even short collapse of venous diameter	Increase in flow velocity towards heart	Increase in flow velocity towards heart

US guidance for internal jugular vein catheterization seems to be preferable over anatomically oriented puncture (Bock et al. 1999; Silberzweig and Mitty 1998; Caridi et al. 1998).

3.4.3 Inferior Vena Cava

In about 89% of patients, technically adequate CDDS examinations of the IVC can be performed (Kazmers et al. 2000). In the remaining patients, direct CDDS investigation may be impossible due to overlying bowel gas and/or marked obesity. However, the hepatic part of the IVC is visible in nearly all US examinations. Anatomic variants of the IVC may be expected in about 1% of patients due to the complex nature of the embryological development of the IVC (Chuang et al. 1974; Pierro et al. 1990; Kubale 1992). The cross-section of the IVC is pulsatile and referred to as the 'double beat' image (Hennerici and Neuerburg-Heusler 1998). In addition to this cardiac pulsation, there is respiratory variability with a decrease or even collapse in IVC diameter during inspiration and maximum distension at end-expiration (Smith et al. 1985). The cross-sectional area is oval with the anteroposterior diameter being smaller than the lateral diameter, the latter ranging between 1.5 and 3 cm. In thin patients, the IVC is easily completely compressed against the spine with the US transducer. The IVC cross-sectional area increases with various pathologic processes associated with decreased right and left cardiac function, inflow obstruction into the right atrium (pericardial effusion, constrictive pericarditis), and hypervolemia, whereas hypovolemia and shock lead to severe 'flattening' of the IVC.

The normal Doppler curve shows clear cardiac pulsatility and respiratory phasicity, with an inspiratory decrease and an expiratory increase in the flow velocity usually being seen (Smith et al. 1985). For details regarding normal and pathologic cardiac pulsatility, see the chapter by Henk et al. in this book. Using CDDS equipment, flow pulsatility within the IVC is easily assessed using frequency-encoded color imaging. Provided that the frame rate of the CDDS unit is high enough, this pulsatility is displayed by a change of color within the IVC during the cardiac cycle. Peak flow velocities towards the heart are usually below 1 m/s (Hennerici and Neuerburg-Heusler 1998).

3.4.4 Renal Veins

The renal veins are formed by fusion of various intrarenal interlobar veins. The right renal vein reaches the IVC directly, the left renal vein crosses the abdominal aorta ventrally. The left renal vein is joined by the left testicular (or ovary) vein. There is marked variability of the renal veins, with a retroaortic left renal vein and a periaortic venous ring being the more common variants.

As the venous valves are missing, the Doppler spectrum shows cardiac pulsatility and respiratory phasicity. As one proceeds with Doppler sampling from the IVC to the more intrarenal veins, cardiac pulsatility decreases and is absent in the peripheral veins of the kidney. Especially in thin persons, the left renal vein may be 'compressed' between the aorta and the superior mesenteric artery, which is referred as the 'nutcracker' phenomenon. Thus, the left renal vein is prominent, and interlobar veins in the renal sinus may have the appearance of grade 1 (Scola et al. 1989) or even grade 2 hydronephrosis. CDDS readily clarifies this situation and reveals this 'hydronephrosis' to be veins (Fig. 3.10).

3.4.5 Hepatic Veins, Splenoportal Axis

Normal CDDS findings are described in detail in the chapters by Seitz, Weskott, Kubale and Henk et al. in this book.

a

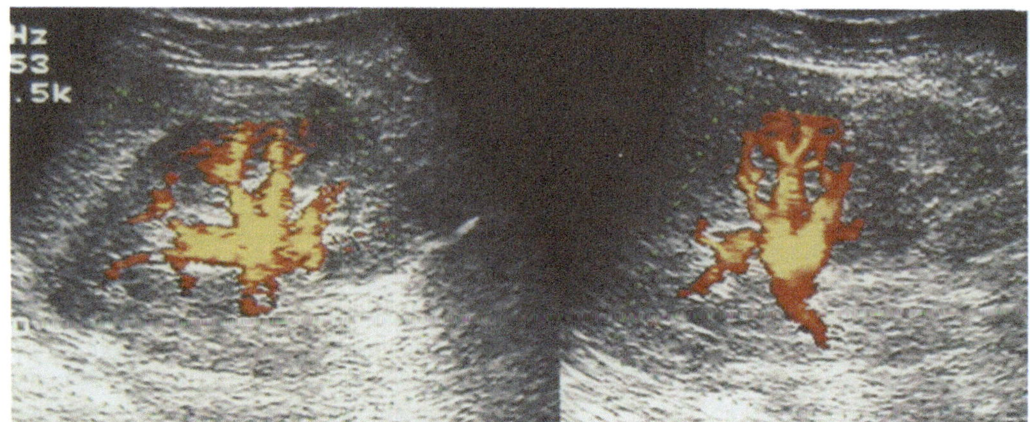

b

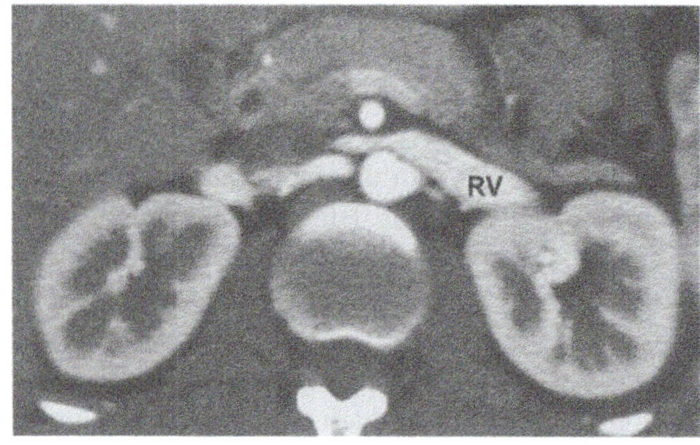

Fig. 3.10a, b. 'Nutcracker' phenomenon. **a** Amplitude-encoded color Doppler images of the left kidney in a young male patient with prominent renal veins. **b** Corresponding contrast-enhanced CT at the level of the left renal vein (*RV*) showing compression of the RV between the abdominal aorta and superior mesenteric artery ('nutcracker') with consecutive increase of distal venous diameter

References

Battino J (1991) Echogenicity of blood. J Mal Vasc 16: 342–345

Battino J (1992) Echogenicity of blood. J Radiol 73:705–708

Benter T, Teichgraber UK, Kluhs L et al (2001) Anatomical variations in the internal jugular veins of cancer patients affecting central venous access. Anatomical variation of the internal jugular vein. Ultraschall Med 22:23–26

Bock U, Mollhoff T, Forster R (1999) Ultrasonography guided versus anatomically oriented puncture of the internal jugular vein for central venous catheterization. Ultraschall Med 20:273–274

Bollinger A, Mahler F, de Sepibus G (1968) Diagnostik peripherer Venenerkrankungen mit Doppler-Strömungsdetektoren. Dtsch Med Wochenschr 46:2197–2201

Bollinger A, Rutishauser W, Mahler F, Grüntzig A (1970) Zur Dynamik des Rückstroms aus der Vena femoralis. Kreisl Forsch 59:963–971

Caridi JG, Hawkins IF Jr, Wiechmann BN, Pevarski DJ, Tonkin JO (1998) Sonographic guidance when using the right internal jugular vein for central vein access. Am J Roentgenol 171:1259–1263

Chuang VP, Mena CE, Hoskins PA (1974) Congenital anomalies of the inferior vena cava. Review of embryogenesis and presentation of a simplified classification. Br J Radiol 47: 206–213

Ganong WF (1991) Review of medical physiology. Section VI. Circulation 30. Dynamics of blood and lymph flow, 15th edn. Appleton and Lange, Norwalk, CT

Gardener AMM, Fox RH (1989) The return of blood to the heart. Libbey, London

Gooding GAW, Hightower DR, Moore EH, Dillon WP, Lipton ML (1986) Obstruction of the superior vena cava or subclavian veins: sonographic diagnosis. Radiology 159:663–665

Hach W, Hach-Wunderle V (1996) Phlebographie der Bein- und Beckenvenen. Schnetztor, Konstanz

Hayashi H, Ootaki C, Tsuzuku M, Amano M (2000) Respiratory jugular venodilatation: its anatomic rationale as a landmark for right internal jugular vein puncture as determined by ultrasonography. J Cardiothorac Vasc Anesth 14:425–427

Hennerici M, Neuerburg-Heusler D (1998) Vascular diagnosis with ultrasound. Clinical references with case studies. With contributions by Karasch T, Rautenberg W. Thieme, Stuttgart

Hugue C (1997) Physiologie et physiopathologie du système veineux. In: Kchouk H (ed) Echo-Doppler Veineux. Masson, Paris, pp 14–24

Kappert A (1976) Lehrbuch und Atlas der Angiologie. Huber, Bern

Kazmers A, Groehn H, Meeker C (2000) Duplex examination of the inferior vena cava. Am Surg 66:986–989

Kubale R (1992) Abdominelle und retroperitoneale Gefäße. In: Rettenmaier G, Seitz K (eds) Sonographische Differentialdiagnostik, vol II. Verlag Chemie, Weinheim

Lichtenstein D, Saifi R, Augarde R, Prin S, Schmitt JM, Page B et al (2001) The internal jugular veins are asymmetric. Usefulness of ultrasound before catheterization. Intensive Care Med 27:301–305

Müller-Lisse UL, Müller-Lisse GU, Holzknecht N, Reiser M (1998) Ultraschalluntersuchungen der Venen. Radiologe 38:560–569

Patel MC, Berman LH, Moss HA, McPherson SJ (1999) Subclavian and internal jugular veins at Doppler US: abnormal cardiac pulsatility and respiratory phasicity as a predictor of complete central occlusion. Radiology 211:579–583

Pierro JA, Soleimanpour M, Bory JL (1990) Left retrocaval ureter associated with left inferior vena cava. Am J Roentgenol 155:545–546

Robbin ML, Gallichio MH, Deierhoi MH, Weber TM, Allon M (2000) US vascular mapping before hemodialysis access placement. Radiology 217:83–88

Scola FH, Cronan JJ, Schepps B (1989) Grade 1 hydronephrosis: pulsed Doppler US evaluation. Radiology 171:519–520

Sigel B, Machi J, Beitler JC, Justin JR (1983) Red cell aggregation as a cause of blood-flow echogenicity. Radiology 148: 799–802

Silberzweig JE, Mitty HA (1998) Central venous access: low internal jugular vein approach under imaging guidance. Am J Roentgenol 170:1617–1620

Smith HJ, Grottum P, Simonsen S (1985) Ultrasonic assessment of abdominal venous return. I. Effect of cardiac action and respiration on mean velocity pattern, cross-sectional area and flow in the inferior vena cava and portal vein. Acta Radiol Diagn 26:581–588

Staubesand J (1980) Ankle joint pump and the prevention of thrombosis. Med Welt 31:1813

Van der Heiden MS, de Kroon MG, Bom N, Borst C (1995) Ultrasound backscatter at 30 MHz from human blood: influence of rouleau size affected by blood modification and shear rate. Ultrasound Med Biol 21:817–826

4 Doppler Imaging of Jugular Vein and Thoracic Inlet Venous Obstruction

N. Gritzmann, T. Rettenbacher, A. Hollerweger, P. Macheiner

CONTENTS

4.1 Introduction

For many years phlebography was the only imaging test for venous obstruction of the internal jugular vein (IJV) and the thoracic inlet (Balestreri et al. 1995). Over the past decade, color duplex Doppler sonography (CDDS) has been widely performed for IJV and subclavian vein (SV) thrombosis. Since incomplete thrombosis of the IJV is often asymptomatic, its real incidence was not known before high resolution ultrasound probes were available. Central venous catheters are the leading cause of IJV thrombosis.

N. Gritzmann, MD
Professor of Radiology, Department of Radiology, Hospital of the Brothers of St. John, Kajetanerplatz 1, 6020 Salzburg, Austria
T. Rettenbacher, MD; A. Hollerweger, MD;
P. Macheiner, MD
Department of Radiology, Hospital of the Brothers of St. John, Kajetanerplatz 1, 6020 Salzburg, Austria

Usually, high resolution transducers with a central frequency of about 7.5 MHz are used for evaluation of the IJV and SV. Especially for incomplete thrombosis and recanalization of thrombosis, CDDS equipment along with B-mode imaging is useful. Mediastinal obstruction can be assessed by CDDS analysis of the Doppler curve.

4.2 Sonoanatomy

All cervical veins have a thin wall with usually one echogenic layer displayed sonographically. The lumen is nearly echo-free. Usually, artifacts are seen from the dependent wall of the jugular vein. By changing the angle of insonation, they are easily recognized as artifacts and can be differentiated from partial thrombosis.

4.2.1 Internal Jugular Vein

The IJV is by far the most important cervical vein. The vein is supplied with blood flow from the brain via the jugular foramen, from the face via the vena angularis, and from the parotid region via the retromandibular vein. Immediately below the base of the skull, the IJV cannot be displayed sonographically due to superposition of bony structures. The IJV lies superficial and lateral to the carotid artery. It can be easily compressed with the transducer. During the Valsalva maneuver, the vein enlarges significantly, and the cross-sectional area is usually more than doubled. Very often, a venous valve can be seen sonographically before the IVC joins the SV. It is found on the left side more regularly than on the right. The IJV can be divided anatomically into four sections in the neck. The first lies immediately below the base of the skull and cannot be investigated by US. The second is the jugulodigastric section from the posterior belly of the digastric muscle to the level of the hyoid bone. The third goes from the hyoid level to the omohyoid muscle, which is fixed to the sheaths of the IJV. The fourth runs from the omohyoid muscle to the confluens with the SV. These sections are important for the nomenclature of the cervical lymph node groups and have a clinical significance in lymph node staging and neck dissection (Hübsch et al. 1989; Gritzmann 1988).

4.2.2 Subclavian Vein

In contrast to the IJV, the SV cannot be compressed with the transducer since the wall is suspended and detracted by surrounding fibrous tissues. The SV is imaged by supra- and infraclavicular positions of the transducer. Usually, it is located superficially to the echogenic lung and can be seen sonographically. Parts of the vein can be overlain by air in the lungs. After the confluence with the IJV, it is called the brachiocephalic vein (BCV). These veins are usually not adequately imaged by B-mode US, and the superior vena cava (SVC) can only be seen if mediastinal masses constitute a sonographic 'window' for parasternal US imaging. However, the SVC can be assessed by intravascular ultrasound (Bolz et al. 1993).

In normal individuals, the Doppler spectra of the IJV and SV show significant cardiac and respiratory phasicities. For details, see Chapter 3.

Variants of the IJVs are rare. There can be a marked difference in the diameter of the IJV from one side to the other mainly due to a difference in size of the bony jugular foramen at the skull base. Doubled IJVs on one side usually unite to one vein before the SV is reached. Congenital ectasia can be found rarely in children (Al-Dousary 1997) and has to be differentiated from venous congestion.

4.3 Thrombosis

The leading cause of IJV thrombosis is central venous access. The incidence is reported to vary between 46% and 63% (Kraybill and Allen 1993; Karnik et al. 1993; Fischer et al. 1993). In children, IJV thrombosis due to central venous access is reported to occur in 4% to 33% of cases (Rand et al. 1994).

It is of interest that catheter size, time of placement, type of catheter material, or presence or absence of anticoagulation are not significant parameters for the development of IJV thrombosis. However, the presence of local hematomas and inflammatory changes are associated with a higher incidence of thrombosis (Karnik et al. 1993). Following neck surgery and local radiation therapy, IJV thrombosis is a rare, but typical complication. Other reasons for IJV thrombosis include i.v. drug abuse with associated thrombophlebitis. Inflammations of the cervical soft tissues only rarely cause IJV thrombosis.

A typical causative agent for thrombosis of the SV is significant exercise with the arms, especially working above the head like painting or screwing. This entity is called 'Schrötter–von Paget' syndrome or 'thrombose par effort'. In patients with thoracic inlet syndrome, obstruction of the SV as well can be found inconsistently. Thromboses can also be seen in mediastinal diseases like bronchial neoplasms, tuberculosis, and Behçet disease. Unclear thrombosis can be paraneoplastic. In particular, tumors like pancreatic carcinoma have a high incidence of thrombosis. Embolism due to cervical vein thrombosis is relatively uncommon. Approximately 8% of patients with thrombosis were reported to present with significant pulmonary embolism. Of these, 25% were fatal (Kerr et al. 1990).

4.3.1 Symptoms

Usually, unilateral thrombosis of the IJV is asymptomatic. In some cases, swelling of the face can be found. If significant thrombophlebitis of the IJV is present, clinical symptoms are present (rubor, color). The vast majority of IJV thromboses are located below the jugular foramen. Therefore, neurologic symptoms are rare, but they have been described in patients with bilateral IJV obstruction. This fact is the main reason that bilateral neck dissections with resection of the IJV during one operation are avoided.

In contrast to the IJV, acute complete thrombosis of the SV presents with significant clinical symptoms like swelling and livid coloration of the arm. In chronic SV obstruction, the symptoms may be more subtle, and often only venous collaterals in the region of the shoulder are found.

4.3.2 US Morphology of Thrombosis

In acute thrombosis of the IJV, hypoechoic structures are found in the lumen. In complete thrombosis, the vessel is enlarged and not compressible by applying pressure via the transducer. The compression should be performed carefully to avoid embolism. In incomplete thrombosis, the IJV dilatation is usually not pronounced or completely missing, and CDDS shows areas of blood flow (Fig. 4.1).

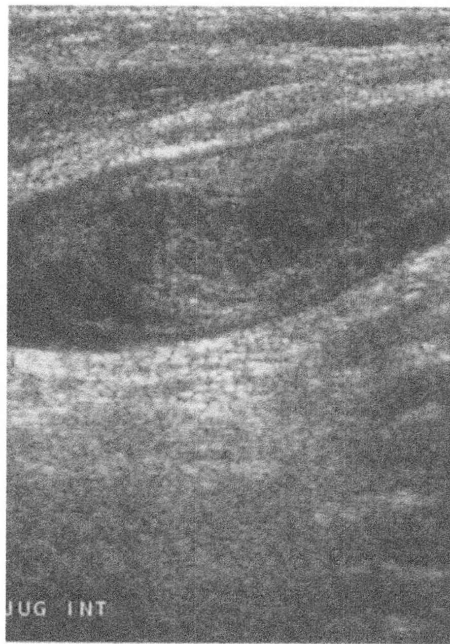

a

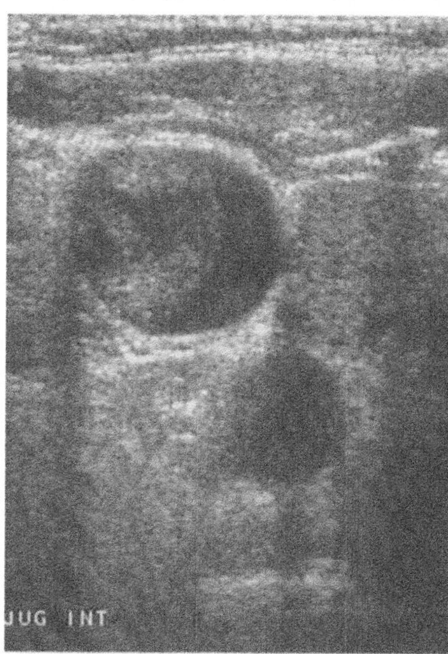

b

Fig. 4.1a, b. Partially occluding thrombus of the right internal jugular vein (IJV). Longitudinal (**a**) and transverse (**b**) scans. The vein is dilated with inhomogeneous thrombotic material in the lumen

There may be difficulty in differentiating incomplete thrombosis from recanalized, long-standing thrombosis. If the time course of clinical symptoms is not helpful, these US findings are in favor of recanalization: Recanalized thrombosis is more inhomogeneous, with mixed highly echogenic and cystic areas, whereas incomplete thrombosis usually presents with a homogeneous, hypoechoic clot.

SV thrombosis presents with the same US findings. However, due to its deep position, there might be some difficulty in investigating the SV by US, especially the part behind the clavicle, depending on the patient's body habitus.

Once thrombosis has been verified by B-mode and CDDS, extension of the clot proximally and distally has to be established. Especially if the proximal extension of thrombosis to the BCV and SVC remains unclear, alternative imaging methods (MR-venography, CT-venography, conventional phlebography) should be performed (Finn et al. 1993). However, the accuracy of sonography in the diagnosis of IJV and SV thrombosis is reported to be high, up to 96% (Koksoy et al. 1995).

The distal part of a central venous catheter is easily visible on US, whereas the central part in the SCV cannot be seen. Thrombotic or fibrotic material adherent to a catheter is a common finding (Fig. 4.2).

4.3.3 CDDS Findings in Thrombosis

Damping of the cardiac pulsations or a continuous flow is characteristic in a perfused vein distal to a thrombosed segment. Furthermore, there is loss of respiratory variability (Burbridge et al. 1993). These indirect signs are of major importance for the diagnosis of proximal, mediastinal obstruction of veins like BCV and SVC. These CDDS findings are accompanied by dilatation of the vein and collateral veins on B-mode US. Blood flow in the collateral veins is more continuous, without significant cardiac and respiratory variability, than in normal cervical veins.

4.3.4 Prethrombosis

Prethrombosis is a dynamic-functional state which can be followed by definitive thrombosis. In this setting, dilatation of the vein, venous flow with very low velocity, and sludging can be seen on real-time

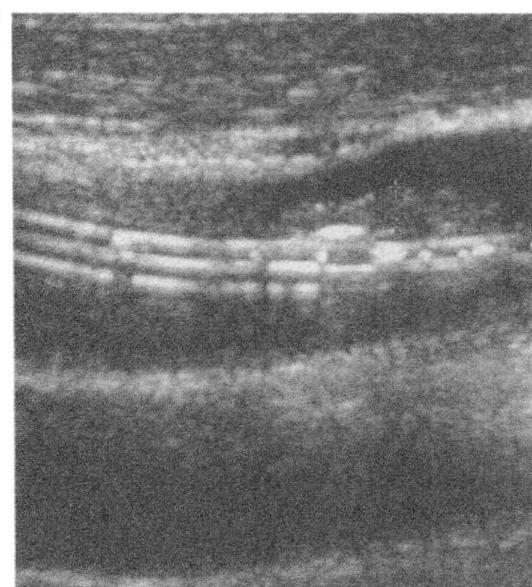

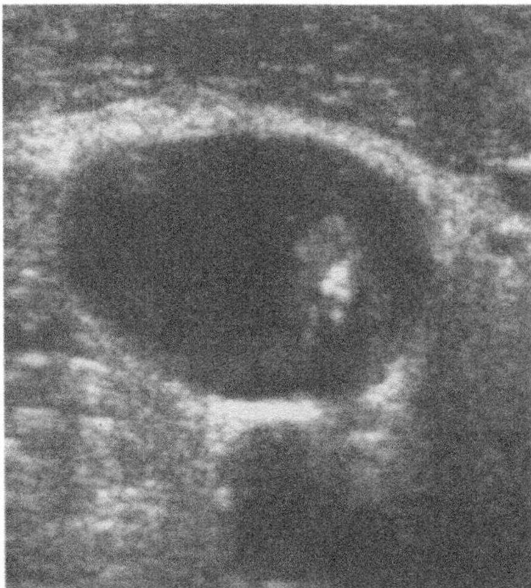

Fig. 4.2a, b. IJV thrombosis adherent to a central venous catheter. Longitudinal (**a**) and transverse (**b**) scans of the right IJV. Central venous catheter (*bright spot* and *bright lines*) surrounded by thrombotic material

US. Sludging is due to aggregation of the corpuscular elements of the blood. This sludging leads to the high echogenicity of blood in this state. The progression to definitive thrombosis or the normalization of blood flow following the prethrombotic state can be documented by follow-up US investigations.

4.3.5 Monitoring of Therapy

CDDS is an excellent modality to monitor and follow up the effects of anticoagulation and thrombolytic therapy in the thrombosed cervical veins. Short-term follow-up CDDS examinations are helpful to document recanalization of thrombosis (Huber et al. 1988; Hübsch et al. 1988; Bloching et al. 1989; Grassi and Polak 1990; Longley 1993).

4.3.6 Postthrombotic Changes

Incomplete or absent thrombolysis after SV thrombosis is followed by chronic swelling of the arm. Subcutaneous collateral veins may be visible in the ipsilateral shoulder region. Sonographically, an irregular wall of the vein and/or permanent obstruction can be found. In this setting, phlebography may have advantages over CDDS in the demonstration of collateral vessels and length of the obstructed vein. In the case of missing thrombolysis, the clot will retract and becomes adherent to the wall. Sonographically, this postthrombotic vein presents as a flat, hypoechogenic stripe (Fig. 4.3).

4.4 US Guidance for Central Venous Access

Real-time US is an excellent modality to guide central venous catheter placement. In our opinion, patients with a history of previous complicated central venous access, a history of previous thrombosis, or clinical signs of postthrombotic syndrome should preferably undergo central venous catheter placement under US guidance to keep complications low. US guidance may also be an advantage for physicians with little expertise in the positioning of central venous catheters. Recently, MR angiography has been suggested for the mapping of potential central venous access sites in patients with advanced venous occlusive disease as an alternative to US (Rose et al. 1996).

4.5 Compression or Obstruction of Veins in the Neck

Compression or obstruction of the IJV and SV by cervical lymph node metastasis is not uncommon. In contrast to the carotid artery and its branches, the clinical significance of compression or even infiltration of the veins of the neck is not that dramatic, as unilateral disease is usually asymptomatic, and the veins can be resected during neck dissection. However, bilateral simultaneous neck dissection with resection of the IJV should be avoided. In patients with bilateral cervical lymph node metastases, US is helpful in deciding which side should be operated on

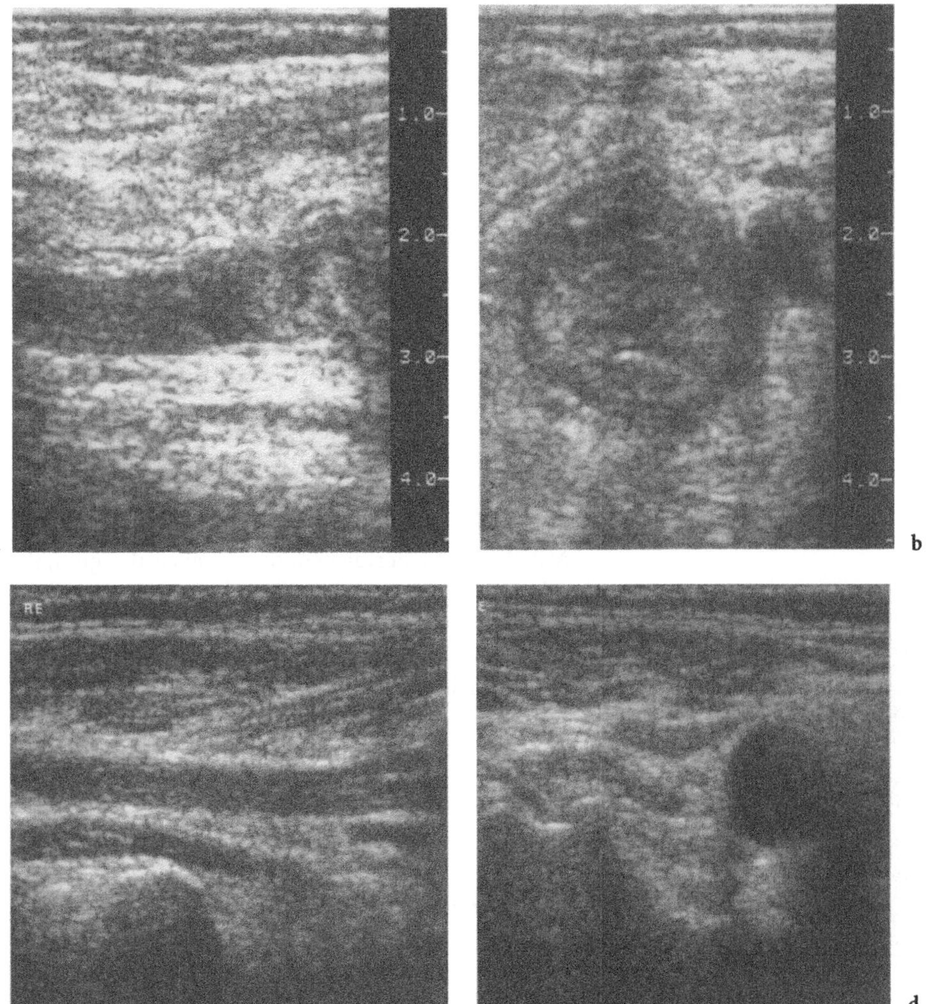

Fig. 4.3a–d. Completely occluding thrombosis of the right IJV and follow-up after 4 months. Longitudinal (**a**) and transverse (**b**) scans at the time of acute thrombosis. The IJV is dilated with totally occluding inhomogeneous thrombus. Longitudinal (**c**) and transverse (**d**) scans after 4 months. There is significant retraction of the thrombotic material, but the lumen is still completely occluded

first (Gritzmann et al. 1987, 1990). Usually, significant prevertebral, epidural, and subcutaneous veins produce sufficient collateralization to allow the second neck dissection to be performed within 2–3 weeks. Sonopalpation, where the investigating physician or sonographer tries to document movement between the node and the thin vascular wall, is a useful tool for the diagnosis of vascular invasion. When movement between the vein and neoplastic node is demonstrated, the IJV may be preserved (functional-modified neck dissection). However, when no movement between the node and venous wall is present or if there is a blurred border to the adjacent node, radical neck dissection with resection of the vein is warranted (Gritzmann et al. 1987) (Fig. 4.4).

However, it may be difficult to image venous obstruction of the SV by tumors arising from the thoracic inlet like bronchogenic carcinoma (Pancoast tumor), due to its deep position.

4.6 Compression or Obstruction of Mediastinal Veins

In complete mediastinal vein obstruction, the cervical veins are dilated. The flow is continuous and shows fewer respiratory phasicities (Fig. 4.5) (Burbridge et al. 1993). Of course these are indirect hemodynamic signs of central obstruction. CT or MR is mandatory for the evaluation of the site and cause of obstruction. MR-angiography can be used for the assessment of the veins of the thoracic inlet (Finn et al. 1993). Phlebography can be indicated for the evaluation of a vein before insertion of a stent and for the follow-up of venous stents within the SVC. Cardiac reasons (e.g., severe pericardial effusion) for altered inflow in the right atrium that cause venous congestion can be diagnosed by cardiac US. Besides primary mediastinal and lymph node malignancies,

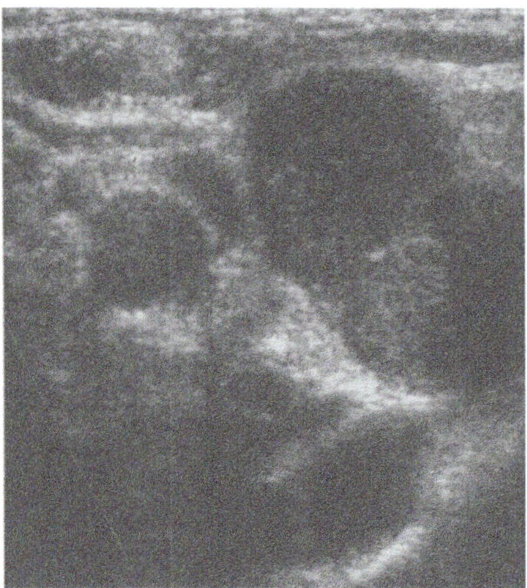

Fig. 4.4. Transverse scan of the left lower neck. Lymph node metastasis. There is a hypoechoic mass compressing the left IJV

a
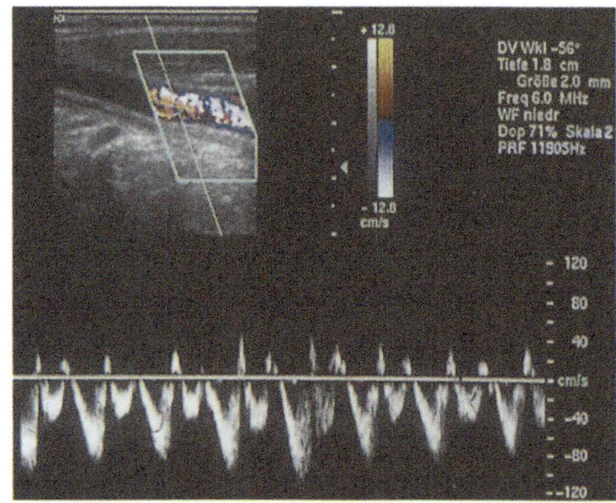

b
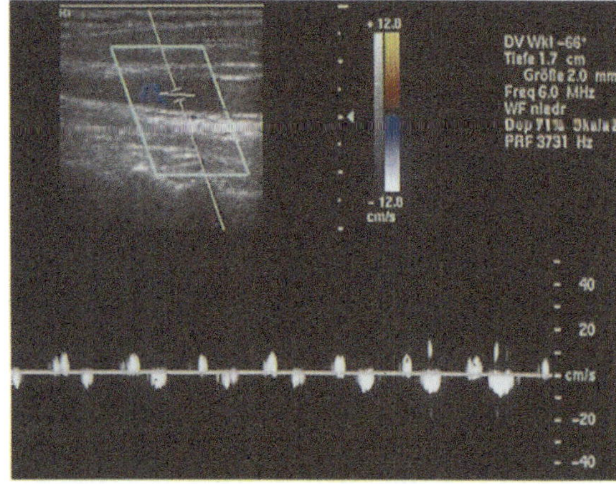

Fig. 4.5a, b. CDDS findings in imaging of both IJVs in a patient with thrombosis of the left BCV. **a** Longitudinal scan of the right IJV. Normal IJV Doppler curve with marked cardiac variability. **b** Longitudinal scan of the left IJV. Note the dampened cardiac variability compared with a

mediastinal fibrosis, tuberculosis, and Behçet syndrome (vasculitis) are the main reasons for stenosis and obstruction of great mediastinal veins.

4.7 Summary

US is the primary investigation for thrombosis of the IJV and for obstructions of the thoracic inlet veins (Koksoy et al. 1995). The accuracy of US for IJV pathology is high. For the thoracic inlet veins, US is sufficient for the diagnosis of thrombosis or obstruction in the majority of patients (Baxter et al. 1991). When all aspects of thrombosis or obstruction cannot be displayed completely by US, phlebography, CT, or MR should be performed. In the cervical region, the relationship between lymph node metastasis and the veins can be assessed with high accuracy. The main disadvantage of US in this area is that not all areas of the thoracic inlet can be visualized sonographically. Furthermore, especially in this area, the skill of the operator is a significant variable, and documentation and overview are still difficult.

References

Al-Dousary S (1997) Internal jugular phlebectasia. Int J Pediatr Otorhinolaryngol 138:273–280

Balestreri L, De Cicco M, Matovic M, Coran F, Morassut S (1995) Central venous catheter-related thrombosis in clinically asymptomatic oncologic patients: a phlebographic study. Eur J Radiol 20:108–111

Baxter GM, Kincaid W, Jeffrey RF, Millar GM, Porteous C, Morley P (1991) Comparison of colour Doppler ultrasound with venography in the diagnosis of axillary and subclavian vein thrombosis. Br J Radiol 164:777–781

Bloching H, Reuss JA, Seitz K, Rettenmaier G (1989) Thrombosen von Vena subclavia und Vena jugularis sowie Vena cava superior: sonographische Diagnostik und Therapiekontrolle bei TPA-Lysetherapie. Ultraschall Med 10:314–317

Bolz KD, Aadahl P, Mangersnes J, Rodsjo JA, Jorstad S, Myhre HO, Angelsen BA, Nordby A (1993) Intravascular ultrsonographic assessment of thrombus formation on central venous catheters. Acta Radiol 34:162–167

Burbidge SJ, Finlay DE, Letourneau JG, Longley DG (1993) Effects of central venous catheter placement on upper extremity duplex US findings. J Vasc Interv Radiol 14:399–404

Finn JP, Zisk JH, Edelman RR, Wallner BK, Hartnell GG, Stokes KR, Longmaid HE (1993) Central venous occlusion: MR angiography. Radiology 187:245–251

Fischer M, Krunes U, Thieme T (1994) Katheterinduzierte Thrombosen-duplexsonographische Untersuchungen zu Häufigkeit und Ausmass. Ultraschall Med 15:304–307

Grassi CJ, Polak JF (1990) Axillary and subclavian venous thrombosis: follow-up evaluation with color Doppler flow US and venography. Radiology 175:651–654

Gritzmann N (1988) Halsanatomie. In: Czembirek H, Frühwald F, Gritzmann N (eds) Kopf-Hals-Sonographie. Springer, Vienna Berlin Heidelberg New York, pp 119–129

Gritzmann N, Czembirek H, Hajek P, Karnel F, Frühwald F (1987) Sonographische Halsanatomie und ihre Bedeutung beim Lymphknotenstaging von Kopf-Hals-Malignomen. Fortschr Röntgenstr 146:1–7

Gritzmann N, Helmer M, Steiner E, Grasl MC (1990) Invasion of the carotid artery and jugular vein by lymph node metastases: detection using sonography. Am J Roentgenol 154:411–414

Huber P, Schmitt HE, Jäger K (1988) Die tiefe Venenthrombose der oberen Extremität. Schweiz Med Wochenschr 118: 1230–1236

Hübsch P, Frühwald F, Gritzmann N (1989) Venen. In: Czembirek H, Frühwald F, Gritzmann N (eds) Kopf-Hals-Sonographie. Springer, Wien Berlin Heidelberg New York, pp 181–188

Hübsch PJ, Stieglbauer RL, Schwaighofer BW, Kainberger FM, Barton PP (1988) Internal jugular and subclavian vein thrombosis caused by central venous catheters. Evaluation using Doppler blood flow imaging. J Ultrasound Med 7: 629–636

Karnik R, Valentin A, Winkler WB, Donath P, Slany J (1993) Duplex sonography detection of internal jugular venous thrombosis after removal of central venous catheters. Clin Cardiol 16:26–29

Kerr TM, Lutter KS, Moeller DM, Hasselfeld KA, Roedersheimer LR, McKenna PJ, Winkler JL, Spirtoff K, Sampson MG, Cranley JJ (1990) Upper extremity venous thrombosis diagnosed by duplex scanning. Am J Surg 160:202–206

Koksoy C, Kuzu A, Kuzu A, Kutlay J, Erden I, Ozcan H, Ergin K (1995) The diagnostic value of colour Doppler ultrasound in central venous catheter related thrombosis. Clin Radiol 50:687–689

Kraybill WG, Allen BT (1993) Preoperative duplex venous imaging in the assessment of patients with venous access. J Surg Oncol 52:244–248

Longley DG, Finlay DE, Letourneau JG (1993) Sonography of the upper extremity and jugular veins. Am J Roentgenol 160:957–960

Rand T, Kohlhauser C, Popow C, Rokitansky A, Kainberger F, Jakl RJ, Ponhold W, Weninger M (1994) Sonographic detection of internal jugular vein thrombosis after central venous catheterization in the newborn period. Pediatr Radiol 24: 577–580

Rose SC, Gomes AS, Yoon HC (1996) MR angiography for mapping potential central venous access sites in patients with advanced venous occlusive disease. Am J Roentgenol 166: 1181–1187

5 Doppler Imaging of Liver Veins

H. P. Weskott

CONTENTS

5.1 Examination Techniques

The three major liver or hepatic veins (left, middle, and right HV) drain the blood into the inferior vena cava (IVC) just underneath the diaphragm. The topography of the vasculature defines the segmental anatomy of the liver.

Different US techniques are used to analyze hepatic venous flow:

- After angle correction, the pulse-wave (PW) Doppler enables an estimation of velocities and flow pattern. The precise correlation of flow phenomena to the cardiac cycle is made possible by simultaneous ECG registration.
- CDDS visualizes hepatic venous flow in a predefined region of interest. Changes in color intensity and aliasing help to detect local changes in flow velocities and to quantify stenosis with PW Doppler thereafter.
- The advantage to displaying blood flow in the amplitude-encoded color Doppler technique lies in demonstrating very slow volume flow in small-sized vessels, even at unfavorable Doppler angles (Weskott 1997), yet detection of the flow direction is not possible. Recently, US devices have become available which add a Doppler signal to the amplitude signal, thus also enabling the recognition of the flow direction (convergent Doppler).

Using pulsed Doppler mode, the size of the sample volume is related to the width of the liver vein investigated and should be about 2/3 of its diameter. The wall filter is adjusted to around 50 Hz, with very slow velocities as low as possible. The position of the baseline should be oriented according to the predominant hepatofugal flow. The same applies to the adjustment of the color bar. To avoid a low frame-rate, the color box should not be chosen too large.

The investigation should be performed in the supine position after a period of at least 4 h of fasting. To standardize the examination procedure, the sample volume should be placed 3–5 cm distant to the IVC. Thus, a sufficiently high velocity tracing of the spectrum curve is achieved with the maximum velocities decreasing towards the peripheral venous branches. Well suited for investigation are the right and middle HV, which can be visualized in a longitudinal plane via an intercostal approach. Due to its small size and because of motion artifacts of the pulsating heart, the left HV is less well suited for the recording of Doppler curves, but has to be included in the investigation, especially in venoocclusive disease and diffuse liver disease.

The hepatic venous flow depends on changes in the right atrial hemodynamics and mirrors atrial pressure changes. The Doppler waveform also depends on the compliance of the liver tissue surrounding the thin hepatic venous wall and the hepatic venous resistance. Intrathoracic pressure variation with respiration (Fig. 5.2b,d), increased intra-abdominal pressure, and patient positioning (Fig. 5.2c) influence the Doppler spectra as well. With deep inspira-

H. P. Weskott, MD
Klinikum Hannover, Städtisches Krankenhaus Siloah, Medizinische Klinik II, Roesebeckstrasse 15, 30449 Hannover, Germany

tion, the intra-abdominal pressure rises, resulting in a decrease of venous return and the phasic oscillation of the velocity curve.

Accordingly, Doppler measurements in HVs should be performed at end expiration. Prior to interpretation of the hepatic venous flow patterns, the patient's cardiac and pulmonary condition should be known.

The normal hepatic venous Doppler spectrum shows a triphasic, W-shaped pattern. It reflects the venous pressure changes during atrial systole, ventricular systole, and ventricular diastole.

Figure 5.1 shows a normal triphasic flow pattern of the middle HV. The terminology of the flow maxima and flow minima accords with that used in cardiology (a, c, x, v and y wave and descent).

The a-wave reflects atrial systole and is the first peak flow from the IVC to the HVs after the p-wave (hepatopetal flow). Reflecting tricuspid valve closure, hepatic venous Doppler signals can sometimes detect a c-wave, having the same direction as the a-wave and occurring concomitantly with tricuspid valve closure. During atrial filling and with a closed tricuspid valve, the right atrial pressure decreases, until the maximum flow velocity of the x-decent is reached with increased blood flow from the HV into the IVC. With the consecutive increase in right atrial pressure, the hepatofugal flow decreases again until the lowest flow velocity of the v-wave is reached at the time of tricuspid valve opening. In some healthy subjects, the v-wave reaches the baseline and may even be reversed with a lower hepatopetal flow velocity than the a-wave. In these cases, a fourth phase can be defined. With the filling of the right ventricle, the hepatofugal flow increases again until the maximum of the y-descent. Thereafter, with right

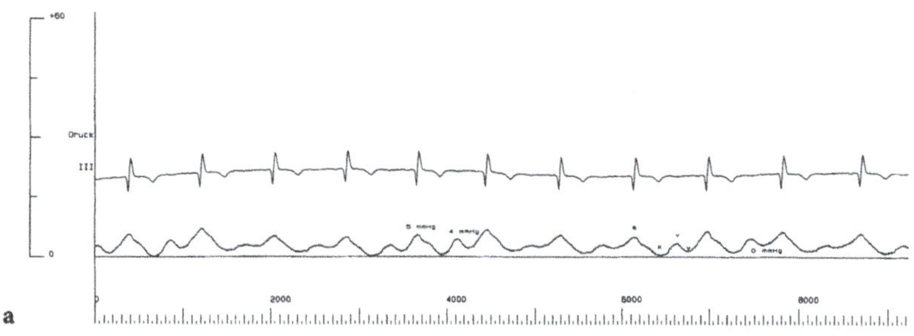

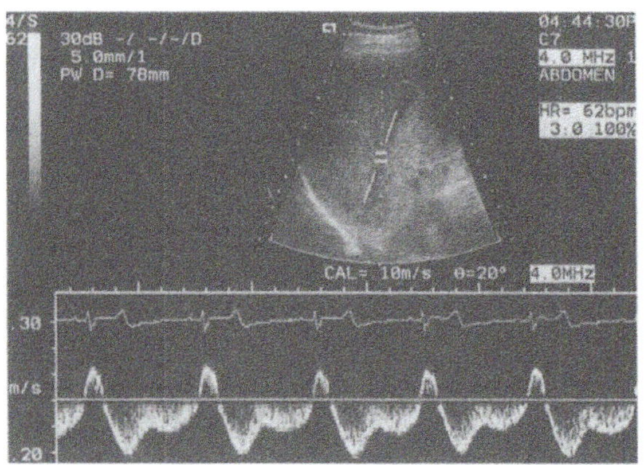

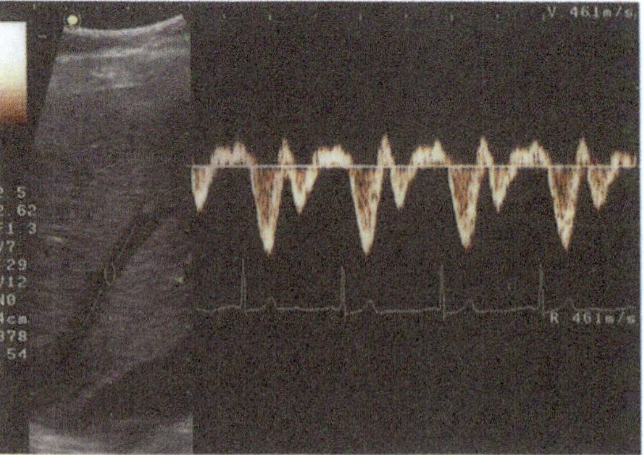

Fig. 5.1. **a** Right atrial pressure curve. **b** Schematic drawing of the three phases from a hepatic venous Doppler curve. *Phase 1* represents the a- and c-wave, *phase 2* the x-descent, and *phase 3* the y-descent. **c** Triphasic flow pattern of the middle hepatic vein (HV) during expiration (same patient as in **a**). **d** The short-term, low-velocity c-wave can only be detected inconstantly. The v-wave shows a reverse flow, thus adding a fourth phase to the Doppler waveform

atrial filling, the right atrial pressure rises again with a consequent decrease of hepatofugal flow velocity (Braunwald 1984). The Doppler curve thus mirrors the right atrial pressure curve. Only infrequently can the a-wave and the c-wave be differentiated from one another in the Doppler spectrum, commonly they are fused to one single wave. During inspiration, the c-wave is sometimes more pronounced. The maximum flow velocities of the x-decent and the y-decent may differ; usually, the diastolic velocity peak is somewhat lower. In around half of the investigations, a short-term, low-velocity, end-systolic reverse flow phenomenon (hepatopetal v-wave) can be observed (Pennestri et al. 1984).

Mean peak flow-velocities during systole (x-decent) are reported to be –29 cm/s in adults and –44 cm/s in children. Mean peak velocities during diastole (y-decent) are reported to be –18 cm/s in adults and–25 cm/s in children (Abu-Yousef 1991; Teichgräber et al. 1997; Meyer et al. 1993). The higher flow velocities in children are probably due to the higher compliance of a child's liver.

With decreasing venous diameter, the flow velocities decrease towards the periphery of the liver (Teichgräber et al. 1997). In inspiration, the phasic oscillation of the blood flow may decrease somewhat, and the a-wave may flatten and even lose its retrograde orientation (Fig. 5.2d). The systolic x-wave flattens during inspiration, leading to a decrease of the x: y ratio from 1.4 to 1.1 (Abu-Yousef 1992) (Fig. 5.2b). Due to the increase in venous pressure of the IVC during the Valsalva maneuver, the hepatic venous waveform turns into a flat monophasic flow pattern.

During pregnancy, phasic oscillation of the Doppler wave curve changes. With increasing duration of pregnancy, the triphasic velocity pattern changes towards a flattened monophasic band-shaped Doppler profile, probably due to an increased intra-abdominal pressure up to 80% in the last trimester (Roobottom et al. 1995).

Depending on the atrial output, atrial flutter or fibrillation can lead to a partial loss of the atrial systolic component (a-wave) of the hepatic venous Doppler profile (Fig. 5.3).

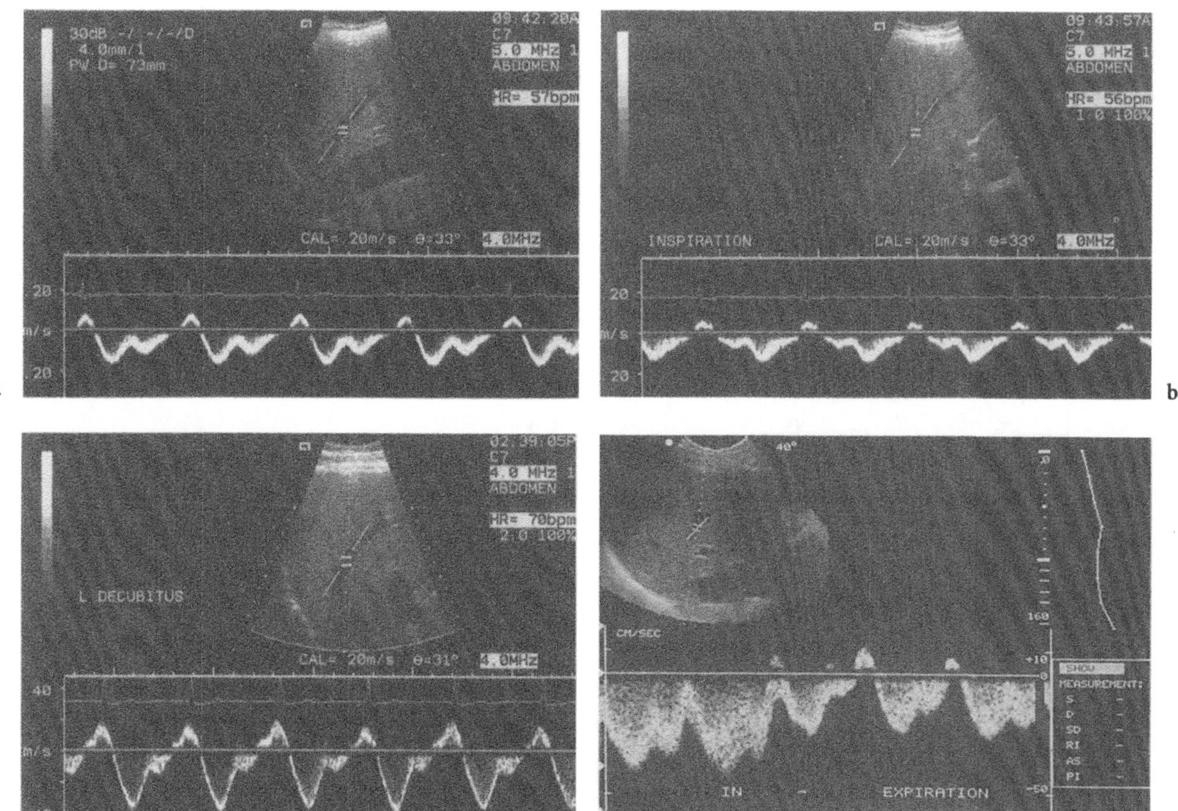

Fig. 5.2. **a** Doppler waveform at expiration. **b** Variation of the hepatic venous Doppler curve at inspiration from supine into a left decubitus position during expiration (**c**). Notice the relative change of the systolic and diastolic peak velocities (a–c: same patient). **d** Biphasic flow pattern at inspiration that changes into a triphasic waveform during expiration

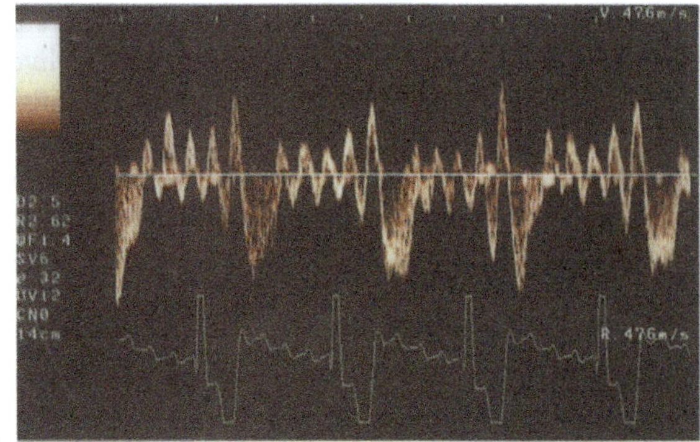

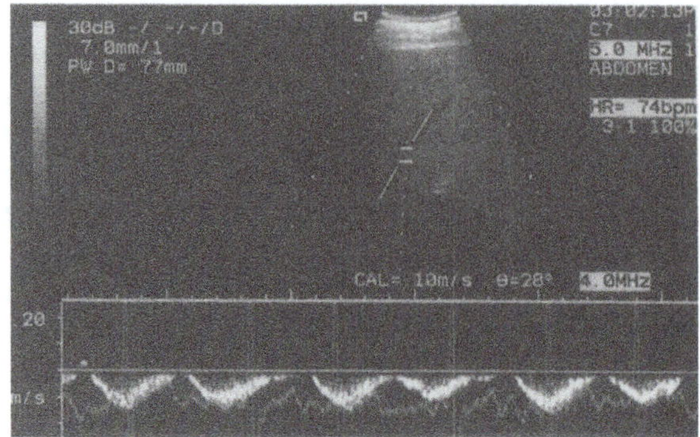

Fig. 5.3a–c. Doppler waveform in patients with atrial flutter (**a**) and fibrillation (**b**). **c** Right atrial pressure curve of the patient with atrial fibrillation

In addition to velocity calculations and assessment of the phasic oscillation, characteristic landmarks of the Doppler waveform can be correlated to the R-wave of the simultaneously recorded ECG (Fig. 5.4). The time interval between the R-wave and x-descent obviously varies with the distance to the cardiac chambers but is also influenced by the elasticity (compliance) of the hepatic parenchyma. According to the first reported data, it may be clinically useful to measure these time intervals in diffuse liver disease as well. Since the time interval between the R-wave and the x-descent is influenced by the heart rate, an index has been suggested. This QXr index represents the quotient of the Rx-time interval and the time interval between two consecutive R-waves, the normal value being 0.34±0.06 (Hamato et al. 1997a,b).

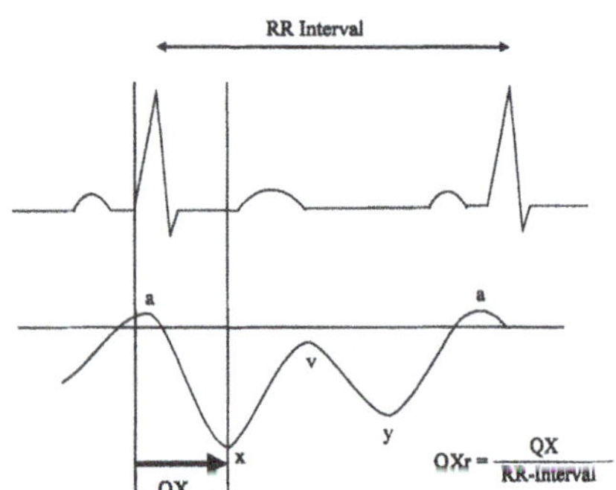

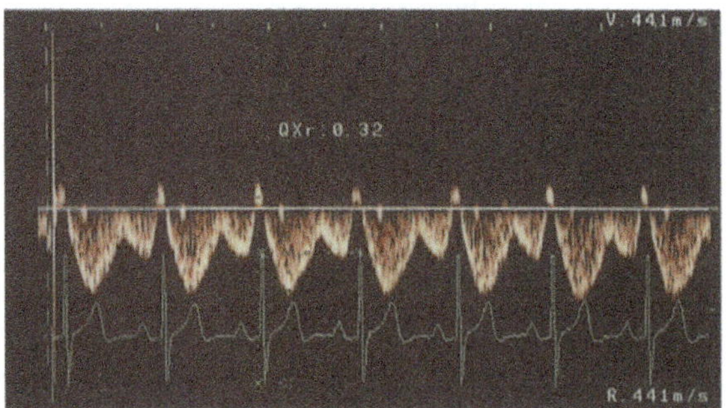

Fig. 5.4. Schematic diagram of the hepatic waveform correlated to the ECG tracing. Measurement of the time interval between R-wave of the ECG and the peak velocity of the x-wave (adapted from: Hamato 1997a,b)

5.2 Influence of Extrahepatic Disease

5.2.1 Right Heart Failure

In the presence of tricuspid valve insufficiency, there is systolic regurgitation of blood into the hepatic venous system: Depending on the degree of valvular regurgitation, there is initially a flattening of the systolic flow curve, until eventually flow reversal may lead to a melting of the systolic flow curve with the a-wave. This results in a M-shaped flow velocity pattern in the HVs. With severe right heart failure, the a-wave may be missing, as right atrial contraction may have hardly any hemodynamic consequences.

In this situation, the hepatic venous flow profile resembles a sinus wave (Fig. 5.5b). In right heart failure, the Doppler curve of the POV mirrors that of the HVs (Fig. 5.6b).

In various heart diseases, supraventricular and ventricular arrhythmias are present that influence the Doppler waveform. In atrial fluttering with regular transconduction, sometimes more than one a-wave can be observed. Because of the low right atrial volume output in patients with atrial fibrillation, the a-wave is very often absent (Fig. 5.5c).

A severe right heart failure leads to a saw-like appearance of the flow profile with changing peak velocities in atrial fibrillation, supraventricular or ventricular arrhythmia. Independent of the heart rhythm, severe right heart failure leads to a pulsatile flow in the portal venous system as well as a hepatopetal (diastolic component) and a hepatofugal (systolic component) flow.

The degree of flow changes in the hepatic venous system and the width of the HVs do not always reflect the degree of right heart failure, and sometimes the portal venous flow characteristic is the only reliable Doppler sonographic evidence for severe right heart failure. As the right atrial pressure curve in patients with dilative cardiomyopathy may be normal, some patients show a normal triphasic flow profile in the HVs as well and still have pulmonary hypertension.

Figure 5.6a, b shows a Doppler curve in a patient with pulmonary valve stenosis with quadrophasic flow within normal-sized HVs due to a relatively high pressure level during the v-wave.

The velocity waveform of the HVs not only depends on the pressure changes of the right atrium, but may be modulated by an increase of liver tissue elasticity. In patients with cardiac failure and diffuse liver disease, the waveform can therefore appear normal (Fig. 5.7).

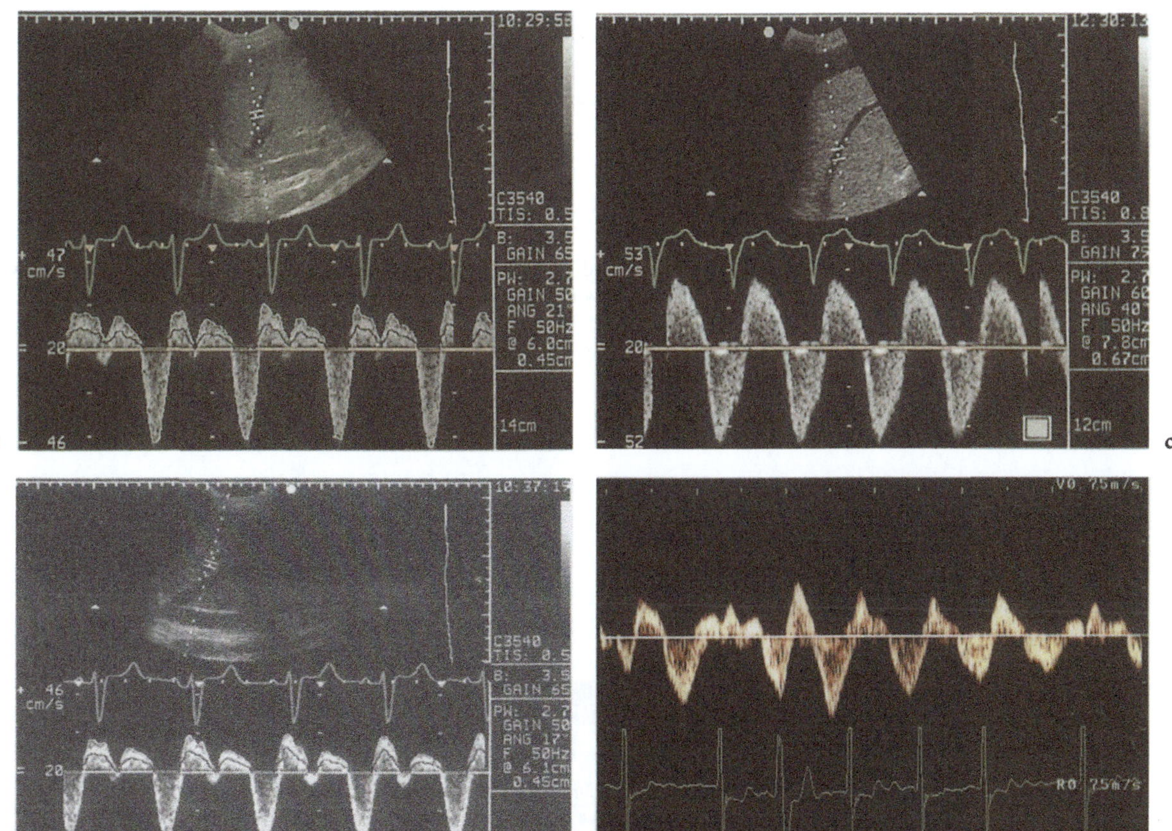

Fig. 5.5a–d. Doppler spectrum curves in patients with tricuspid regurgitation. **a** Relatively high a-wave followed by a c-wave and a reverse flow during systole. Only the diastolic flow component has a hepatofugal direction towards the vena cava. **b** Right atrial pressure curve of the same patient. **c** Sinus wave-like shape of the Doppler waveform with a highly reversed flow during systole. An a-wave cannot be detected. **d** Patient with dilated cardiomyopathy and atrial fibrillation. Analyzing the simultaneously registered ECG, the reverse flow during ventricular systole can easily be identified and indicates tricuspid regurgitation

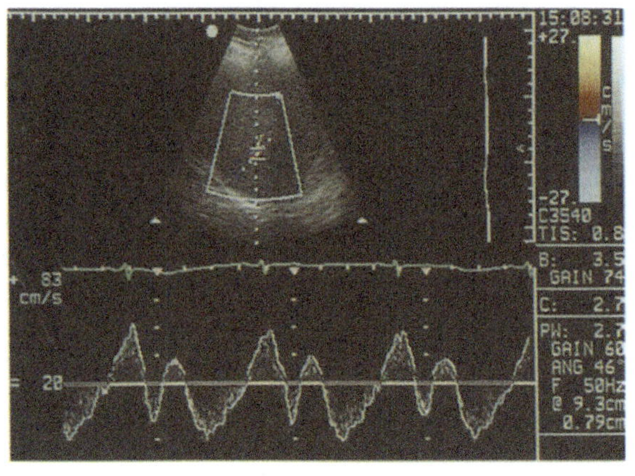

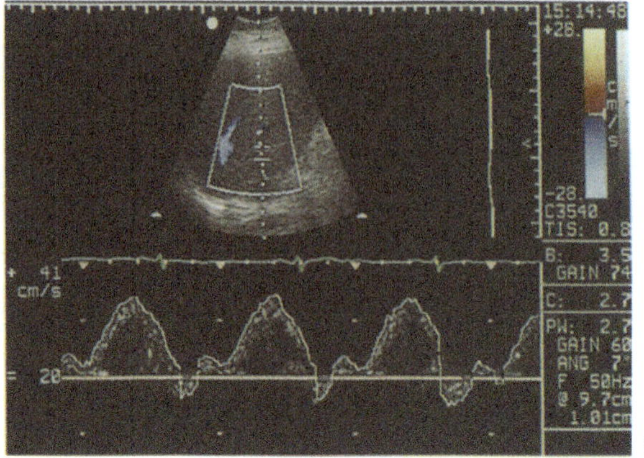

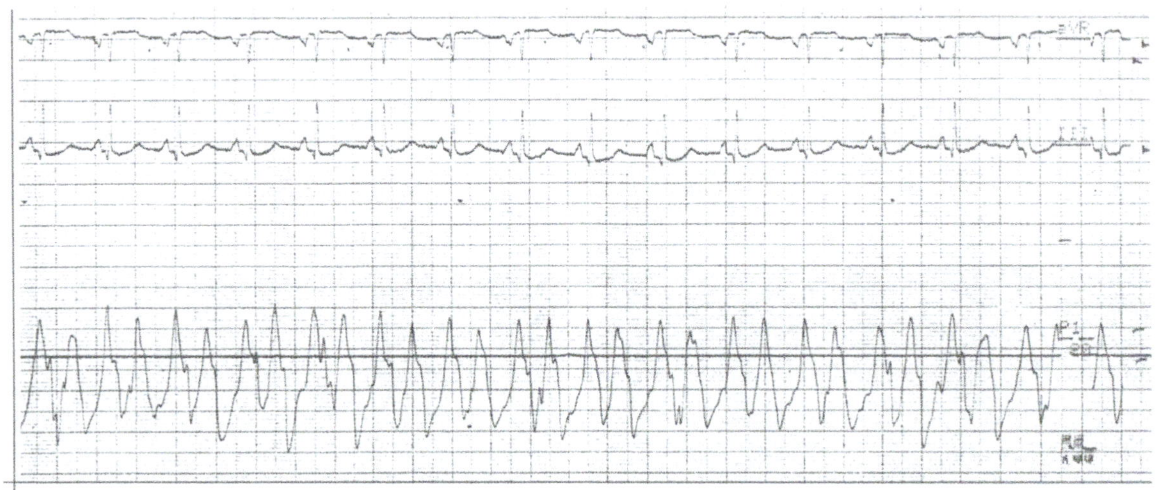

Fig. 5.6a–c. Spectral Doppler tracing of the middle HV (**a**) and right portal vein (**b**) in a 23-year-old woman with pulmonary valve stenosis. **c** Right atrial pressure curve. Note pulsatile flow in the main portal vein (hepatopetal and hepatofugal)

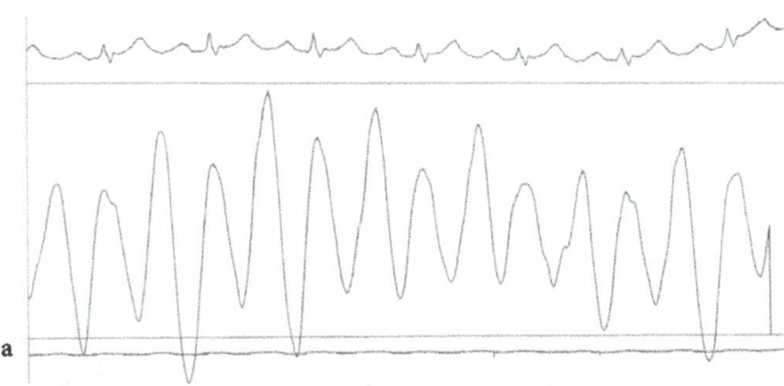

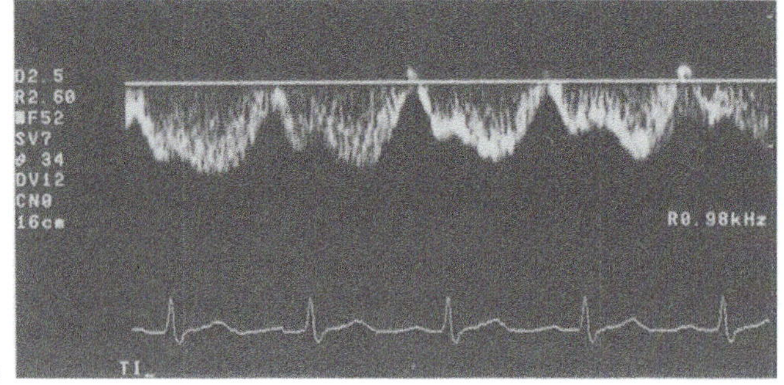

Fig. 5.7a, b. Patient with dilated cardiomyopathy and hepatic steatosis. **a** Right atrial pressure curve. **b** Normal velocity waveform from the middle HV

5.2.2 Pulmonary Hypertension

Pulmonary hypertension may lead to changes in the spectral curve of the hepatic and portal venous system even in the absence of typical signs of right heart failure. One characteristic feature of pulmonary hypertension is an elevated a-wave in the atrial pressure curve; compared with the x-wave, the flow-velocity profile of the HVs shows a relatively high retrograde flow during atrial systole (Fig. 5.8).

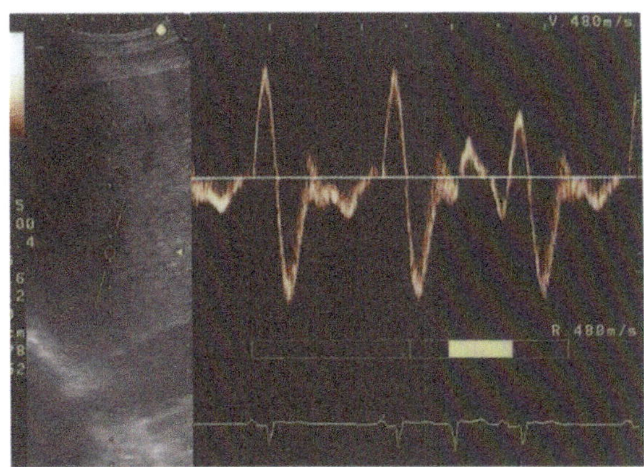

Fig. 5.8. Patient with pulmonary hypertension. Doppler waveform from hepatic venous flow shows an a-wave that is slightly higher than x-descent (28 cm/s and –30 cm/s). Due to an extrasystole after two regular heart beats, the 4th waveform shows a decreased a-wave, while the peak velocity of the x-descent remains unchanged

5.3 Status of Increased Abdominal Pressure

Intra-abdominal pressure is increased for example in the presence of ascites and in the postoperative state and is often accompanied by an elevation of the diaphragm. Invasive measurements in patients with liver cirrhosis have shown that an elevation of the intra-abdominal pressure is accompanied by an increase of the free hepatic venous pressure and the wedged hepatic venous pressure, while the gradient between the two remains constant (Luca et al. 1993).

5.4 Diffuse Liver Disease

Aside from changes in the course and diameter, diffuse liver disease may lead to alterations in the Doppler waveform of the HVs. Because diffuse liver disease does not affect all liver segments to the same extent, it is necessary to investigate all three major HVs. CDDS helps to detect regional flow changes.

Changes in the phasic oscillation of the HV flow-velocity profile are caused by alterations of the compliance of the hepatic parenchyma or by local venous stenosis. Local stenosis may not only be due to external compression, but can also be caused by focal thrombosis, e.g., in the vicinity of parenchymal nodes (Wanless et al. 1994). Irrespective of focal venous stenosis, hepatic cirrhosis leads to an increased stiffening of the hepatic tissue (Bolondi et al. 1991). Due to organ atrophy and venous compression caused by surrounding parenchymal changes, the HV diameter decreases, thus making it more difficult to depict continuous hepatic veins in gray scale imaging. In these instances, color flow imaging is better suited to detect the longitudinal course of the hepatic veins (Fig. 5.9)

a

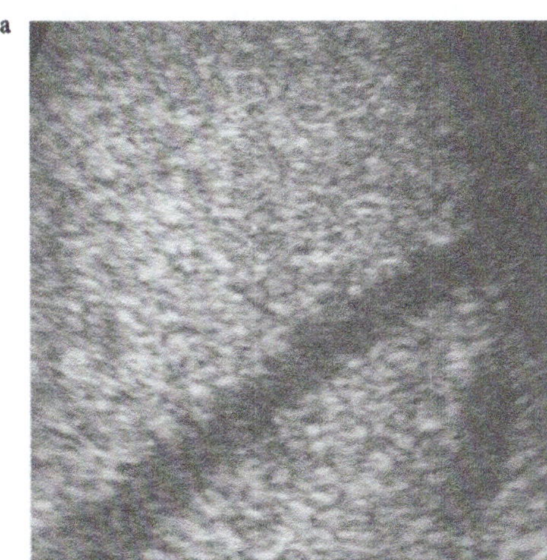

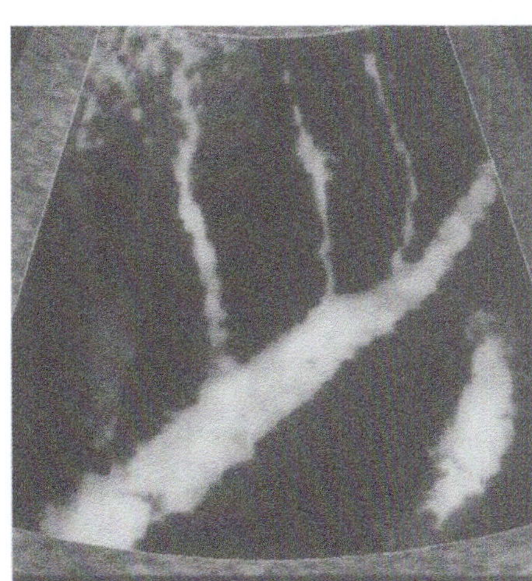

b

Fig. 5.9a, b. Patient with liver cirrhosis. In gray-scale imaging, the branches of the middle HV cannot be depicted (**a**), whereas amplitude Doppler imaging demonstrates the tiny irregular veins flowing into the middle HV (**b**)

and to assess Doppler curves with the appropriate angle correction.

With CDDS, local HV stenosis can easily be evaluated (Fig. 5.10). Stenosis may vary in length from a few millimeters up to 4 cm (Lorenz and Winsburg 1997). Distal to the stenosis, the flow is always bi- or monophasic.

With increasing area stenosis, the flow profile distally is attenuated until eventually only a monophasic, band-shaped flow is recognized. After correction of the stenosis, e.g., with stenting, a triphasic flow can be re-established (Ohta et al. 1994).

Aside from local stenosis, a decrease in compliance of the liver tissue influences the Doppler waveform as well. In order to characterize the change in flow pattern, Bolondi et al. (1989, 1991) suggested three and Ohta et al. (1994) suggested five typical flow patterns in patients with diffuse liver diseases (Fig. 5.11).

Bolondi et al. (1989, 1991) found a relationship between the disappearance of the characteristic phasic HV waveform and the severity of liver cirrhosis. In 25% of the patients with liver cirrhosis, the phasic oscillation of the hepatic venous flow is completely lost and in a further 25%, significantly reduced.

However, a monophasic hepatic venous flow is not specific for hepatic cirrhosis, but with the exception of its occurrence in late pregnancy, it is considered to be a pathological feature: A monophasic venous flow pattern may be observed when fatty hepatic infiltration has already caused a reduction of the compliance (Colli et al. 1994) or when tissue edema and inflammation in organ rejection are present in a transplanted liver (Britton et al. 1992). In addition, a monophasic flow in all three HVs is suggestive but not specific for the presence of a Budd-Chiari syndrome (Bolondi et al. 1991).

On the other hand, acute inflammatory or necrotic liver diseases do not cause significant alterations in the hepatic venous flow profile. In acute hepatitis, the peak HV velocities tend to increase (Teichgräber 1998).

Since hepatic venous stenosis and/or advanced alterations of the parenchymal compliance are necessary to flatten the Doppler curve with eventually complete loss of phasic oscillation, about 30–50% of

a

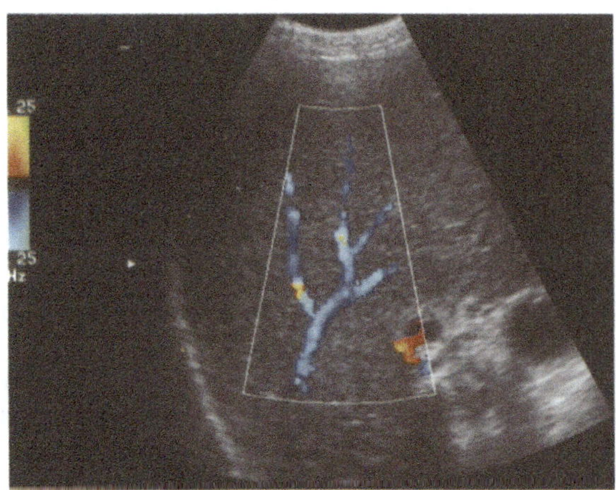

b

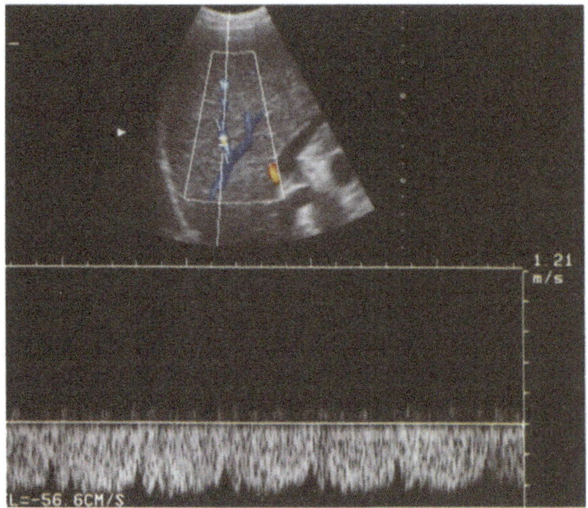

c

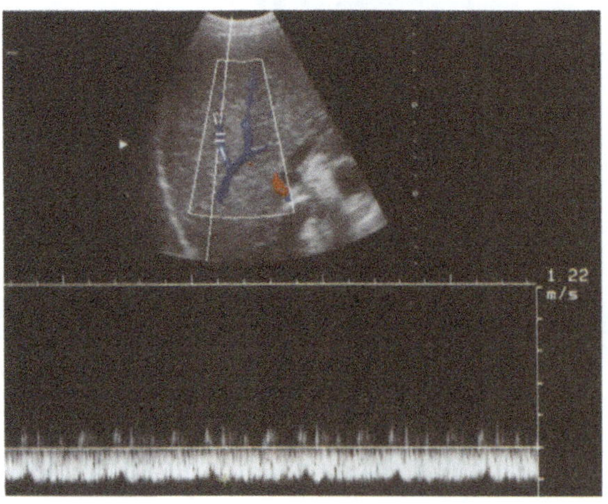

Fig. 5.10a–c. Patient with liver cirrhosis. **a** CDI demonstrates irregular hepatic venous flow with two focal stenoses at the site of color aliasing. **b** Flat Doppler waveform with increased velocity at the site of stenosis. **c** Peak velocity decreased just peripheral from the stenosis

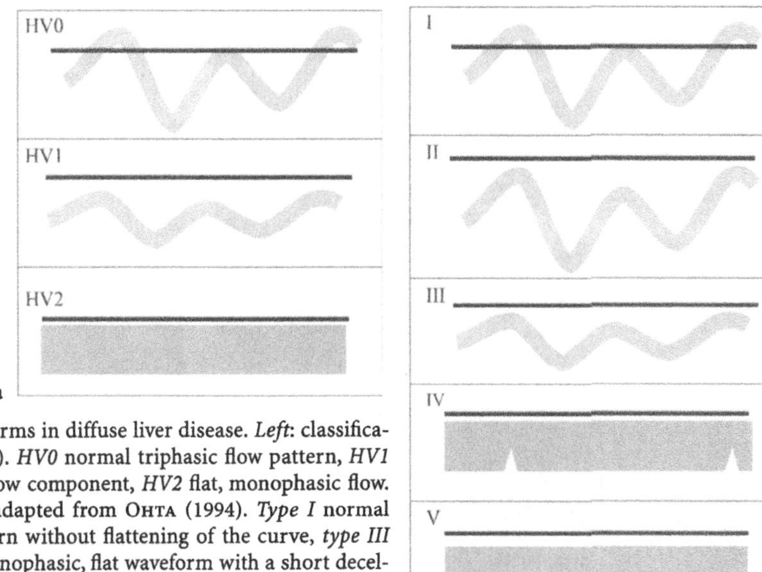

Fig. 5.11a, b. Classification of HV waveforms in diffuse liver disease. *Left*: classification adapted from Bolondi et al. (1991). *HV0* normal triphasic flow pattern, *HV1* biphasic flow pattern without reverse flow component, *HV2* flat, monophasic flow. *Right*: Classification of HV flow types adapted from Ohta (1994). *Type I* normal flow pattern, *type II* biphasic flow pattern without flattening of the curve, *type III* flattened biphasic waveform, *type IV* monophasic, flat waveform with a short deceleration indicating atrial systole, *type V* completely flat waveform without oscillation caused by cardiac pressure changes

patients with liver cirrhosis have a normal triphasic hepatic venous flow profile (Ohta et al. 1994). With progression of the parenchymal changes in cirrhosis, the triphasic flow pattern loses first its atrial component, leading to a biphasic flow pattern; with further progression, the flow velocities equalize until only a band-shaped flow pattern is detectable.

According to Colli et al. (1994), a pathological hepatic venous flow pattern has a diagnostic accuracy of 0.77 and a specificity of 0.78 in detecting Child A hepatic cirrhosis in patients with chronic hepatitis C.

The degree of flattening of the hepatic venous flow profile is correlated to the Child classification and thus is a prognostic factor in patients with hepatic cirrhosis (Fig. 5.12).

In a CDDS study of 120 patients with hepatic cirrhosis, Ohta et al. (1995) found that patients with a band-shaped hepatic venous flow profile died of hepatic failure within less than 2 years (sensitivity 0.41, specificity 0.99).

Difficulties in the interpretation of HV Doppler waveforms arise when liver cirrhosis and cardiac insufficiency coexist, particularly in patients with alcohol-induced liver cirrhosis, who may develop congestive cardiomyopathy with tricuspid regurgitation. In these patients, a biphasic or triphasic flow pattern may be re-established in the presence of cardiac insufficiency again or never become bi- or monophasic.

As mentioned above, the time delay between the R-wave in the ECG and the x-wave in the HV flow profile is influenced by the elasticity of the hepatic parenchyma. In liver cirrhosis, the QXr-value decreases to 0.20±0.03, but with fatty infiltration of the liver, it increases to 0.39±0.07. In case of a triphasic flow in liver cirrhosis, this index may be the only hint of a decreased tissue compliance (Fig. 5.13b). In patients with chronic hepatitis, the QXr-value was 0.27±0.03 (Hamato 1997a,b). Further evaluation of the diagnostic potential of the QXr-value has to be awaited; it does not represent a substitute for invasive diagnostic procedures.

5.5 Focal Liver Disease

Focal liver disease may lead to distortion of the HVs, local venous stenosis (Fig. 5.14), and/or thrombotic occlusion. Lesions with a similar echogenicity to the liver parenchyma are sometimes only detected by US because of the displacement of an adjacent HV or portal vein (POV) branch.

5.6 Hepatic Venous Outflow Obstruction

Hepatic venous obstruction may occur at different levels and can be caused by various diseases. Venous occlusions may affect the small HVs (venoocclusive disease), the large HVs, or the IVC. Possible causes include spontaneous thrombosis due to coagulation disorders, fibrinous webs, primary membranous

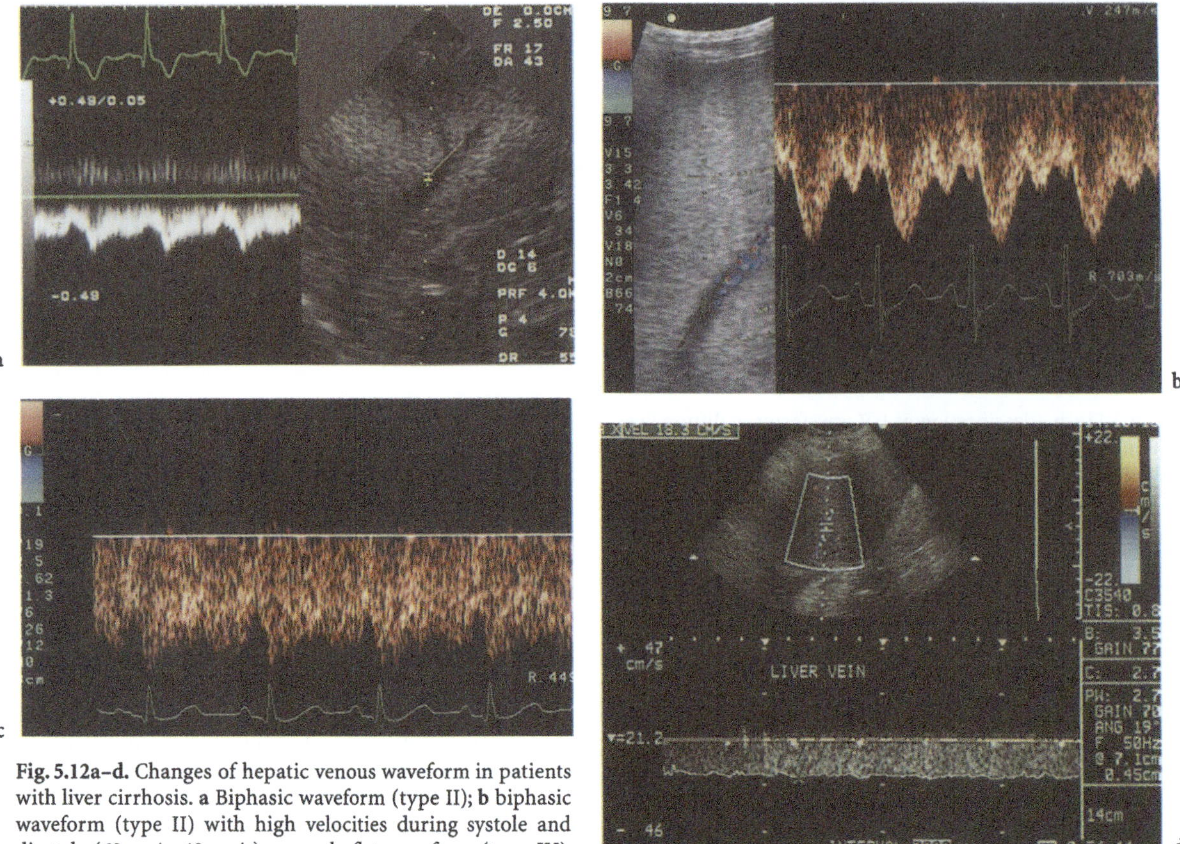

Fig. 5.12a–d. Changes of hepatic venous waveform in patients with liver cirrhosis. **a** Biphasic waveform (type II); **b** biphasic waveform (type II) with high velocities during systole and diastole (62 cm/c, 42 cm/s); **c** nearly flat waveform (type IV). Note the short time interval between R-wave and x-descent (QXr: 0.18). **d** Completely flat waveform

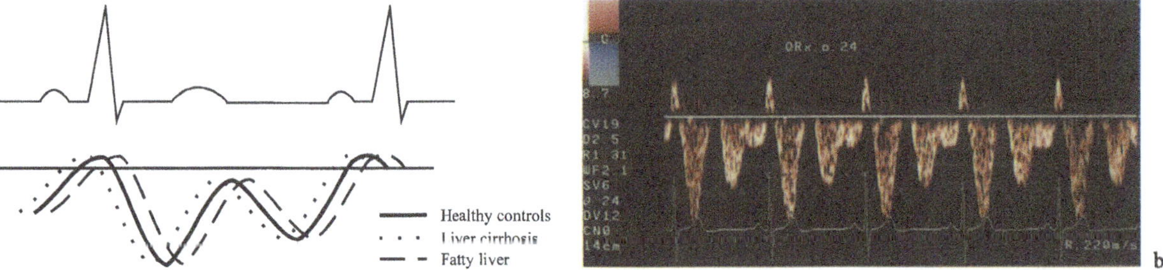

Fig. 5.13. a Schematic drawing of the QXr calculation in patients with liver cirrhosis and fatty liver compared with a normal control group (adapted from HAMATO 1997a,b; see also Fig. 5.11c). **b** Patient with liver cirrhosis and esophageal varices. Hepatic venous flow shows a triphasic flow pattern but a decreased Qxr value

obstruction, space-occupying lesions, or tumor thrombus.

5.6.1 Budd-Chiari Syndrome

This disorder represents a partial or complete obstruction of the HVs, with the clinical features of hepatomegaly, ascites, and upper abdominal pain. The gray-scale US appearance is that of an enlarged left hepatic lobe and a massively enlarged caudate lobe. The HVs present with various, but definitely increased echogenicity or cannot be detected by gray-scale US at the venous confluence. Apart from thrombus formation, underlying causes may be tumor invasion or–rarely–a congenital web that obstructs the IVC or HVs, most frequently seen in patients of Asian origin. Increased echogenicity of the venous lumen on gray-scale US is highly suggestive for the presence

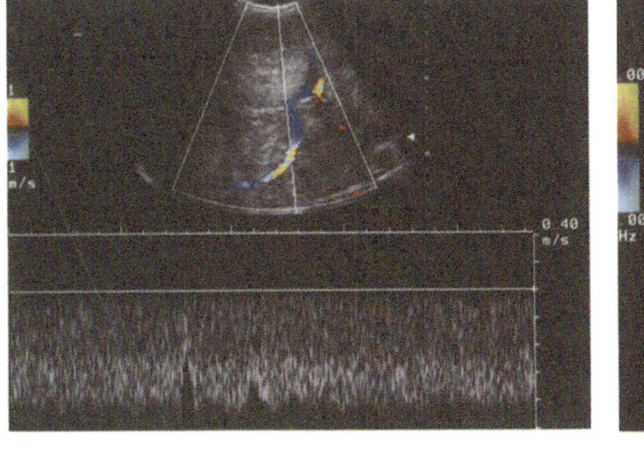
a

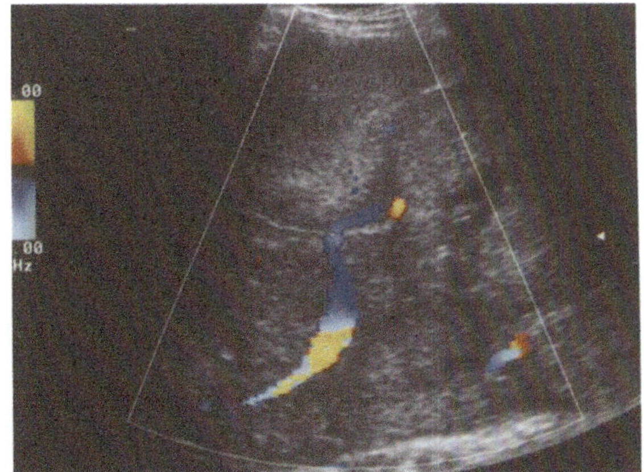
b

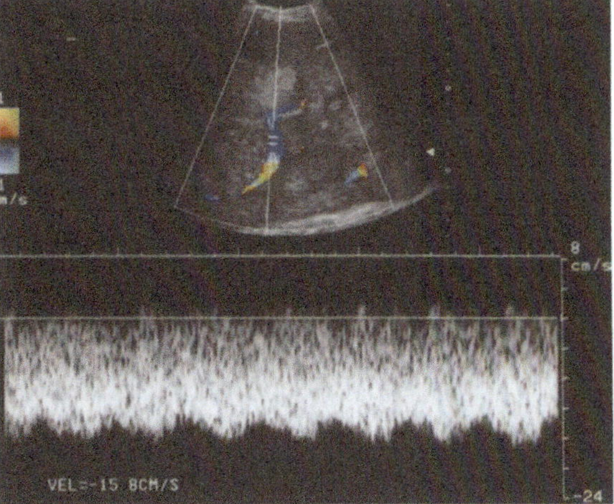
c

Fig. 5.14a–c. Focal stenosis caused by liver metastasis. Aliasing indicates the site of stenosis in CDI mode, that can be verified by estimating local velocity by using PW Doppler

of thrombotic occlusion. In two-thirds of the patients, the underlying cause is never determined.

Duplex Doppler US and especially CDDS are important aids to establish the diagnosis (GRANT et al. 1989); in the presence of hepatic enlargement, real-time imaging may suggest hepatic venous occlusion due to compression by the surrounding hepatic tissue, while CDDS may still show HV patency. Due to a stenosis (Fig. 5.15) or thrombosis of the hepatic venous outflow, a reversed flow in the remaining patent HVs and intrahepatic collaterals are important CDDS findings.

5.6.2 Venoocclusive Disease

Thrombotic occlusion of small HVs is a well-known complication after bone marrow transplantation (McDONALD et al. 1984; JONES et al. 1987). The causative (therapy-induced) endothelial damage affects predominantly the small terminal HVs. The clinical features are well correlated to the histopathological findings and include: weight loss, hepatic enlargement and/or tenderness in the right upper abdominal quadrant, jaundice or elevation of the bilirubin level in the first 20 days after bone marrow transplantation. The clinical course may range from mild to fulminant with liver necrosis and death due to multiorgan failure (HOMMEYER et al. 1992). US features include hepatosplenomegaly, ascites, thickening of the gallbladder wall, hepatic venous compression, and increased echogenicity of the hepatic parenchyma. In addition, flow in the POV is also altered up to the occurrence of flow reversal. Shortly after transplantation, pathological CDDS findings are only found in 50% of the patients with clinical signs of venoocclusive disease (VOD), and similar CDDS features may be observed in patients without VOD. Thus, sonography is not particularly helpful in the management of patients with VOD after bone marrow transplantation (HOMMEYER et al. 1992).

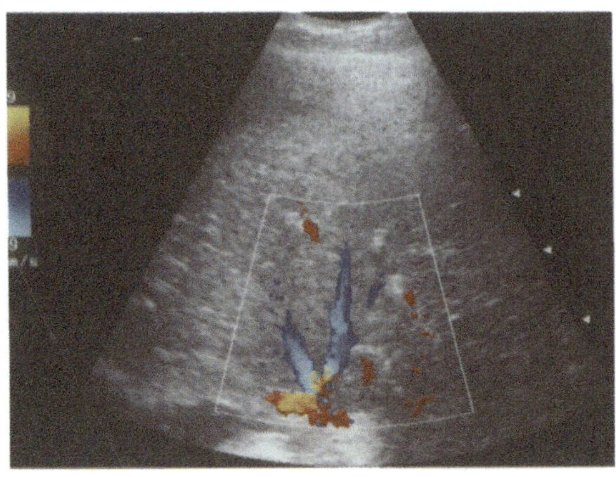

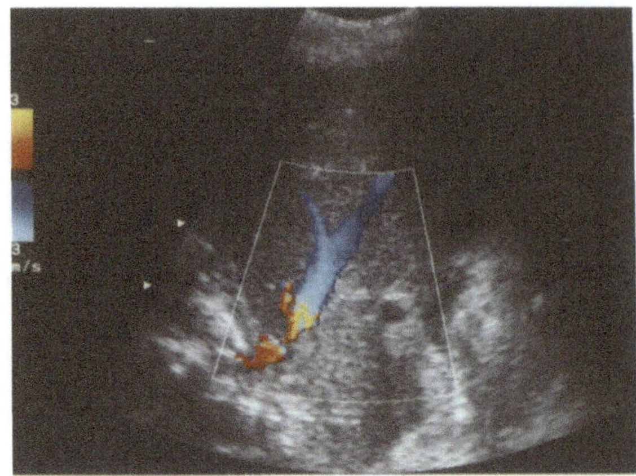

a b

Fig. 5.15a, b. Color aliasing due to a stenosis at the hepatic venous confluence: **a** intercostal scan plane, **b** subcostal scan plane

5.7 Doppler of Liver Veins in the Clinical Follow-up After Liver Transplantation

In the follow-up after liver transplantation, CDDS of the hepatic veins should document venous patency and a triphasic hepatic venous flow pattern. In none of the patients with a triphasic hepatic venous flow profile after liver transplantation was there early acute rejection (Coulden et al. 1990). Britton et al. reported on 50 children with liver transplantation, in whom the Doppler investigation of the HVs within the first 2 weeks after transplantation detected an acute rejection with a sensitivity of 0.92 and a specificity of 1.0 (Britton et al. 1992).

Acknowledgements: I gratefully acknowledge Dr. H. Klempt and Mrs. Bali Bassan for their help with the manuscript, Dr. K. Schäfer for supporting me with the right atrial pressure measurements and Prof. v. Leitner for his valuable critical comments.

References

Abu-Yousef MM (1991) Duplex Doppler sonography of the hepatic vein in tricuspid regurgitation. Am J Roentgenol 156:79–83

Abu-Yousef MM (1992) Normal and respiratory variations of the hepatic and portal venous Duplex Doppler waveform with simultaneous electrocardiographic correlation. J Ultrasound Med 11:263–268

Bolondi L, Gaiani S, Li Bassi S (1989) Changes in the hepatic vein waveform detected by Doppler ultrasound in liver cirrhosis. Hepatology 9:S117

Bolondi L, Li Bassi S, Gaiani S, Zironi G, Benzi G, Santi V, Barbara L (1991) Liver cirrhosis: changes of Doppler waveform of hepatic veins. Radiology 178:513–516

Braunwald E (1984) Heart disease. A textbook of cardiovascular medicine. Saunders, Philadelphia

Britton PD, Lomas DJ, Coulden RA et al (1992) The role of hepatic vein Doppler in diagnosing acute rejection following paediatric liver transplantation. Clin Radiol 45:228–232

Colli A, Cocciolo M, Riva C et al (1994) Abnormalities of Doppler waveform of the hepatic veins in patients with chronic liver disease: correlation with histologic findings. Am J Roentgenol 162:833–837

Grant EG, Perrella R, Tessler FN, Lois J, Busuttil R (1989) Budd-Chiari syndrome: the results of duplex and color Doppler imaging. Am J Roentgenol 152:377–381

Hamato N, Moriyasu F, Someda H, Nishikawa K, Chiba T, Okuma M (1997a) Clinical application of hepatic venous hemodynamics by Doppler ultrasonography in cirhotic liver disease. Ultrasound Med Biol 23:829–835

Hamato N, Moriyasu F, Someda H, Nishikawa K, Chiba T, Okuma M (1997b) Phase shift of the hepatic vein flow velocity waveform in cirrhotic liver disease: experimental and clinical studies. Ultrasound Med Biol 23:821–828

Hommeyer SC, Teefey SA, Jacobson AF, Higano CS, Bianco JA, Colacurio CJ (1992) Venocclusive disease of the liver: prospective study of US evaluation. Radiology 184: 683–686

Jones RJ, Lee KS, Beschorner WE et al (1987) Venocclusive disease of the liver following bone marrow transplantation. Transplantation 44:778–783

Lorenz J, Winsberg F (1997) Focal liver stenoses in diffuse liver disease. J Ultrasound Med 15:313–316

Luca A, Cirera I, Garcia-Pegan JC, Feu F, Pizcueta P, Bosch J, Rodes J (1993) Hemodynamic effects of acute changes in intra-abdominal pressure in patients with cirrhosis. Gastroenterology 104:222–227

McDonald GB, Sharma P, Matthews DE, Shulman HM, Thomas ED (1984) Venocclusive disease of the liver after bone marrow transplantation: diagnosis, incidence, and predisposing factors. Hepatology 4:116–122

Meyer RJ, Goldberg SJ, Donnerstein RL (1993) Superior

vena cava and hepatic vein velocity patterns in normal children. Am J Cardiol 72:238–240

Ohta M, Hashizume M, Tomikawa M, Ueno K, Tanoue K, Sugimachi K (1994) Analysis of hepatic waveform by Doppler ultrasonography in 100 patients with portal hypertension. Am J Gastroenterol 89:170–175

Pennestri F, Loperfido F, Salvatori MP et al (1984) Assessment of tricuspid regurgitation by pulsed Doppler ultrasonography of the hepatic veins. J Cardiol 54: 363–368

Roobottom CA, Hunter JD, Weston MJ, Dubbins PA (1995) Hepatic venous Doppler waveforms: changes in pregnancies. J Clin Ultrasound 23:477–482

Teichgräber UKM, Gebel M, Benter T, Manns MP (1997) Duplexsonographische Charakterisierung des Lebervenenflusses bei Gesunden. Ultraschall Med 18:267–271

Teichgräber UKM, Gebel M, Manns MP (1998) Doppler measurements of hepatic venous flow in patients with liver disease and healthy subjects. Ultrasound Med 16:S83

Wachsberg RH, Angyal EA, Klein KM, Kuo HR, Lambert WC (1997) Echogenicity of hepatic versus portal vein walls revisited with histologic correlation. J Ultrasound Med 16:807–810

Wanless IR, Wong F, Blendis LM et al (1994) Hepatic and portal thrombosis in cirrhosis: possible role in development of parenchymal extinction and portal hypertension. Hepatology 20:105A

Weskott HP (1997) Amplitude Doppler ultrasound: slow flow detection level tested with a flow phantom. Radiology 201:125–130

6 Doppler Imaging of Abdominal Veins

R. Kubale and H.-P. Weskott

CONTENTS

R. Kubale, MD
Institut für Radiologie, Sonographie und Nuklearmedizin, Ringstrasse 60–62, 66953 Pirmasens, Germany
H.-P. Weskott, MD
Innere Medizin 2, Krankenhaus Siloah, Roesebeckstrasse 2, Hannover, Germany

6.1 Introduction

The venous system is subject to numerous disorders that involve the vessels either primarily or secondarily. Most important are thromboses, which may originate in the abdominal veins or ascend from deep venous thrombosis in the lower extremity. The clinical symptoms depend on the location and size of the vessel and the speed of the process. Slowly progessive occlusions with good collateralization or immediate recanalization may remain asymptomatic. Acute thrombosis of the pelvic veins, IVC, and the porto-spleno-mesenteric axis could be life-threatening.

6.2 Normal Anatomy

6.2.1 Inferior Vena Cava, Renal and Gonadal Veins

The IVC is formed at the level of the fourth vertebra, normally running along the right side of the aorta. Its diameter ranges from 2 to 3 cm depending upon abdominal and thoracic pressure due to respiratory and cardiac activity. Its tributaries are the iliac veins, the renal veins, the right ovarian/testicular vein, and at least 3 to 6 liver veins (Fig. 2.11). The left gonadal vein empties directly into the left RV. Several connection channels and collaterals can develop to the vertebral plexus and to the ascending lumbar veins.

Using B-mode US, the upper portion of the IVC is best seen on a longitudinal view, using the liver as an acoustic window, or on a lateral view. The lumen should appear echo-free with a completely homogenous filling of color in apnea using CDDS (Fig. 6.1a). The renal veins can be observed laterally on intercostal or ventrally on transverse scans for at least 8–10 cm (Fig. 6.1b,c), showing a homogeneous color pattern. The ovarian or testicular veins can be identified on a lateral view. Normally, the flow

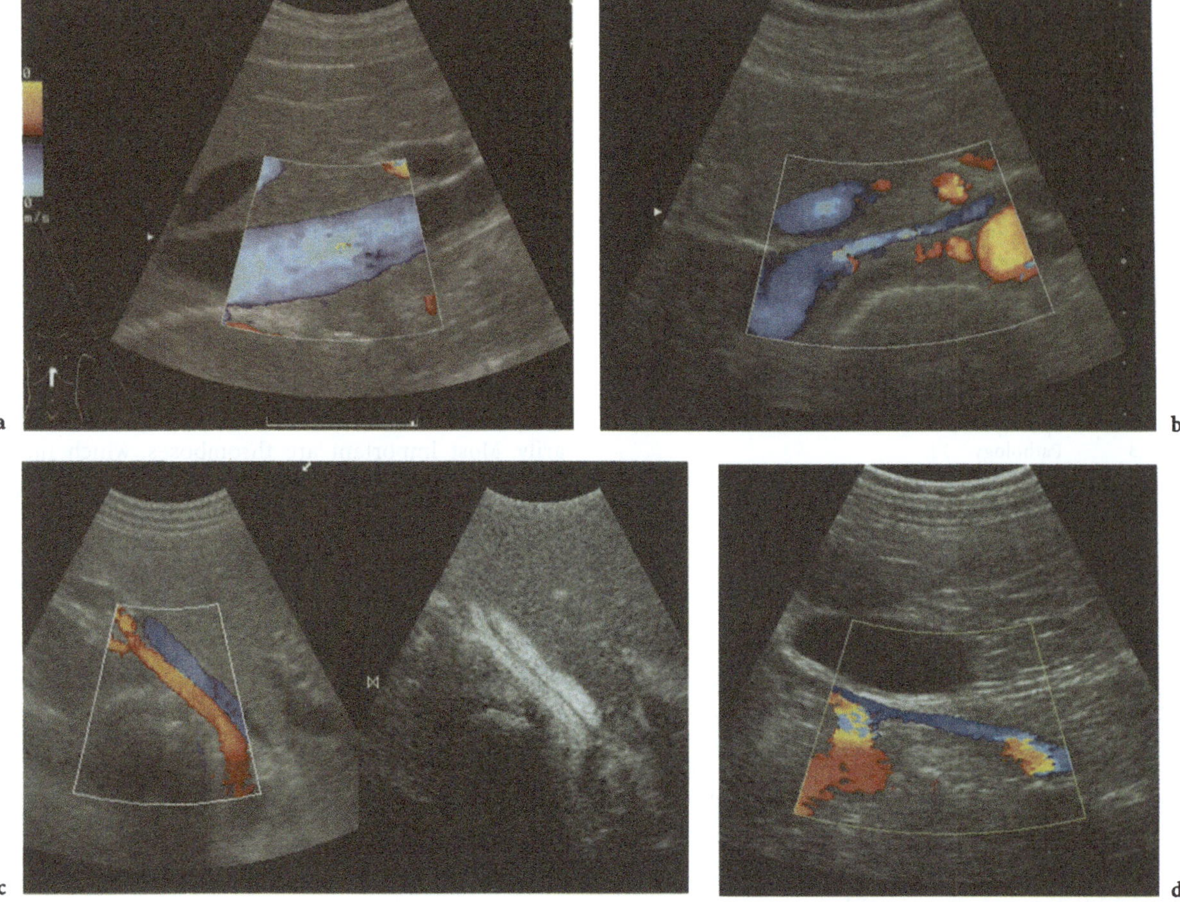

Fig. 6.1a–d. Normal inferior vena cava, renal and gonadal veins (CDDS). **a** Longitudinal view of the IVC with complete, homogenous filling of the lumen. **b** Transverse scan with normal left RV. **c** Right RV from a ventrolateral view. With CDDS, the renal artery is coded in *red*, the RV in *blue* (*left half* of the picture). B-flow is helpful for better delineation of the vessel border (*right half* of the picture). **d** Left testicular vein (view from lateral) with psoas muscle (*), distended ureter (>), and aorta with left renal artery showing an aliasing due to low PRF (with permission from Kubale and Stiegler 2002)

direction is upwards to the IVC or the RV (Fig. 6.1d). Reverse flow can be depicted during high abdominal pressure or in patients with varicoceles. The examination technique and normal anatomy are discussed thoroughly in Chapter 2.

6.2.2
Splenoportal Axis and Mesenteric Veins

The POV is formed by the union of the SPV and the SMV at the level of the 12th thoracic or 1st to 2nd lumbar vertebra (Fig. 2.11). The normal POV has a length of 5–6.5 cm. The diameter has been reported to be 9–11 mm as measured by US (Rahim and Adam 1985). It runs from its initial position behind the head of the pancreas at the inferior margin of the hepatoduodenal ligament to the porta hepatis. It lies between or behind the hepatic artery and the bile duct. At the porta hepatis, it divides into segmental branches. Within the sinusoids, blood from the terminal portal venule merges with hepatic arterial blood. Blood flows from the sinusoids into the HVs, which drain into the IVC.

The most important tributaries of the POV are the SPV, the SMV, the IMV and the gastric veins (Fig. 2.11).

The SPV runs from the hilum of the spleen, dorsal to the pancreas, emptying into the confluence together with the SMV. The SMV ascends on the right side of the corresponding artery in front of the pars horizontalis of the duodenum, collecting branches from both sides. The IMV is a continuation of the superior hemorrhoidal vein; it receives the drainage from the left colon through the left colic and sigmoid veins (Fig. 2.11). It lies in the retroperitoneal space to the left of the spine and empties after passing behind the pancreas into either the SPV or the SMV.

On CDDS, the POV is seen either from a lateral or from a ventral view (Fig. 6.2a,b). The flow profile is variable, showing an eccentric jet or a helical flow pattern (Fig. 6.3). If the peak velocity is not located in the center of the portal vein, higher settings of the PRF and/or wall filter may mimic a partial thrombosis.

The splenic vein is best seen on lateral or ventral views (Fig. 6.2c,d). In thin patients, forced compression with the US transducer could mimic an occlusion. The SMV is best seen on longitudinal and transverse scans from a ventral approach, showing several tributaries from the jejunal and ileal veins (Fig. 6.4). The inferior mesenteric vein can only rarely be seen sonographically due to its small diameter (<0.6 cm) and its variable course. Its cranial portion could be depicted with CDDS emptying into the SPV or crossing the SMA anteriorly before draining into the SMV in more than 75% of cases.

6.3 Pathology

6.3.1 Inferior Vena Cava, Renal and Gonadal Veins

6.3.1.1 Variants and Malformations

The IVC originates from three paired embryologic veins: The paired posterior and anterior cardinal veins collect blood from the embryologic body with its primitive kidneys and unite to form a common trunk. The subcardinal veins develop medially as a new system. As the mesonephroi enlarges, they become larger and develop intersubcardinal anastomoses. Last to appear are the supracardinal veins which anastomose with the subcardinal veins. After further development, the posterior cardinal veins are obliterated and the left supracardinal vein disappears

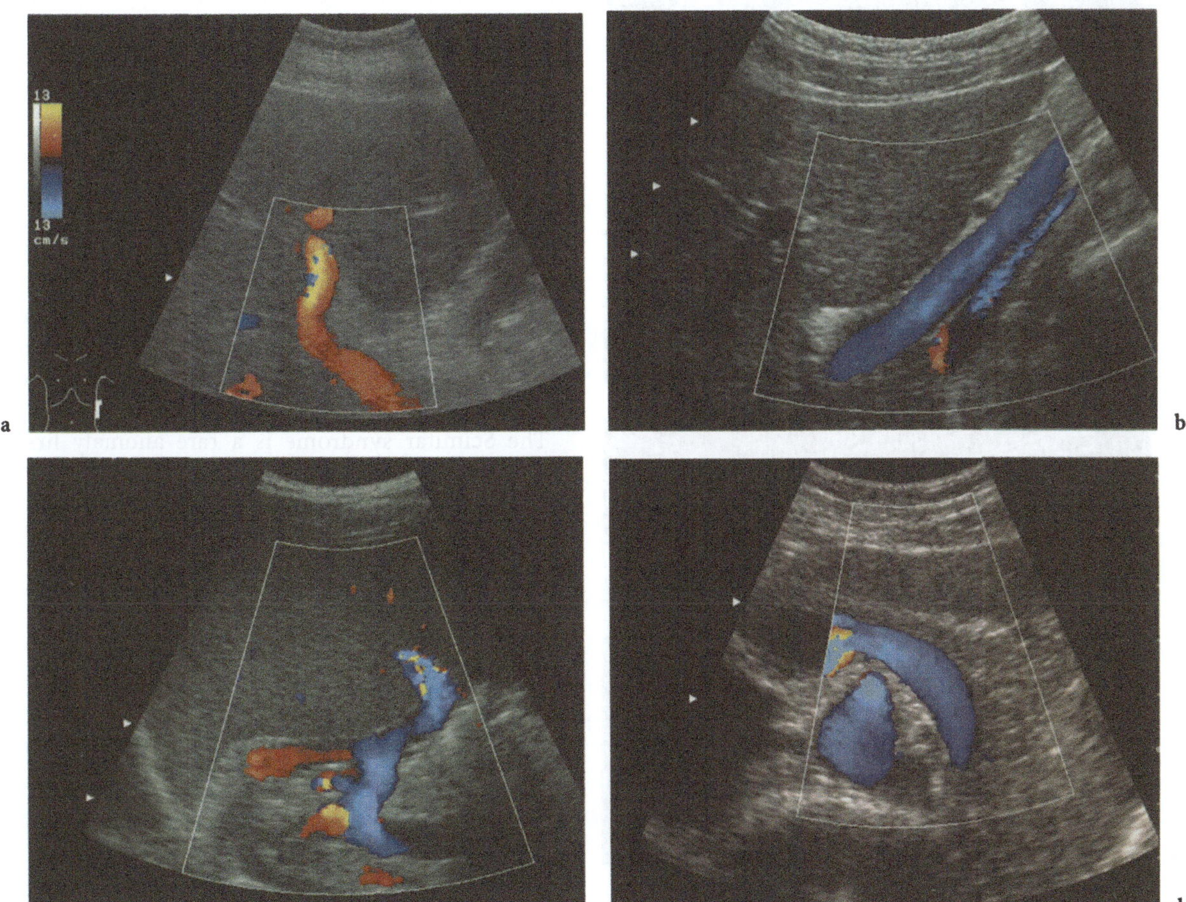

Fig. 6.2a–d. Normal portal and splenic veins in a healthy subject. **a** Longitudinal scan from intercostal lateral (*red* means flow towards the transducer). **b** Ventral view with PV, IVC (*), and hepatic artery. **c** Longitudinal view from left lateral with hilum of the spleen and SPV. **d** Transverse scan with aorta, origin of the mesenteric artery, and SPV

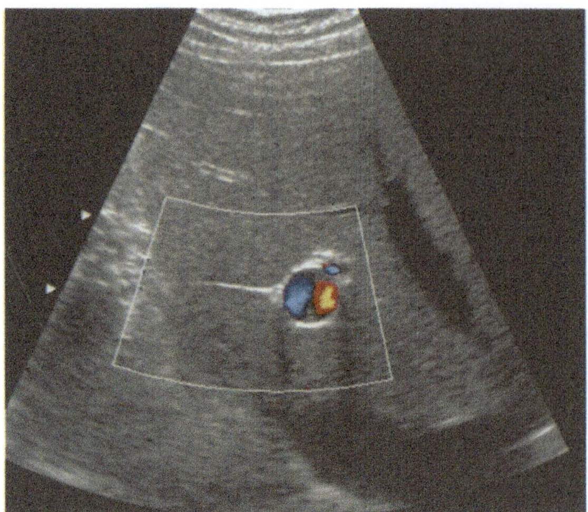

Fig. 6.3. Spiral flow pattern in the POV. At a 90° angle of insonation, flow is indicated in *blue* and *red* because of a helical flow pattern

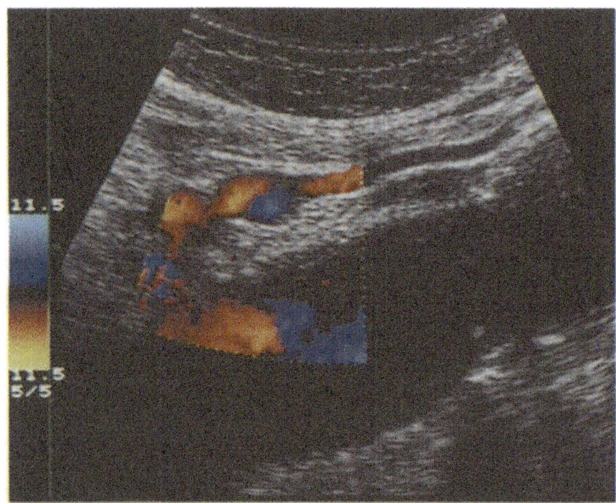

a

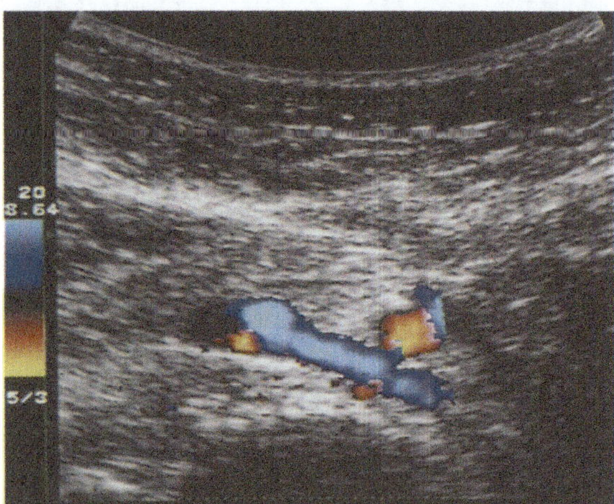

b

Fig. 6.4a, b. Normal SMV with tributaries (CDDS). **a** Longitudinal scan with SMV. Changes in caliber and turbulence due to inflow effect from the jejunal tributaries. **b** Transverse scan with jejunal branches crossing dorsally to the SMA (with permission from Kubale and Stiegler 2002)

'due to degeneration'. The right supracardinal vein remains and finally becomes the postrenal segment of the IVC. The other segments arise from the right subcardinal vein and from anastomoses between the supracardinal and subcardinal veins.

Due to this complex embryology, numerous anatomic variations and malformations can be seen: The variety of findings range from partial or complete aplasia to duplication of the IVC and variations of renal and ovarian or testicular veins (Table 6.1). Most of these anomalies are asymptomatic, but their detection can be of great importance for surgical and radiological vascular interventions, e.g., diagnosis of a left retroaortal renal vein (Fig. 6.5).

The persistent right posterior cardinal vein (type A) is known as a retrocaval or circumcaval ureter. The ureter lies in its proximal portion dorsal to the IVC, showing a medial displacement on intravenous pyelography. In CDDS, this anomaly is seen only in cases of obstruction with compression of the ureter by the IVC. A persistent right supracardinal vein results in a normal right-sided IVC (type B). The persistence of the right and left supracardinal vein leads to the so-called double postrenal IVC (0.2–3.0%). The persistent left supracardinal vein alone results in a left-sided IVC (type C: 0.2–0.5%).

Other anomalies are characterized by the absence of the prerenal segment of the IVC with azygos or hemiazygos continuation. These anomalies can be associated with complex collateral vessels (Fig. 6.6). Patients with partial or complete aplasia of the IVC should be examined for associated cardiac disease and further malformations. Vice versa, especially in young patients with recurrent DVT, anomalies of the IVC should be considered (Gayer et al. 2003).

The Scimitar syndrome is a rare anomaly first described in 1836 which is characterized by an

Table 6.1. Congenital anomalies of the IVC and renal veins

I Post-renal segment of the IVC
Type A: Persistence of the right posterior cardinal vein (retro- or circumcaval ureter)
Type B: Persistence of the right supracardinal vein (normal position of IVC)
Type C: Persistence of the left supracardinal vein (left-sided position of IVC)
Type BC: Persistence of the right and left supracardinal veins (duplication of IVC)
II Renal segment of IVC
Persistence of renal venous ring leading to circumaortic venous ring
III Prerenal segment of the IVC
Absence of the hepatic segment with drainage by azygos or hemiazygos system

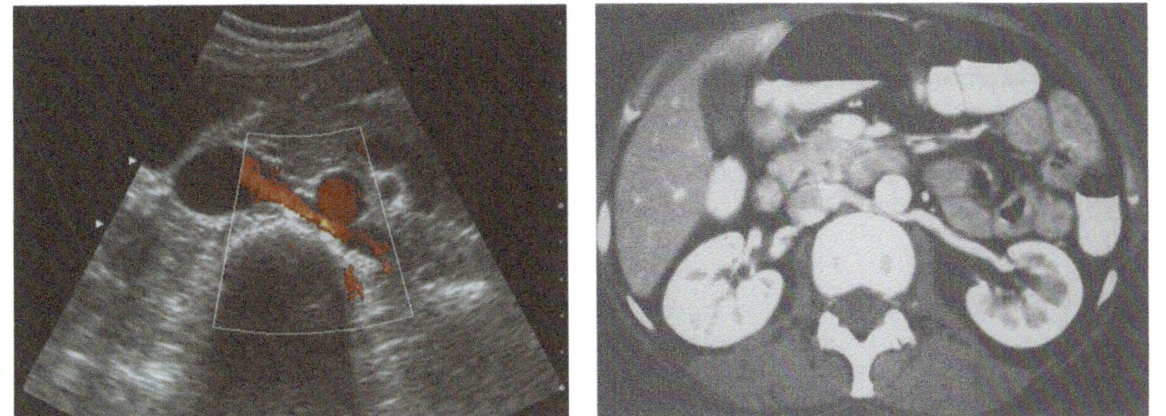

Fig. 6.5a, b. Retroaortal RV (CDDS and CT). Retroaortal renal vein on CDDS (a) and CT (b) crossing behind the aorta

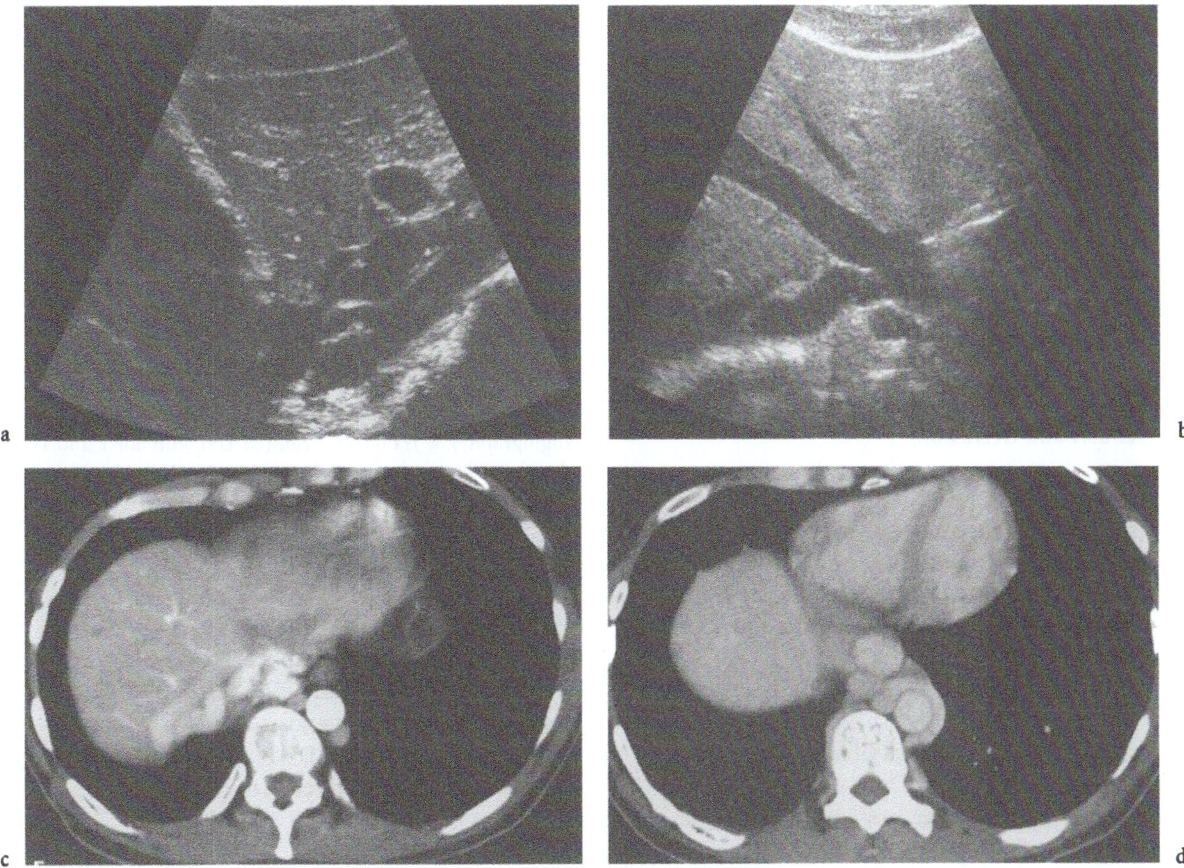

Fig. 6.6a–d. Complex anomaly of the IVC with hemiazygos continuation and multiple cavoportal and portocaval shunts. a Longitudinal scan with interruption of the IVC and hemiazygos continuation (B-mode). b Subcostal view with multiple collaterals and middle hepatic vein showing a wide caliber. c Corresponding image to b on CT with multiple collaterals best shown immediately after administration of contrast. d CT scan taken more cranially with multiple collaterals via hemiazygos system and atypical veins curling around the aorta

anomalous pulmonary vein, passing downwards through the diaphragm and emptying into the IVC. Complex malformations have additional connections to the left atrium (Tortoriello et al. 2002).

Chest X-ray shows a crescent-shaped paracardiac vessel running down to the diaphragm. CDDS shows an atypical vein connected to the IVC.

6.3.1.2
Arteriovenous Fistulae

Arteriovenous fistulae are rare. They are mostly due to aneurysm erosion, iatrogenic injury, blunt trauma, or tumor erosion (Davidovic et al. 2002; Szucs-Farcas et al. 2002). The interval from presumed occurrence to symptoms ranges from 6 h to 2 years [9]. The presence of an abdominal bruit is the most reliable clinical sign. In a study of 16 patients, congestive heart failure was present in 18.7%. Lower extremity edema, scrotal edema, and renal insufficiency are further clinical symptoms. Surgical repair is mandatory to prevent serious complications. Recently, endovascular placement of covered stents has been reported as an alternative treatment (Duxbury et al. 2002; Sprouse and Hamilton (2002).

Signs of an AV fistula in CDDS can include a dilatation of the vein, an increase of flow velocity especially with a high diastolic flow component due to shunting and low resistance, and a jet in the fistula (Fig. 6.7).

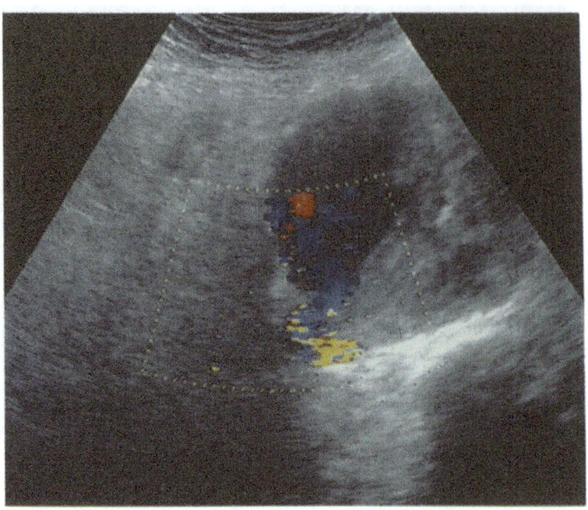

a

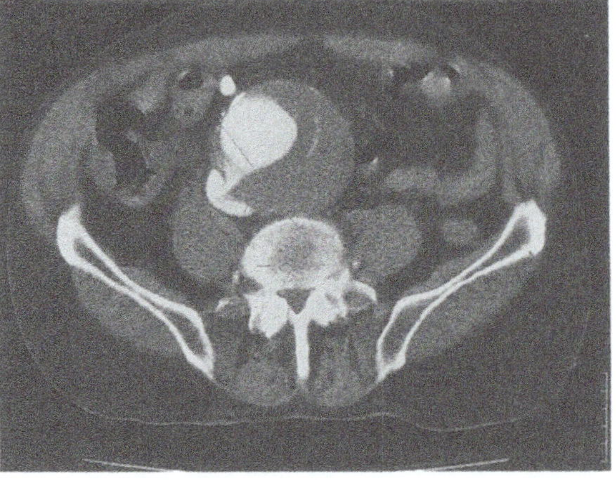

b

Fig. 6.7a, b. AV fistula between aorta and IVC (CDDS and angiography). **a** Transverse scan (CDDS) with aorta and IVC showing a high velocity jet between an aortic aneurysm and the IVC. **b** CT with contrast (arterial phase) showing early enhancement in the IVC immediately after appearance of contrast in the lumen of the aorta (with permission from Dr. Güttner, Bremen; Kubale and Stiegler 2002)

6.3.1.3
Stenosis and Occlusion

Stenoses and occlusions of the IVC and their tributaries can be caused extrinsically by compression or intrinsically by thrombosis or intraluminal tumors (Ferris and Shah 1998). The clinical features are dependent upon the extent, localization, and acuteness of the obstruction.

6.3.1.3.1
Extrinsic Compression and Obstruction of the IVC

Extrinsic compression can occur along the entire perimeter of the vessel at any level due to lymph nodes, renal and adrenal neoplasms, hepatic and pancreatic tumors, aneurysms, retroperitoneal fibrosis, massive ascites, or pregnancy. Other causes include indentations by the celiac ganglion and the crus of the diaphragm.

Sonographically, lymph nodes and neoplasms are easily appreciated on B-mode US, if the examination quality is good to excellent. The persistence of a hyperechoic fat layer adjacent to the IVC or RV is helpful in distinguishing between simple compression and tumor invasion of the vessel wall. Smoothly marginated, tubular stenosis suggests a fibrotic or inflammatory process. CDDS is helpful in identifying the residual lumen and relevant collaterals.

6.3.1.3.2
Intrinsic Obstruction of IVC, Renal and Ovarian Veins

Intrinsic obstructions may be caused by thrombosis and tumors or by tumor thrombi in the IVC, renal or gonadal veins.

Infrarenal occlusions of the IVC are mostly caused by phlebothrombosis of the iliofemoral venous system extending upwards (Fig. 6.8). Thrombus formation is also seen in stasis due to long-standing extrinsic pressure.

The most common cause of midcaval occlusion is renal cell carcinoma with tumor thrombosis of the RV and the IVC (Fig. 6.9). Due to the detection of renal cell carcinoma by US at an early stage, vascular involvement is rare nowadays.

Upper IVC occlusions are rare. Usually, there are abnormalities in the liver causing compression or invasion of the IVC which dispose to thrombus formation. Other reasons are HV occlusions that extend into the IVC and RV tumor thrombi ascending into the upper portion of the IVC.

On CDDS, a thrombus is characterized by a lack of flow. Fresh thrombus material appears voluminous with a pattern of low or mixed echogenicity (Fig. 6.8a). In later stages, the thrombus retracts. Calcifications can be seen. The extent of thrombotic vessels and their tributaries can be analyzed (Fig. 6.8b). In tumor thrombosis, arterial flow in the thrombus can be detected by CDDS, showing vascularization especially in renal cell carcinoma (Fig. 6.9).

Primary RV thrombosis tends to develop in nephrotic syndrome, glomerulonephritis, collagen diseases, amyloidosis, and dehydration. Evaluation should be performed whenever flank pain and renal enlargement are observed.

While acute thrombi are of low echogenicity, older thromboses and tumor thrombi often can already be depicted in a gray-scale image (Fig. 6.10). Acute and partial thromboses can only be identified on CDDS by lack of flow in the vessel lumen.

Ovarian vein thrombosis is a rare but serious postpartum complication. It develops mostly during or shortly after pregnancy, causing nonspecific symptoms usually localized to the lower abdomen. The

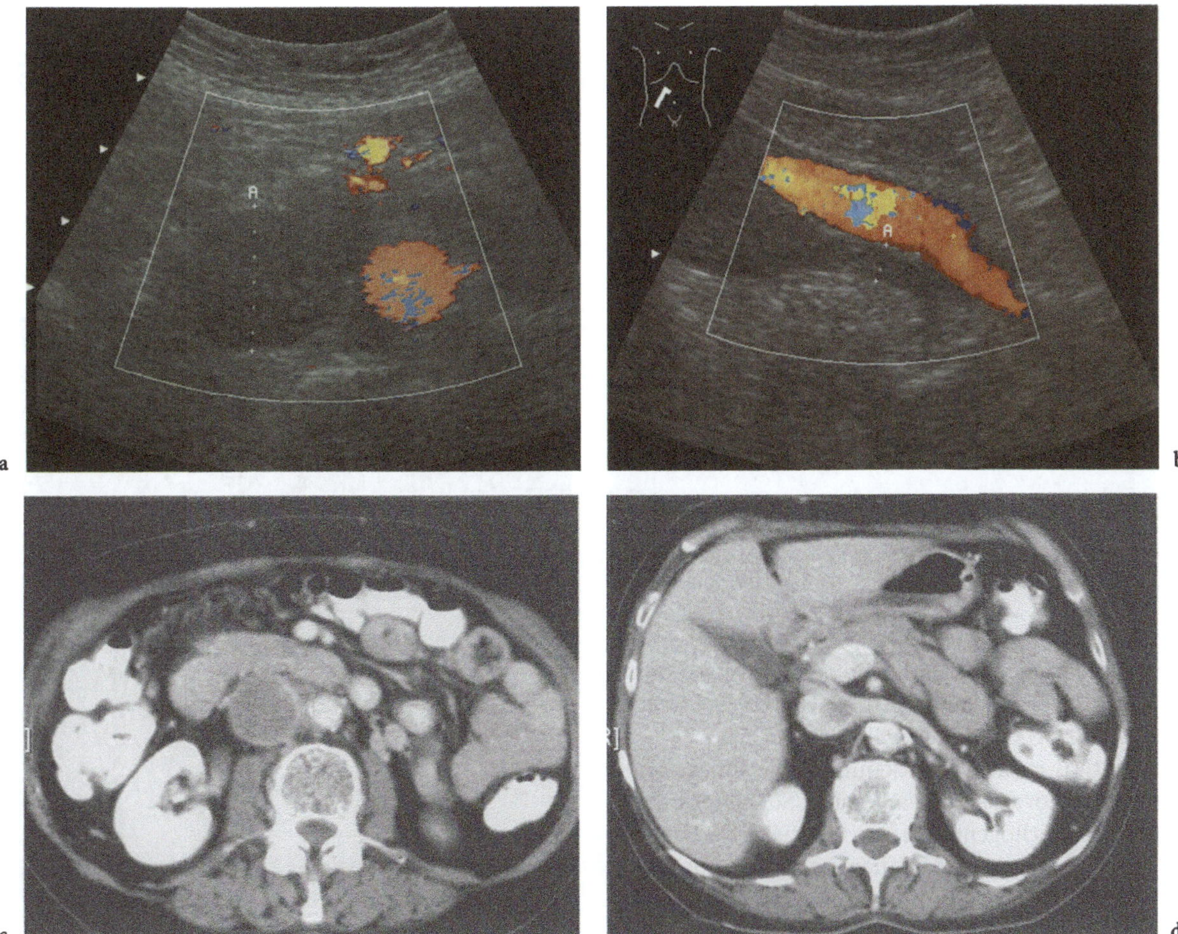

Fig. 6.8a–d. Ascending thrombosis with involvement of the right iliac vein and IVC (CDDS, CT). **a** Transverse scan with thrombus in the IVC (*) and aorta (coded in *red*). **b** Longitudinal scan with old thrombotic material in the iliac vein and fresh, voluminous material in the IVC (CDDS). **c** CT scan corresponding to **a** with complete occlusion of the IVC. Slight enhancement of the vessel wall due to vasa vasorum. **d** Tip of the thrombus at the level of the RV; the RV is patent

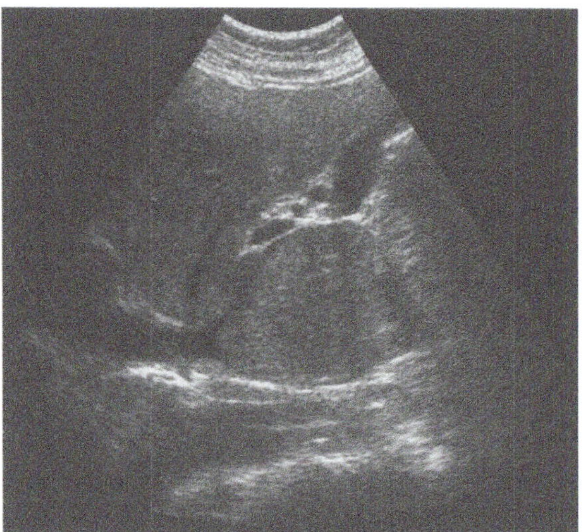

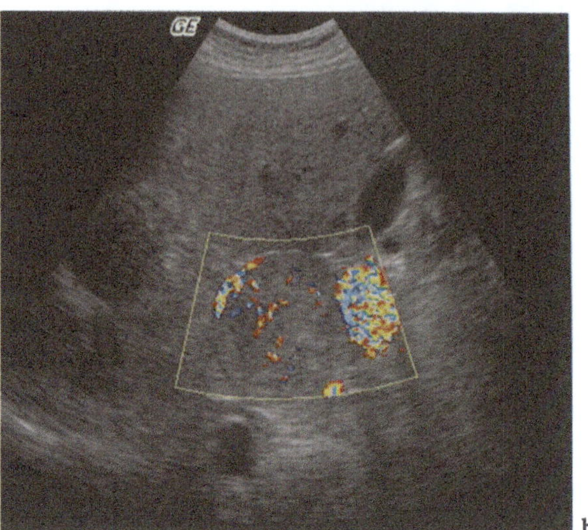

Fig. 6.9a, b. Tumor thrombosis invading the IVC (renal cell carcinoma). **a** Longitudinal B-mode US with tumor thrombus. **b** Transverse scan with aorta and IVC. On CDDS, vessels within the tumor thrombus could be identified due to tumor vascularization

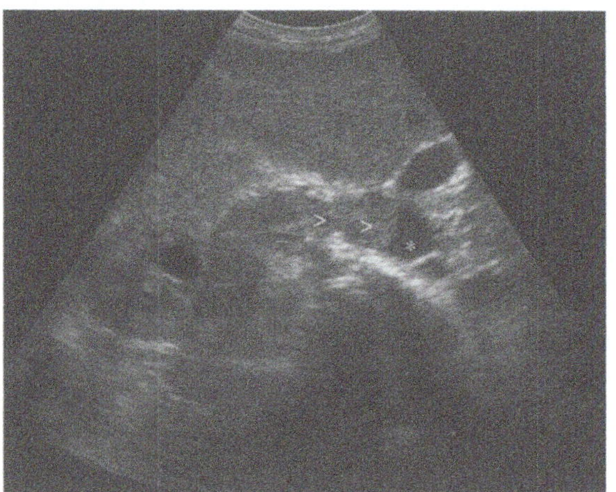

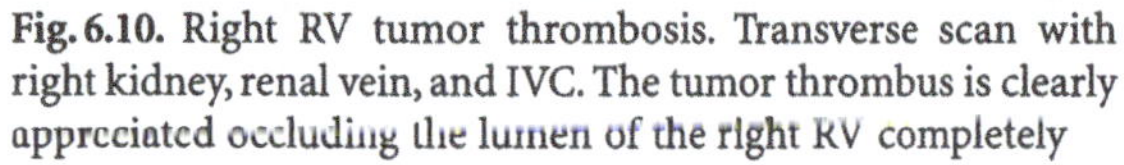

Fig. 6.10. Right RV tumor thrombosis. Transverse scan with right kidney, renal vein, and IVC. The tumor thrombus is clearly appreciated occluding the lumen of the right RV completely

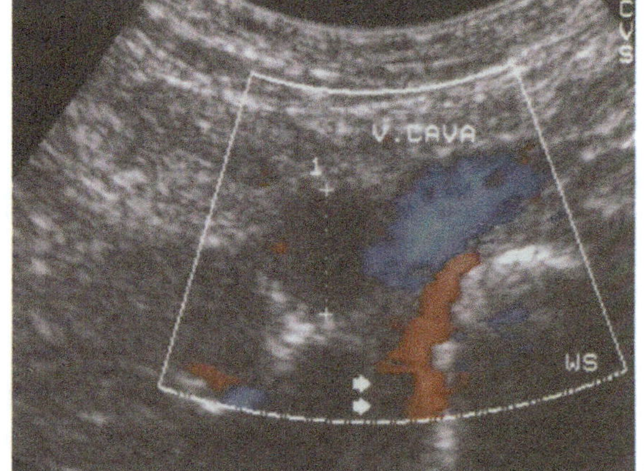

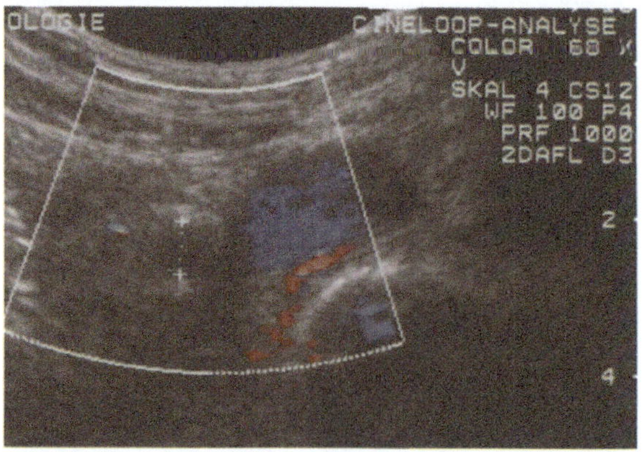

Fig. 6.11a, b. Ovarian vein postpartum thrombosis. **a** Transverse scan from ventral approach with enlarged vessels on the right side (5th day postpartum) with IVC (*blue*) and paravertebral vein (*red*) **b** Follow-up examination 4 weeks later with organized thrombus showing a reduced vessel diameter

right ovarian vein is predominantly involved, mimicking acute appendicitis (Baka et al. 1989; Dessole et al. 2003; Nasser and Spellacy 1968).

With B-mode US, thickening of the adnexa and a distended ovarian vein are found. Sometimes thickened, low-echogenic, perivascular tissue can be seen due to an associated inflammatory response. On CDDS, ovarian vein thrombosis could be depicted very early on due to distension of the vessel and lack of flow (Fig. 6.11).

Primary tumors of the IVC, iliac and renal veins are rare. They can occur in every segment of the IVC and iliac veins. Most likely are leiomyoma and leiomyosarcoma, which should be surgically resected. In the early stages, they can be misinterpreted as thrombosis (ARMSTRONG and FRANKLIN 2002). Thorough evaluation of iliocaval thrombosis by CDDS or CT with bolus contrast administration is recommended before endovascular management.

6.3.1.4
Collateral Circulation and Varices

A slowly progressive occlusion of the IVC evokes the development of collaterals, as first recognized by Morgagni in 1769 (MORGAGNI 1769). Their categorization is based on the level of obstruction (MORGAGNI 1769; PLEASANTS 1911).

In *infrarenal IVC obstructions,* there are four main pathways: The central channels comprise the ascending lumbar veins, including the internal and external venous plexus, the azygos-hemiazygos system, and the IVC above the obstructed segment. The intermediate channels include the ureteric veins, the left renal-azygos system, and the gonadal veins. The distended ovarian-parametrial veins could be mistaken on B-mode US and CT as lymph nodes. CDDS can differentiate clearly by depicting the flow and flow direction. Portal pathways, filled via the superior hemorrhoidal anastomoses to the plexus of the internal iliac venous system, and superficial channels are rare alternative routes.

In *middle IVC obstruction,* the collateral routes are similar to those in infrarenal obstruction: The central routes and the portal system gain more importance. Because the RVs cannot drain directly into the obstructed IVC, there is a spill-over to the azygos and hemiazygos system (intermediate system). Retrograde filling of the ureteric and gonadal veins, particularly on the left side, can drain to the iliac and sacral plexus. Adrenal-phrenic vein anastomoses are rarely seen using CDDS and CT.

Upper IVC obstruction is rare. Drainage is possible via the central and superficial systems and, to a lesser extent, via the intermediate system. In patients with additional occlusion of the HVs, a hepatofugal flow in the portal system could be observed.

6.3.2
Splenoportal Axis and Mesenteric Veins

6.3.2.1
Variants and Malformations

Anomalies of the POV system are rare but clinically important because they may cause hemorrhage, liver dysfunction, or complicate hepatobiliary surgery due to unexpected branching of the vessels.

The veins of the portal system develop out of paired embryonic veins (SAITO et al. 1999). The vitelline veins drain the yolk sac. In the 5th week, cross-anastomoses develop between the vitelline veins in a figure-of-eight configuration. They occur both ventrally and dorsally. After obliteration of the left limb of the cranial ring, the right limb of the caudal limb, and the ventral anastomosis, the S-shaped portal vein is formed lying behind the duodenum (Fig. 6.12).

The right umbilical veins develop from the chorionic villi and supply the embryo with oxygen-rich blood from the mother. The right umbilical vein is obliterated early in embryonal life, while the left one communicates with the right vitelline vein by the ductus venosus. Both are obliterated after birth, remaining in postnatal life as the ligamentum teres and ligamentum venosum.

The parabiliary venous system develops from pancreaticoduodenal and pyloroduodenal veins along the common bile duct and the hepatic artery. They invade the liver in a later stage, when the intrahepatic distribution of the portal vein branches are already established.

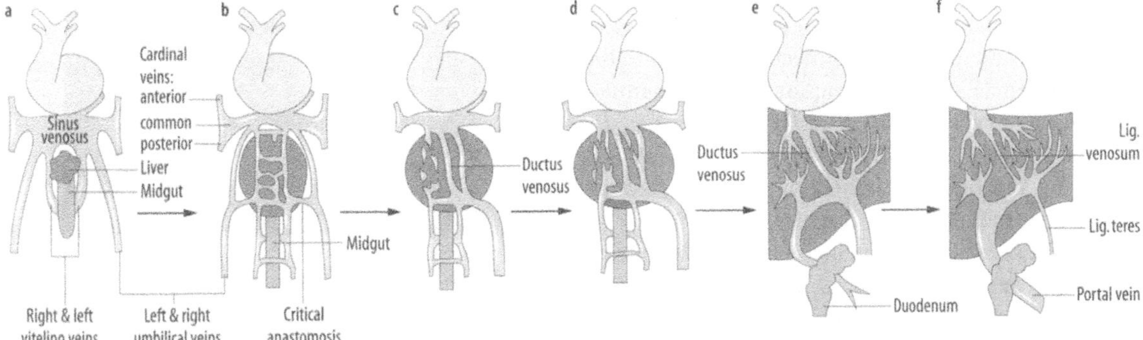

Fig. 6.12. Development of the portal system (according to SAITO et al 1997)

Due to this complex embryological development, numerous anomalies can be seen. They can be classified according to their embryological origin.

6.3.2.1.1
Anomalies Derived from the Vitteline Veins

Atresia may be partial or complete and can involve extra- and intrahepatic branches. In partial atresia, a fibrous string runs from the confluence to the intrahilar portion. In 15% of patients, splenomesenteric vessels are involved. From the patent segment of the portal vein, branches may arise, curling around the stenoses or occlusion, and communicate with the intrahepatic branches of the portal vein.

The congenital portocaval shunt (c-pcs) is a rare disease frequently leading to encephalopathy and laboratory changes. It was described first by Abernethy in 1791, and 21 cases have been published up to now (Ishii et al. 2000; Kerleau et al. 1995; Kubale 1984; Kubale et al. 1999; Raskin et al. 1984). Liver tumors are reported in cases with complete deprivation of portal venous blood (Kubale 1984; Vonnahme et al. 1984; Yonemitsu et al. 2000; Yoshidome and Edwards 1999). Most of them were adenomas and focal nodular hyperplasia. The enterohepatic circulation is disrupted, and the portal venous blood shunts systemically. Park et al. 1990) classified c-pcs into four different types:

- I A single large vessel connects the tributaries of the POV with the IVC. No intrahepatic branches are seen (Fig. 6.13).
- II A peripheral shunt is seen with single or multiple connections between the POV and the HVs.
- III An aneurysm connects the peripheral portal branches with the HVs.
- IV Multiple communications between the peripheral and portal branches and HVs are seen in both lobes.

In type I, B-mode US and CDDS show a mismatch of the diameter of the IVC at the same level proximally and distally of the shunt, a missing main stem of the POV, and ideally the connection channel to the systemic vein (Fig. 6.13). Depiction of those channels is quite easy by a systematic approach. Intrahepatic shunts (types II and III) can be depicted only in CDDS by showing the connection and the effect on blood flow and blood flow direction (Fig. 6.14).

A preduodenal POV is an incidental finding during surgery or autopsy. It is a developmental variant with persistent ventral anastomoses and obliteration of the dorsal anastomoses. It is important in the planning of liver transplantation.

If the vein remains doubled, one trunk is the continuation of the SPV, the other of the SMV. Rarely, the POV divides after union again into 2 to 4 branches. Accessory POVs are small vessels entering the liver. They can be divided into cystic, omental, phrenic, and paraumbilical groups branching into capillaries similar to the main trunk.

6.3.2.1.2
Anomalies Derived from the Umbilical Vein

Within minutes after birth, the pressure in the umbilical vein falls, resulting first in an incomplete functional closure. Complete occlusion with oblitera-

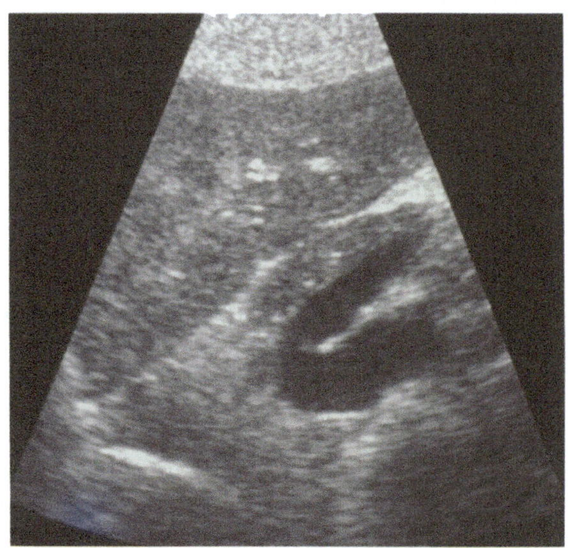

a

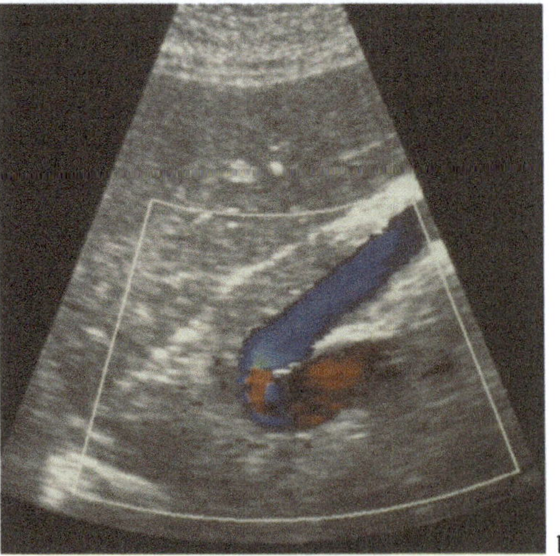

b

Fig. 6.13a, b. Congenital extrahepatic portocaval shunt. Longitudinal scan from ventrolateral approach with the mesenteric vein joining the IVC. The anastomosis is best seen on the B-mode image (**a**). Turbulence and flow reversal in the IVC (**b**) (with permission from Kubale and Stiegler 2002)

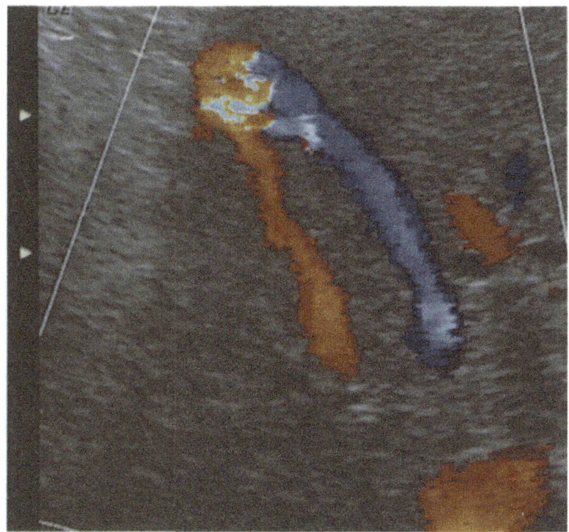

Fig. 6.14. Congenital intrahepatic portocaval shunt. Lateral view with intrahepatic connection between portal branch (*red*) and hepatic vein (*blue*)

tion follows between 3 and 21 days after birth. Patent ductus venosus is considered to be of congenital origin or remains patent as a bypass channel because of high vascular resistance due to poor development of the intrahepatic portal system. Originally thought to be rare, the patent ductus venosus is now reported increasingly often (Barsky et al. 1989; Ikeda et al. 1999; Jacob et al. 1999; Kamata et al. 2000).

A patent ductus venosus can be best seen by CDDS as a vascular channel running parallel to the IVC.

6.3.2.1.3
Anomalies Derived from the Parabiliary Venous System

The veins of the parabiliary venous system run along the common bile duct and the hepatic artery, dividing into a network that anastomoses with the cystic vein. Variations include a large vein that drains directly into the left POV. An aberrant gastric vein draining directly into the quadrate lobe results in focal fatty sparing of the quadrate lobe of the liver (Saito et al. 1999; Weskott and Kubale 2002).

6.3.2.2
Aneurysms and Arteriovenous Fistulae

6.3.2.2.1
Venous Aneurysms

Aneurysms of the splenoportal system once considered rare have been reported more frequently since the advent of CT and especially US (Arda et al. 2002; Ascenti et al. 2001; Nangou et al. 2000). Congenital and iatrogenic causes are being discussed. There is also evidence that portal hypertension is an additional factor for aneurysms. Aneurysms can be seen at any age and can occur in the SPV or in the POV just above the confluence or further distally in its branches (Yang et al. 2003).

B-mode US demonstrates a fusiform or saccular cystic lesion that is often mistaken for a hepatic or choledochal cyst or pancreatic pseudocyst depending on its localization. CDDS shows turbulent flow in the lumen (Fig. 6.15). A complete examination should include demonstration of inflow and outflow, possible thrombi within, and the relation of the aneurysm to the biliary tract.

6.3.2.2.2
Arteriovenous Fistulae

AV fistulae can be caused by trauma, by surgery, or spontaneously due to infection. They can lead to an elevation of pressure in the portal venous system. A high flow fistula can cause aneurysmal dilatation of the POV. Flow volumes of more than 2 l/min can cause dyspnea. Angina abdominalis is reported in rare cases due to inflow obstruction of the mesenteric system. Operative or percutaneous interventional treatment with coils was helpful in two of our own cases and is reported as the therapeutic method of choice Denys et al. 1989; Sing et al. 1997).

High flow fistulae can be depicted by CDDS by demonstrating a mosaic-like vibration artifact and a

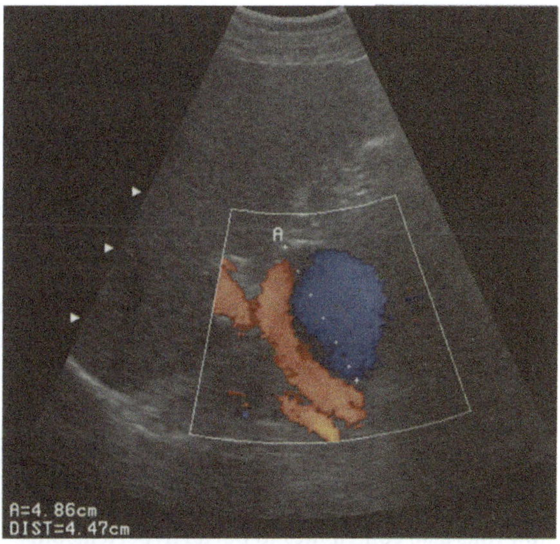

Fig. 6.15. Portal vein aneurysm. Lateral view demonstrating POV filling an aneurysm 4.8 cm in diameter. CDDS demonstrating turbulent flow

flow jet in the fistula best seen with a system setting with high PRF. Secondary effects are an increased inflow with thickened arteries and abundant varices in cases with splenic AV fistulae or a fusiform dilatation of the POV in arterioportal fistulae (Fig. 6.16).

6.3.2.3 Portal Hypertension

6.3.2.3.1 Causes and Pathophysiology

The pressure in the POV is normally 2–3 mmHg higher than in the IVC. It is influenced by inflow from the splanchnic vessels, the intrahepatic resistance, and the outflow through HVs and IVC. Any imbalance of these factors leads to portal hypertension, which is defined by a portal pressure gradient of 12 mmHg.

Portal hypertension can be caused by several diseases leading to an increased vascular resistance (=hepatic resistance), volume flow, or a combination of both factors. Among the hepatic causes for portal hypertension, one can differentiate presinusoidal from sinusoidal and postsinusoidal diseases (Table 6.2).

In industrialized nations, cirrhosis is by far the most common cause of portal hypertension, although schistosomiasis predominates in some tropical and subtropical regions. Vascular resistance depends on a number of factors, of which vessel diameter is the most important (Poiseuille law: $R = 8\eta l/\pi r^4$, where η is the viscosity of blood, l is the length of the blood vessel, and r is the radius of the blood vessel). In the cirrhotic liver, vascular destruction and distortion are caused by architectural disorganization, regenerating nodules, and fibrosis (less than 3% of the liver by weight is normally made up of collagenous material). This results in a decrease in the number and cross-sectional area of venous vessels, due to which flow resistance increases greatly. It is not only the increase in vascular resistance that contributes to portal hypertension. An excessive release of endogenous vasodilators increases blood flow in the POV. In patients with portal hypertension, a hyperdynamic circulation status is often found, characterized by increased cardiac output, expanded blood volume, and decreased systemic vascular resistance with relative hypotension. Although it appears that increased resistance is the primary factor in cirrhosis, increased flow thus also contributes to portal hypertension.

Portal hypertension is usually asymptomatic. Clinical findings and prognosis result from its complications. Over time, portosystemic venous collaterals

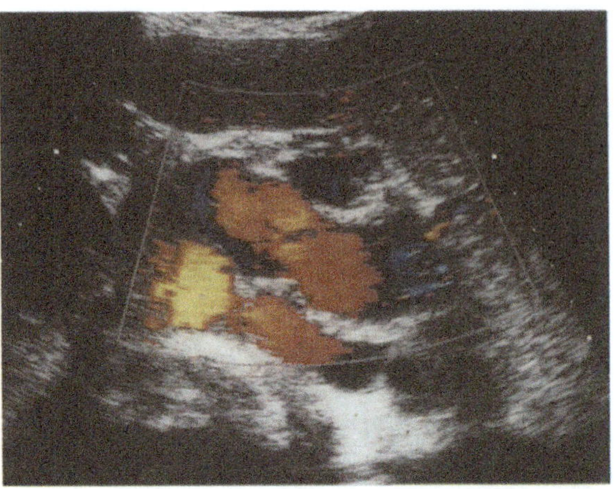

a

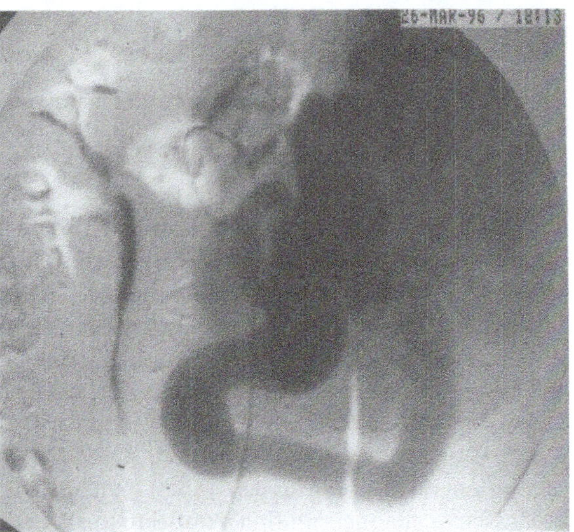

b

Fig. 6.16a, b. Splenic AV fistula. **a** Angiography with catheter in the splenic artery showing a thickened artery and abundant varices. **b** CDDS with varices and enlarged spleen

Table 6.2. Causes of portal hypertension

Prehepatic causes:
Portal or splenic vein thrombosis
Massive splenomegaly from hematologic or tropical disease
Arteriovenous fistula
Presinusoidal causes:
Schistosomiasis
Primary biliary cirrhosis
Congenital hepatic fibrosis
Sarcoidosis
Sinusoidal causes:
Cirrhosis (all etiologies)
Postsinusoidal causes:
Veno-occlusive disease
Posthepatic causes:
Budd-Chiari syndrome
Membranous obstruction of the IVC
Cardiac causes (constrictive pericarditis, restrictive cardiomyopathy)

appear. The most critical collaterals develop in the distal esophagus and gastric fundus. These varices can rupture, causing sudden gastrointestinal hemorrhage.

CDDS provides information about the presence, direction, and characteristics of blood flow (Fig. 6.17). It also helps to evaluate the hemodynamic effects of drugs in the treatment of portal hypertension (PISCAGLIA et al. 1999). Like other abdominal veins, the main POV shows a broad variety of velocities: Due to a helical flow character (Fig. 6.3), its peak velocities are often not found in the center of the vessel. In children and young adults, the peak velocities show a cardiac modulation that decreases with age. Portal hypertension leads to a monophasic band-like flow pattern. The POV diameter increases and flow velocity and volume flow decrease depending on the stage of the disease.

With the development of ascites, mean velocity and volume flow are significantly lower ($p<0.01$) compared with patients without ascites. The rise of postprandial portal flow is significantly lower in patients with portal hypertension and is inversely related to its severity und thus the stage of liver cirrhosis (LIMBERG 1991; LUDWIG et al. 1998). Due to the increased pressure, the cross-sectional areas of the POV, SMV, and SPV change from an oval to a circular shape.

Hepatic arteries and portal venous branches have the same color coding because both show hepatopetal flow direction. A hepatofugal flow can be seen in one or several portal venous branches or the main POV. In the presence of hepatofugal portal flow, the risk of bleeding is significantly reduced. The reason is likely to be the presence of portosystemic collaterals (GAIANI et al 1991). A reverse flow in the main POV or in one of its branches usually indicates a poor prognosis. A diameter of more than 6 mm (WACHSBERG and SIMMONS 1994) and a reverse flow in a dilated left gastric vein (Fig. 6.18) are in most cases associated with esophageal varices (Table 6.3).

Stenoses of the POV can be caused by regenerating nodules or tumors. They can be easily found by CDDS (aliasing) and confirmed by an increase in velocity when using PW Doppler (Fig. 6.19).

Table 6.3. Flow direction and presence of varices in the left gastric vein (MATSUTANI et al. 1993)

Varices	*n*	Hepatopetal flow (%)	Hepatofugal flow (%)
No. of varices	40	88	22
F1 varices	48	31	69
F2 varices	63	3	97
F3 varices	37	0	100

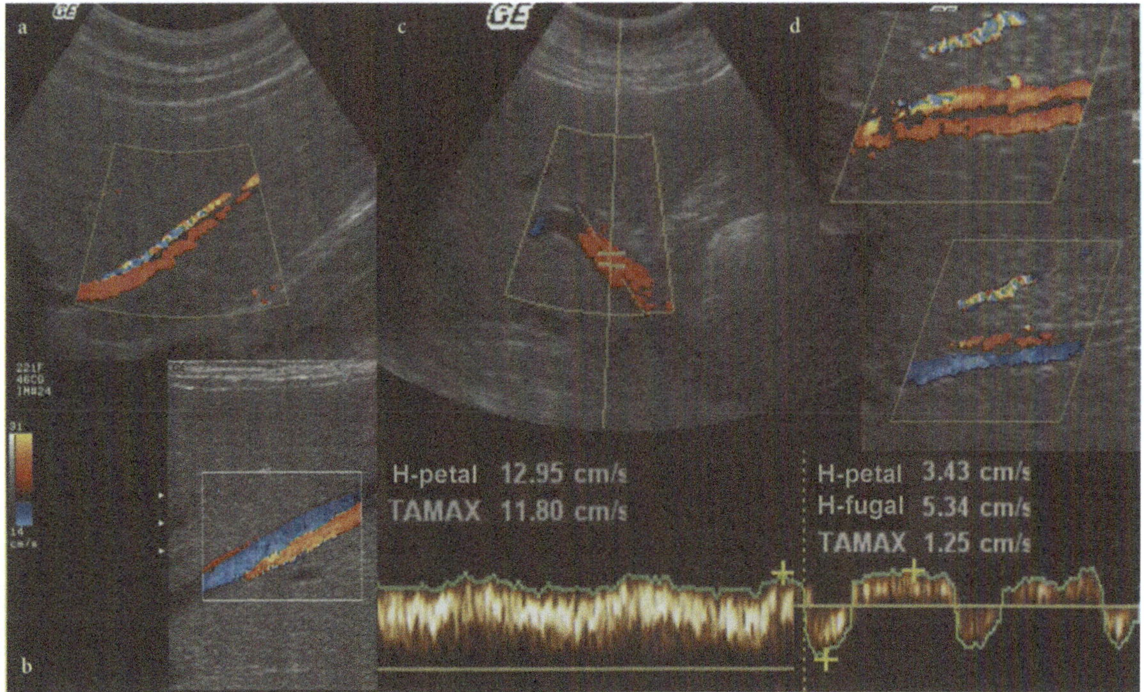

Fig. 6.17a–d. Flow variation in a normal subject (**a**) and in portal hypertension (**b–d**) demonstrated by CDDS. **a** Normal patient with hepatopetal flow in a peripheral POV. The corresponding hepatic artery shows aliasing due to low PRF. **b** Reverse flow of a left intrahepatic portal venous branch (*blue* color coding). **c** Main POV shows continuous hepatopetal flow. **d** A left portal venous branch of the same patient shows pulsatile hepatopetal and hepatofugal flow (to-and-fro flow)

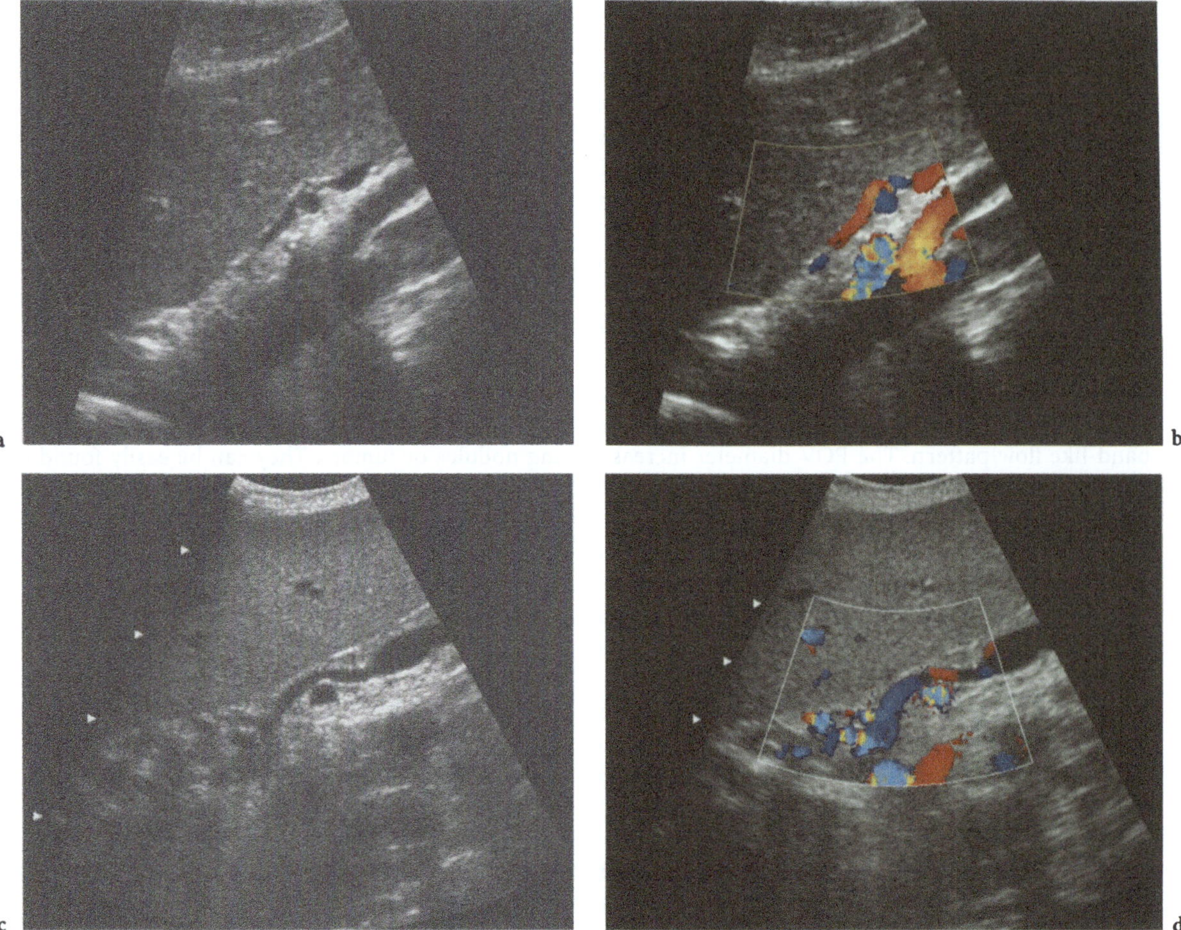

Fig. 6.18a–d. Flow pattern in the coronary vein in normal subjects and patients with portal hypertension. The coronary vein, which runs along the lesser curvature of the stomach, receives blood from distal esophageal veins and drains to the SPV. **a** B-mode demonstrating normal caliber. **b** Orthograde flow demonstrated by CDDS. **c** Dilatation of the coronary vein in a patient with portal hypertension. **d** Reverse flow draining blood to the esophageal veins (with permission from Kubale and Stiegler 2002)

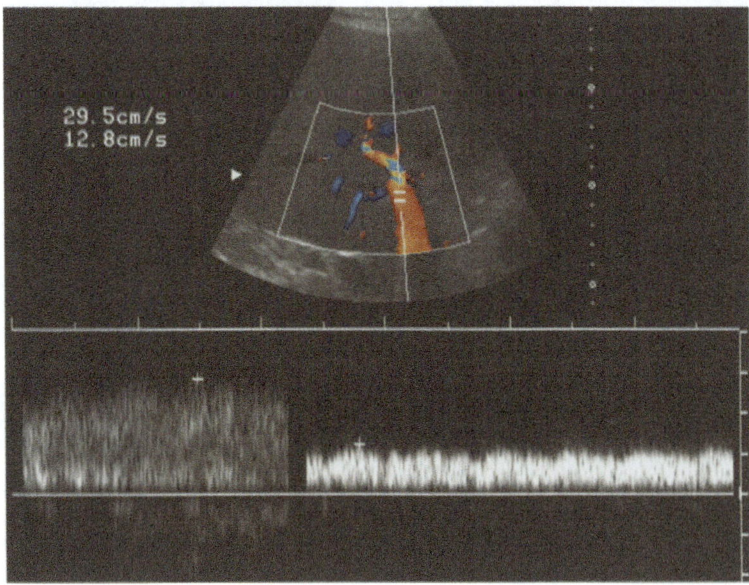

Fig. 6.19. Mild POV stenosis. Increase of flow velocity in the POV indicating mild stenosis of the main POV caused by a liver metastasis. Note: Stenosis indicated by aliasing (ACD, *top*) and by an increase in blood flow velocity (*left side* of the Doppler spectrum) compared with normal flow velocity 2 cm below the stenosis (*right side* of the Doppler spectrum)

Thrombosis of a portal venous branch or even in the main POV can be a complication of a severely reduced portal blood flow or tumor invasion. Hepatocellular carcinoma is the most suggestive cause in patients with liver cirrhosis. Therefore, it is most important to evaluate the underlying disorder that causes a thrombosis of the POV.

Typical sonographic features are initially hypoechoic or heterogeneous thrombotic masses with dilatation of the affected portal segment. As in other veins, CDDS confirms complete thrombosis by complete absence of flow, or partial thrombosis by visualization of residual flow channels. Later the thrombotic material becomes more echogenic and decreases in volume (Fig. 6.20). The thrombosis can resolve, organize, or lead to a worm-like collateralization in the porta hepatis. Although only a few studies have been published, US contrast agents may play a role in differentiating benign from malignant POV thrombosis (Fig. 6.21) (Ricci et al. 2000).

6.3.2.3.2 Effects of Portal Hypertension on Extrahepatic Veins

In advanced portal hypertension, the collateral circulation may carry more than 90% of the blood entering the portal system. The function of collaterals is to decompress the hepatic circulation and divert splanchnic blood flow from the portal to the systemic circulation. The most relevant pathways terminate in the SVC via esophageal, gastric, and azygos veins. Also important are pathways entering the IVC via renal, iliac, and hemorrhoidal veins. Analyzing the anatomical sites and amount of portosystemic collaterals is essential to evaluate the risk of bleeding.

The major sites of collateral formation are reported for:

a Epithelial junction collaterals (gastroesophageal and anorectal)
b Recanalized umbilical vein communicating with the paraumbilical plexus in the abdominal wall
c Retroperitoneal collaterals communicating frequently with the left renal vein
d Spontaneous collaterals at sites of previous abdominal surgery or trauma

The collateral vessels reflect the site of venous occlusion. When the SPV is occluded but the POV remains patent, collaterals will attempt to bypass the occlusion in order to reconstitute the POV. If both the POV and SPV are occluded, drainage from the spleen may be via esophagogastric, splenorenal, or retroperitoneal collateral vessels.

CDDS is very helpful in the search for collateral vessels. Flow in a patent umbilical vein (Fig. 6.22a) can be seen in about one-third of patients with liver cirrhosis, with an increasing number in advanced stages of the disease (56.8% in Child C (Sacerdoti et al. 1995)). Splenorenal, splenoparietal, left gastric, and short gastric veins are effective extrahepatic collaterals. In CDDS, they can be imaged most easily as tortuous veins in the hilum and lower pole of the spleen. In the case of splenorenal shunting, a reverse flow in the splenic vein indicates a change of the intravenous pressure level.

Gallbladder varices (Fig. 6.22b) are not a common finding in portal hypertension but can be seen especially in patients with POV thrombosis (West et al. 1991). Other collaterals can be found adjacent to the pancreas and duodenum.

a 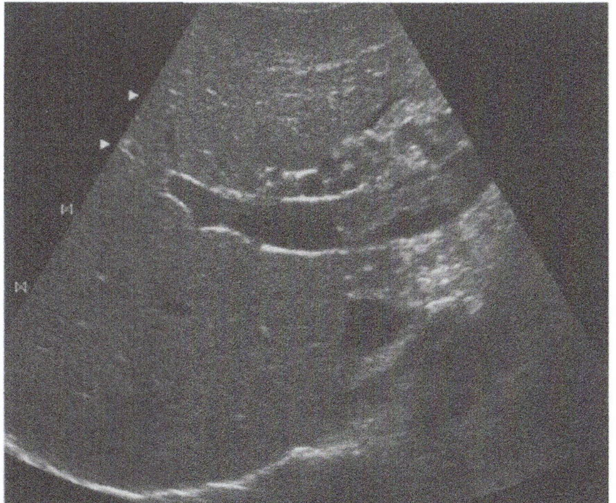

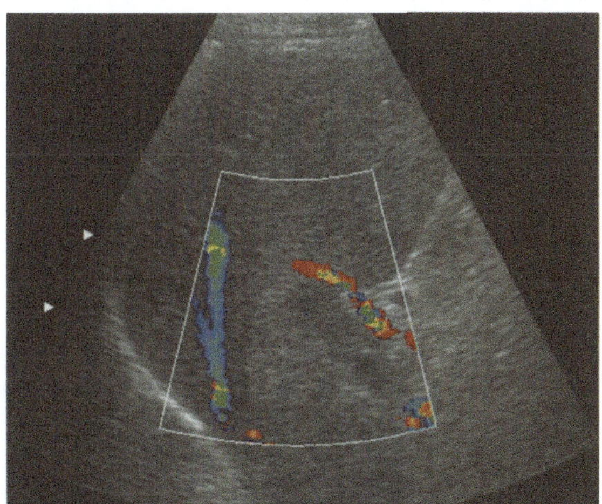 b

Fig. 6.20a, b. POV thrombosis. **a** B-mode image of a POV thrombus in a patient with pancreatitis. **b** CDDS demonstrating occlusion of the main POV (below hepatic artery encoded in *red*) due to hepatocellular carcinoma

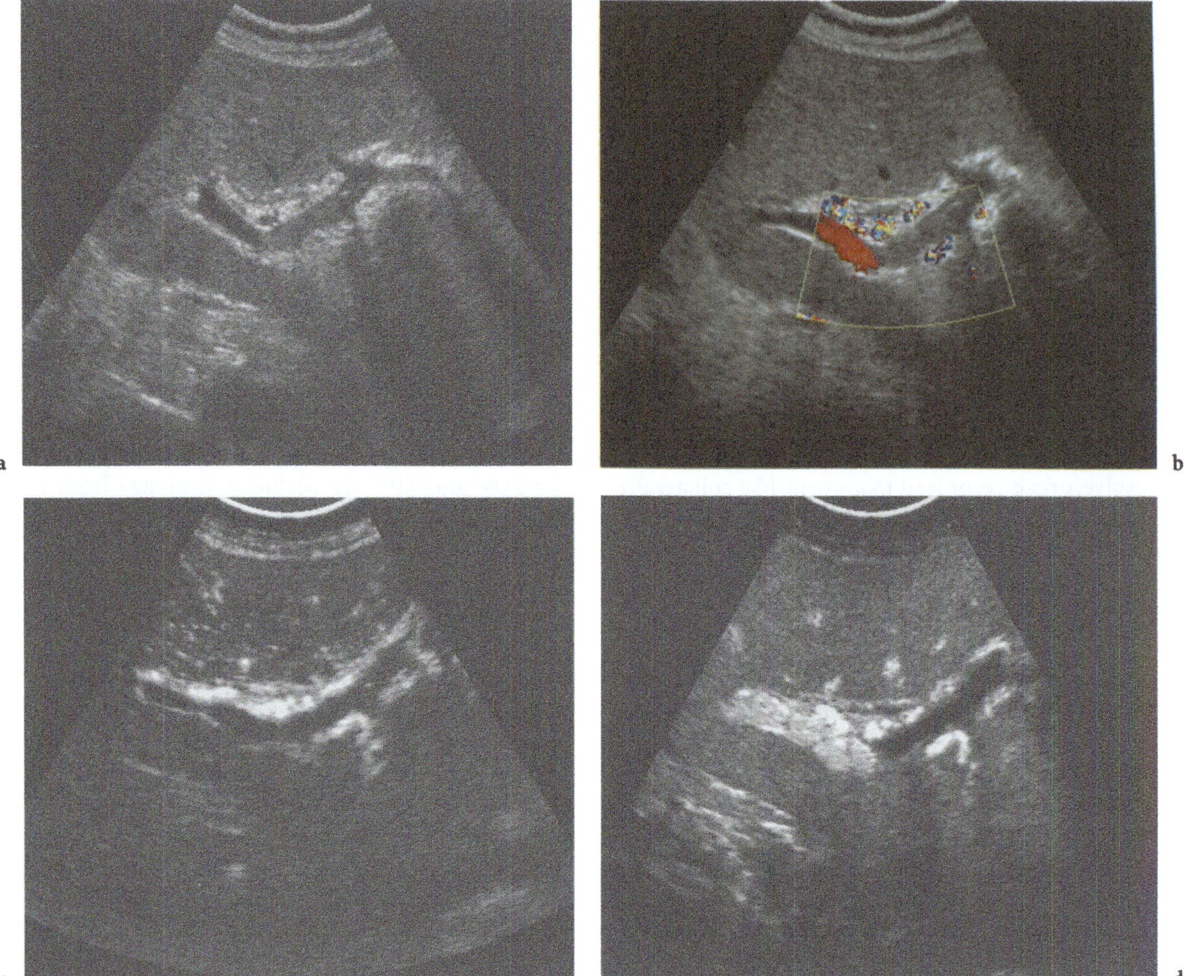

Fig. 6.21a–d. Value of US contrast media administration in POV thrombosis. Thrombosis of the left POV in B-mode (**a**) and CDDS (**b**). Note echogenic material within left POV branch and lack of color flow. After administration of an US contrast agent (Sonovue, Bracco), no enhancement of the POV during the arterial phase (**c**) is seen. At 50 s after administration of contrast material (bolus application), only the right POV branch enhances. The left branch shows no enhancement (**d**). The absence of an early enhancement within the thrombus is suggestive of a thrombotic occlusion (clot)

A portal hypertensive gastropathy correlates in most cases to the stage of liver cirrhosis. It can be imaged best by endoscopic US demonstrating an enhancement of the gastric wall after administration of US contrast agents and in B-flow mode (Fig. 6.23). Some patients may develop varices at unusual sites known as ectopic or aberrant varices. These ectopic varices are predominantly located in the digestive tract including duodenum, jejunum, ileum, colon, rectum, prostate veins and less commonly in the peritoneum, vagina, and urinary bladder. Visible abdominal wall collaterals are common; veins radiating from the umbilicus (caput medusae) are much rarer and indicate extensive flow in the umbilical and periumbilical veins. When using CDDS, varices in the abdominal wall can be detected much more frequently. Collaterals around the rectum can produce rectal varices, often confused with hemorrhoids. Bleeding is occasionally the result.

Unusual causes of portal hypertension are AV fistulae developing between the POV and hepatic artery, mesenteric or splenic arteries and veins. They can result in huge varices and recurrent bleeding (Fig. 6.24).

6.3.2.4 Stenosis and Occlusion of the Splenomesenteric Axis

Obstruction of the POV and its tributaries can occur either extrinsically by tumor mass effect or intrinsi-

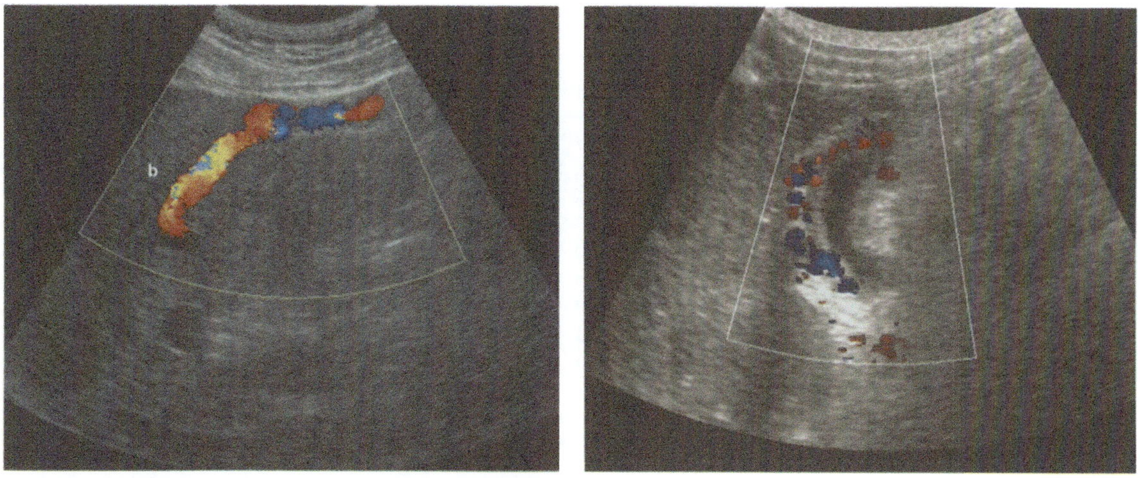

Fig. 6.22a–c. Portosystemic collateral vessels in portal hypertension (CDDS). **a** Recanalized umbilical vein (arising from the left POV branch). **b** Gallbladder varices demonstrated as speckles of color flow within a thickened gallbladder wall. **c** Cavernous transformation after complete occlusion of the POV. Normal main POV in the hepatoduodenal ligament is missing. There is collateral vessel flow indicated in *red* and *blue*

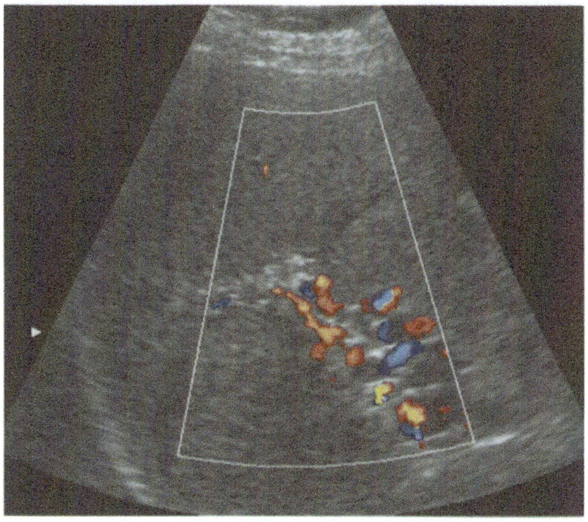

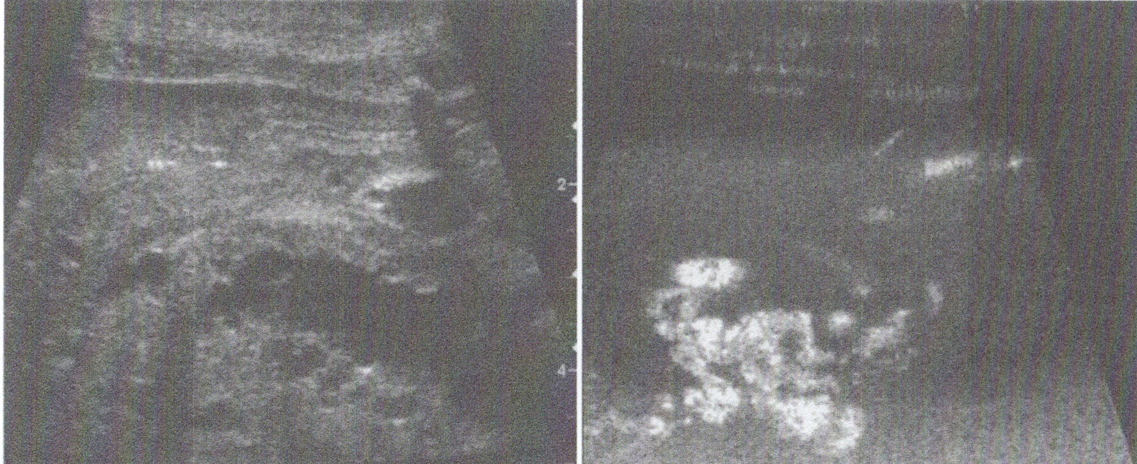

Fig. 6.23. Peripancreatic varices demonstrated by B-flow US technique. A patient with liver cirrhosis and chronic pancreatitis. Transverse B-mode US scan demonstrating the pyloric region of the stomach and irregular vessels surrounding the head and body of the pancreas (*left image*). These peripancreatic varices appear as vessels with bright signal (*right image*) in B-flow technique

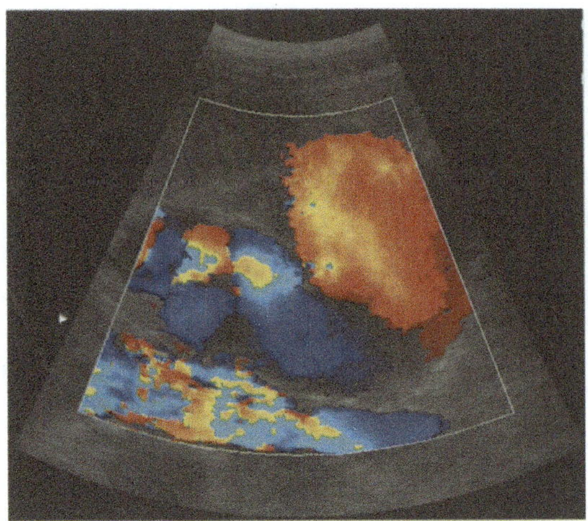

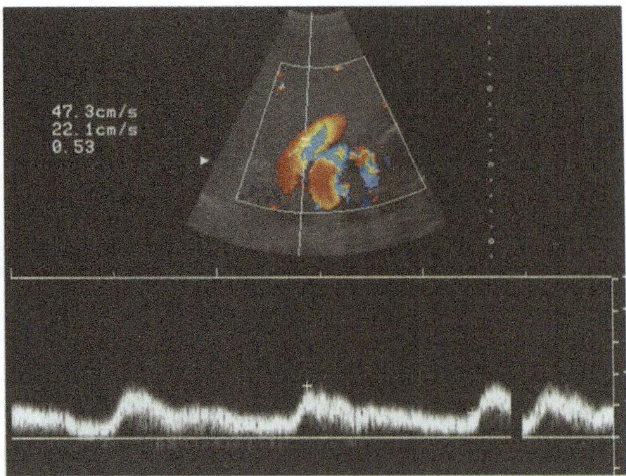

Fig. 6.24a, b. Massive varices in splenosplenic fistula. **a** Longitudinal lateral CDDS scan with spleen, aorta (aliasing), and ectatic vessels. **b** Transverse CDDS scan with splenic artery showing high flow volume (more than 2.5 l/min)

cally by thrombosis due to low flow in the portal system, congenital malformations, coagulation disorders, or infections. Its therapeutic management requires an early diagnosis that can be achieved by CDDS, CT, and MRI. This chapter deals mainly with the splenic and mesenteric veins. Occlusions of the POV are discussed in the previous chapter on portal hypertension.

6.3.2.4.1 Extrinsic Obstruction of the Splenomesenteric Axis

The most import reason for extrinsic obstruction of the splenomesenteric axis is tumor of the pancreas. Tumors arise from ductal, acinar, or endocrine cells, with 80–90% of all pancreatic tumors being ductal adenocarcinomas (Baert and Delorme 1999). Complete surgical resection is the only curative treatment. While the indications for surgical management of pancreatic carcinoma are still controversial, it is clear that the degree of tumor extension and especially vascular involvement are important factors in determining the prognosis and the likelihood of benefit from surgery. The following criteria can be used to define irresectability (Diehl et al. 1998):

- Tumor diameter of more than 5 cm
- Extrahepatic invasion of nonduodenal adjacent tissues
- Stenosis, semicircular encasement of major peripancreatic vessels, or occlusion

These criteria are based on dual-phase CT, but they can be helpful for sonographic evaluation too. Using B-mode US, most neoplasms are hypoechoic compared with the normal pancreas. An additional sign is dilatation of the pancreatic duct. Vascular invasion is best seen by CDDS showing turbulence and an increase in flow velocity. In severe stenosis, collaterals can be depicted around the pancreas. An abnormal Doppler spectrum with a stenosis of more than 50% is suspicious for involvement of the portal and/or splenomesenteric axis. Sensitivity and specificity are reported to be 53% and 89%, respectively Van Delden et al. 1996).

6.3.2.4.2 Intrinsic Obstruction of the Splenomesenteric Axis

Thrombosis of the POV and its splanchnic tributaries is often unsuspected clinically and may be recognized only after imaging studies of the abdomen that are performed for other reasons (Abbitt 1992). Clinical symptoms depend on the amount and acuteness of the occlusion as well as the collateralization. An early diagnosis is essential for the therapy and prognosis.

SPV thrombosis is predominantly caused by acute or chronic pancreatitis. Other reasons are coagulation disorders, gastrointestinal infections, and splenectomy showing splenic thrombosis in at least 7%. About 50% of patients will develop a hemorrhage from gastric or esophageal varices or from other sources in the abdominal cavity. Splenectomy is the procedure of choice in the management of the hemorrhage in these cases (Colum et al. 2001; Kishikawa et al. 2002; Mortele et al. 2001; Smith and Brand 2001).

Although SMV and IMV thrombosis is responsible for 5–15% of cases with intestinal ischemia, it was not recognized as a clinical entity distinct from arterial occlusions until 1935. Early reports emphasized the difficulty of diagnosing it before surgery. With the advent of CT and US, an increasing number of cases with mesenteric vein thrombosis are being reported (MATOS et al. 1986). The most feared complication is intestinal gangrene, in which some or all of the intestine dies because of poor blood supply due to blocked mesenteric veins. Immediate therapy prior to the onset of intestinal gangrene along with the treatment of the underlying cause are essential for a good prognosis.

Early sonographic features of SPV and mesenteric vein thrombosis are hypoechoic or inhomogeneous masses with dilatation of the affected vessel. Reduced or absent compressibility by applying pressure via the scan head may be helpful. CDDS confirms a complete thrombosis by demonstrating absence of flow (Fig. 6.25). In mesenteric vein thrombosis, dilated side branches can be observed upstream due to congestion or thrombus material in the jejunal or ileal branches. Within 6–12 h, collaterals can develop that prevent bowel necrosis.

a

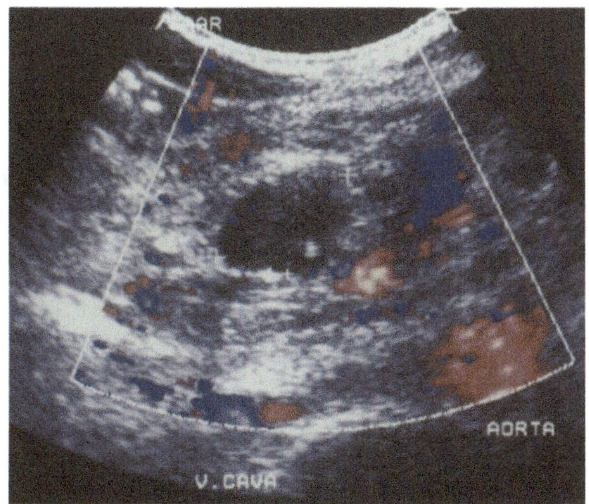

b

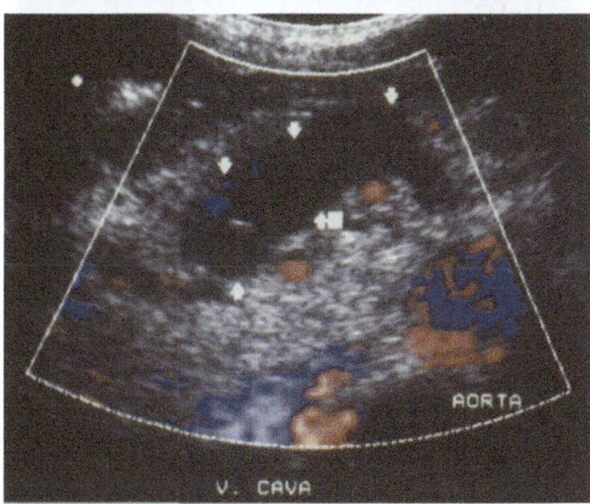

Fig. 6.25a, b. Complete thrombosis of the SMV and IMV (CDDS and CT). **a** Acute thrombosis with complete occlusion of the SMV. Transverse CDDS scan shows an enlarged SMV without flow signal. Branches of the SMA and the aorta are coded in *red*. **b** Transverse scan demonstrating thrombus in the IMV (>)

Follow-up studies in 45 patients (KUBALE et al. 1996) showed a complete recanalization in 15% of cases. In some patients, a remaining wall-adherent thrombus was present at follow-up (Fig. 6.26a). In most patients, the thrombus persists, showing a retraction after 3 weeks (Fig. 6.26b). After 6 months, only a tiny string-like band can be seen on the right side of the SMA. Thirty-six patients could be treated by anticoagulation alone. Six patients had to be operated on with resection of ischemic bowel segments. Four patients died. One late complication was recurrent bleeding due to intramural varices in the duodenum and jejunum (Fig. 6.26c).

6.4 Clinical Value of CDDS in Comparison with Other Imaging Modalities

For diseases of the abdominal veins, different modalities can be used to image the patient with malformations and thrombosis. Each has its strengths and drawbacks:

The traditional procedures of choice for evaluating the IVC and its tributaries has been venography for the lower extremity veins and cavography for the IVC. Both methods require injection of contrast medium into the veins. The hepatic and renal veins can be identified only indirectly by influx phenomenon or directly by selective catheterization.

Direct percutaneous, transjugular, or umbilical vein approaches are invasive methods for evaluating the portal system. Direct splenoportography provides the best opacification of the SPV and POV. Its disadvantages include its inability to visualize the SMV. The late-phase of intraarterial angiography (celiac trunk, mesenteric artery) is helpful to show the splenoportal axis and the mesenteric veins. Nonvisualization of the portal vein may be difficult to interpret because it is not always possible to differentiate thrombosis from inflow effects of unopacified blood out of other pathways and collaterals or retrograde flow in portal hypertension. All methods are invasive.

CT and MRI are gaining increasing importance. Spiral-CT and multislice spiral-CT are excellent techniques for depicting mesenteric, splenic, and portal malformations (BADLER et al. 2002) and thrombosis (FLEISCHMANN 2003; GROVES and DIXON 2002;

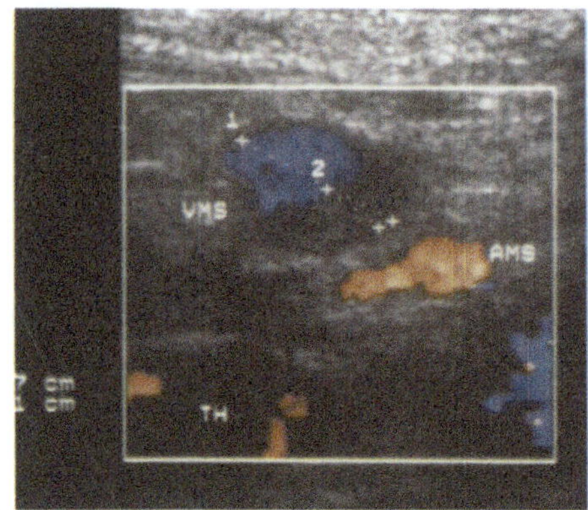

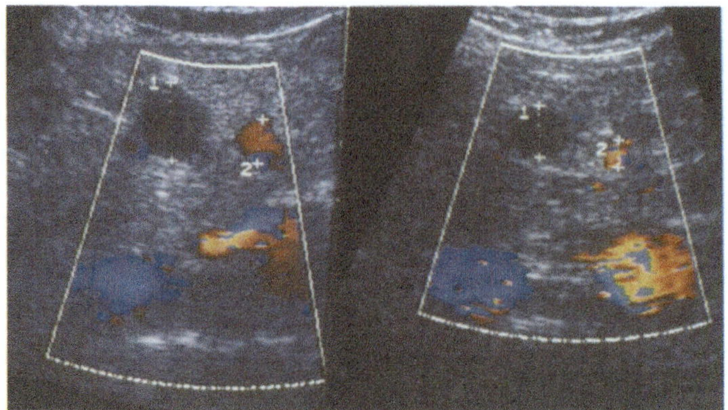

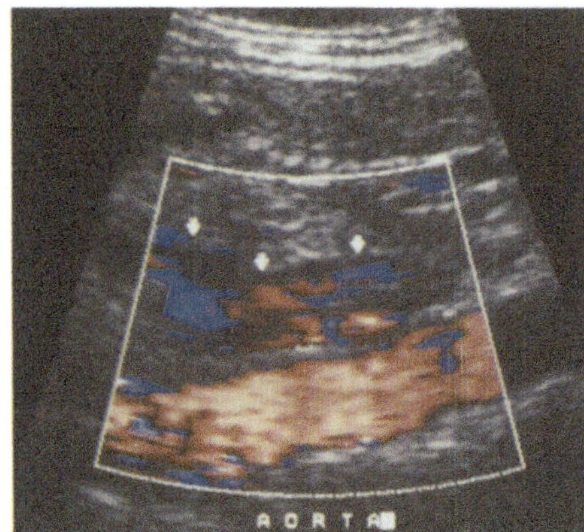

Fig. 6.26a–c. Mesenteric vein thrombosis follow-up. **a** Resolving thrombus with remaining wall-adherent material in the SMV. The SMA and ileal branches are marked in *red*. Additional thrombus in the IVC (*TH*). **b** Complete occlusion of the SMV with thrombus retraction (2 days after first clinical symptoms and follow-up 4 weeks later). **c** Duodenal varices in a patient with persistent occlusion of the SMV and IMV. Transverse scan along the duodenum with tram-line-like ectatic veins in the duodenal wall (with permission from Kubale and Stiegler 2002)

Wilson et al. 2002). CT is the most reliable method for diseases in the pelvis and for AV fistulae that can be depicted after contrast administration. Thrombi and intraluminal tumors appear as filling defects. MR-angiography is gaining increasing acceptance.

Ultrasound has emerged as a safe and effective tool in the evaluation of the venous system of the abdomen. B-mode images show the morphology, CDDS and Doppler measurements provide qualitative, semiquantitative, and quantitative information of flow enabling a systematic analysis of hemodynamic problems.

For venous thrombosis and occlusion, CDDS is the method of choice. Its accuracy depends upon the examination quality, individual skill of the operator, and quality of the US equipment. Ultrasound contrast media provide additional information like transit times, intrahepatic shunting, and parenchymal perfusion, enabling new aspects in functional US imaging.

References

Abbitt PL (1992) Portal vein thrombosis: imaging features and associated etiologies. Curr Probl Diagn Radiol 21: 115–147

Arda K, Kizilkanat KT, Tosun O, Ogdum D (2002) Portal vein aneurysm; CT, MR and MR angiography appearances. Acta Gastroenterol Belg 65:136–138

Armstrong PJ, Franklin DP (2002) Pararenal vena cava leiomyosarcoma versus leiomyomatosis: difficult diagnosis. J Vasc Surg 36:1256–1259

Ascenti G, Zimbaro G, Mazziotti S, Visalli C, Lamberto S, Scribano E, Gaeta M (2001) Intrahepatic portal vein aneurysm: three-dimensional power Doppler demonstration in four cases. Abdom Imaging 26:520–523

Badler R, Price AP, Moy L, Katz DS (2002) Congenital portacaval shunt: CT demonstration. Pediatr Radiol 32:28–30

Baert AL, Delorme GVHL (1999) Pancreas. Springer, Berlin Heidelberg New York

Baka JJ, Lev-Toaff AS, Friedman AC, Radecki PD, Caroline DF (1989) Ovarian vein thrombosis with atypical presentation: role of sonography and duplex Doppler. Obstet Gynecol 73: 887–889

Barsky MF, Rankin RN, Wall WJ, Ghent CN, Garcia B (1989) Patent ductus venosus: problems in assessment and management. Can J Surg 32:271–275

Culum J, Maric Z, Trkulja N (2001) [Segmental portal hypertension as a rare cause of gastric hemorrhage—case report]. Acta Chir Iugosl 48:85–87

Davidovic LB, Kostic DM, Cvetkovic SD, Jakovljevic NS, Stojanov PL, Kacar AS, Pavlovic SU, Petrovic PL (2002) Aortocaval fistulas. Cardiovasc Surg 10:555–560

Denys A, Hammel P, de Baere T, Vilgrain V, Bernades P, Roche A, Menu Y (1998) Arterioportal fistula due to a ruptured pancreatic pseudocyst: diagnosis and endovascular treatment. Am J Roentgenol 170:1205–1206

Dessole S, Capobianco G, Arru A, Demurtas P, Ambrosini G (2003) Postpartum ovarian vein thrombosis: an unpredictable event: two case reports and review of the literature. Arch Gynecol Obstet 267:242–246

Diehl SJ, Lehmann KJ, Sadic M, Lachmann R, Georgi M (1998) Pancreatic cancer: value of dual-phase helical CT in assessing resectibility. Radiology 206:373–378

Duxbury MS, Wells IP, Roobottom C, Marshall A, Lambert AW (2002) Endovascular repair of spontaneous non-aneurysmal aortocaval fistula. Eur J Vasc Endovasc Surg 24:276–278

Ferris EJ, Shah HR (1998) The inferior vena cava. In: Baum S (ed) Abrams' Angiography, 4th edn. Little, Brown, Boston

Fleischmann D (2003) Multiple detector-row CT angiography of the renal and mesenteric vessels. Eur J Radiol 45 [Suppl 1]:S79–S87

Gaiani S, Bolondi L, Bassi S, Siringo S, Barbara L (1991) Prevalence of spontaneous hepatofugal portal flow in liver cirrhosis. Clinical and endoscopic correlation in 228 patients. Gastroenterology 100:160–167

Gayer G, Luboshitz J, Hertz M, Zissin R, Thaler M, Lubetsky A, Bass A, Korat A, Apter S (2003) Congenital anomalies of the inferior vena cava revealed on CT in patients with deep vein thrombosis. Am J Roentgenol 180:729–732

Groves AM, Dixon AK (2002) Superficial collateral veins on abdominal CT: findings in cirrhosis and systemic venous obstruction. Br J Radiol 75:645–647

Ikeda S, Yamaguchi Y, Sera Y, Ohshiro H, Uchino S, Ogawa M (1999) Surgical correction of patent ductus venosus in three brothers. Dig Dis Sci 44:582–589

Ishii Y, Inagaki Y, Hirai K, Aoki T (2000) Hepatic encephalopathy caused by congenital extrahepatic portosystemic venous shunt. J Hepatobiliary Pancreat Surg 7:524–528

Jacob S, Farr G, De Vun D, Takiff H, Mason A (1999) Hepatic manifestations of familial patent ductus venosus in adults. Gut 45:442–445

Kamata S, Kitayama Y, Usui N, Kuroda S, Nose K, Sawai T, Okada A (2000) Patent ductus venosus with a hypoplastic intrahepatic portal system presenting intrapulmonary shunt: a case treated with banding of the ductus venosus. J Pediatr Surg 35:655–657

Kerlean JM, Heron F, Manrique A, Janvresse A, Bourreille J (1995) [Late manifestation of congenital intrahepatic portacaval shunt in a healthy liver]. Rev Med Interne 16: 616–618

Kishikawa H, Nishida J, Nakano M, Hosoe N, Iguchi T, Tanaka T, Terayama K, Tanaka Y, Ishii H (2002) [Idiopathic splenic vein thrombosis with thrombocytopenia and marked splenomegaly]. Nippon Shokakibyo Gakkai Zasshi 99:843–847

Kubale R (1984) Histologische Veränderungen beim portokavalen kongenitalen Shunt. Dissertation, Hannover

Kubale R, Schneider G, Koehler M, Roth R, Kramann B (1996) Mesenteric venous thrombosis: diagnostic and therapeutic management of mesenteric veins. Radiology 201:318

Kubale R, Stiegler H (2002) Farbkodierte Duplexsonographie, interdisziplinärer vaskulärer Ultraschall - Thieme, Stuttgart

Limberg B (1991) Duplexsonographische Diagnose der portalen Hypertension bei Leberzirrhose. Einfluss einer standardisierten Testmahlzeit auf die portale Hämodynamik. Dtsch Med Wochenschr 116:1384–1387

Ludwig D, Schwarting K, Korbel CM, Brunig A, Schiefer B, Stange EF (1998) The postprandial flow is related to the severity of portal hypertension and cirrhosis. J Hepatol 28:631–638

Matos C, Van Gansbeke D, Zalcman M, Ansay J, Delcour C, Engelholm L, Struyven J (1986) Mesenteric vein thrombosis: early CT and US diagnosis and conservative management. Gastrointest Radiol 11:322–325

Matsutani S, Furuse J, Ishii H, Mizumoto H, Kimura K, Ohto M (1993) Hemodynamics of the left gastric vein in portal hypertension. Gastroenterology 105:513–518

Morgagni JB (1769) The seats and causes of disease investigated by anatomy. Millar and Cadell, London

Mortele KJ, Mergo PJ, Taylor HM, Ernst MD, Ros PR (2001) Splenic and perisplenic involvement in acute pancreatitis: determination of prevalence and morphologic helical CT features. J Comput Assist Tomogr 25:50–54

Nangou P, Bertrand P, Samann I, Filali A, el Hassani R, Benabdellah C, Elhadj R, Boulakia C, Icard P (2000) [Portal vein aneurysm]. Ann Chir 125:476–478

Nasser N, Spellacy WN (1968) Ovarian vein thrombosis. A rare cause of pelvic pain. Report of a case and review of the literature. J Lancet 88:306–308

Park JH, Cha SH, Han JK, Han MC (1990) Intrahepatic portosystemic venous shunt. Am J Roentgenol 155:527–528

Piscaglia F, Gaiani S, Donati G, Masi L, Bolondi L (1999) Doppler evaluation of the effects of pharmacological treatment of portal hypertension. Ultrasound Med Biol 25:923–932

Pleasants JH (1911) Obstruction of the inferior vena cava with a report of 18 cases. John Hopkins Hosp Rep 16:363–548

Rahim N, Adam EJ (1985) Ultrasound demonstration of variations in normal portal vein diameter with posture. Br J Radiol 58:313–314

Raskin NH, Bredesen D, Ehrenfeld WK, Kerlan RK (1984) Periodic confusion caused by congenital extrahepatic portacaval shunt. Neurology 34:666–669

Ricci P, Cantisani V, Biancari F, Drud FM, Coniglio M, Di Filippo A, Fasoli F (2000) Contrast-enhanced color Doppler US in malignant portal vein thrombosis. Acta Radiol 41:470–473

Sacerdoti D, Bolognesi M, Bombonato G, Gatta A (1995) Paraumbilical vein patency in cirrhosis: effects of hepatic hemodynamics evaluated by Doppler sonography. Hepatology 22:1689–1694

Saito H, Ishibashi T, Zuguchi M, Sato A, Yamamoto R, Tsuboi M, Takahashi S, Yamada S (1999) Embryology, anatomic variation and pathology of the portal venous system. RSNA, Chicago

Sing TM, Le SD, Wong KP, Young N (1997) Transcatheter embolization of a congenital intrahepatic arterioportal venous malformation: a case report. Australas Radiol 41: 292–296

Smith TA, Brand EJ (2001) Pancreatic cancer presenting as bleeding gastric varices. J Clin Gastroenterol 32: 444–447

Sprouse LR, Hamilton IN Jr (2002) The endovascular treatment of a renal arteriovenous fistula: placement of a covered stent. J Vasc Surg 36:1066–1068

Szucs-Farkas Z, Toth J, Szollosi Z, Peter M, Bartha I (2002) Pseudoaneurysm and ilio-caval fistula caused by malignant fibrous histiocytoma of the aorta—CT diagnosis and angiographic confirmation. Eur Radiol 12:450–453

Tortoriello TA, Vick GW III, Chung T, Bezold LI, Vincent JA (2002) Meandering right pulmonary vein to the left atrium and inferior vena cava: the first case with associated anomalies. Tex Heart Inst J 29:319–323

Van Delden OM, Smts MJ, Bemelman WA, Reeders JWRJ (1996) Comparison of laparoscopic ultrasound and transabdominal ultrasound in staging of cancer of the pancreatic head region. J Ultrasound Med 16:207–212

Vonnahme FJ, Dubuisson L, Kubale R, Klempnauer R, Grun M (1984) Ultrastructural characteristics of hyperplastic alterations in the liver of congenital portacaval-shunt rats. Br J Exp Pathol 65:585–596

Wachsberg RH, Simmons MZ (1994) Coronary vein dia-meter and flow direction in patients with portal hypertension: evaluation with duplex sonography and correlation with variceal bleeding. Am J Roentgenol 162:637–641

Weskott HP, Kubale R (2002) Leber und portalvenöses System. In: Kubale R, Stiegler H, Baert AL (eds) Farbkodierte Duplexsonographie. Thieme, Stuttgart, pp 298–341

West MS, Gara BS, Horii SC, Hayes WS, Cooper C, Silverman PM, Zeman RK (1991) Gall bladder varices: imaging findings in patients with portal hypertension. Radiology 154:495–498

Wilson MW, LaBerge JM, Kerlan RK, Martin AJ, Weber OM, Roberts T, Vitalich C, Higgins CB, Gordon RL (2002) MR portal venography: preliminary results of fast acquisition without contrast material or breath holding. Acad Radiol 9:1179–1184

Yang DM, Yoon MH, Kim HS, Jin W, Hwang HY, Cho SW, Kim HS (2003) Portal vein aneurysm of the umbilical portion: imaging features and the relationship with portal vein anomalies. Abdom Imaging 28:62–67

Yonemitsu H, Mori H, Kimura T, Kagawa K, Tsuda T, Yamada Y, Kiyosue H, Matsumoto S (2000) Congenital extrahepatic portocaval shunt associated with hepatic hyperplastic nodules in a patient with Dubin-Johnson syndrome. Abdom Imaging 25:572–575

Yoshidome H, Edwards MJ (1999) An embryological perspective on congenital portacaval shunt: a rare anomaly in a patient with hepatocellular carcinoma. Am J Gastroenterol 94:2537–2539

7 Quantitative Assessment of Splanchnic Venous Hemodynamics by Doppler Techniques

K. H. Seitz and M. Merz

CONTENTS

7.1 Introduction

The seemingly simple duplex Doppler approach of blood flow measurement was established in the mid-1980s after numerous comparisons with other methods (Bru et al. 1983; Kurz et al. 1985; Moriyasu et al. 1984; Nakayama et al. 1983; Ohnishi et al. 1985; Seitz and Kubale 1988; Walter et al. 1986; Dauzat et al. 1989). The breakthrough for a broad clinical use failed to appear because the examination technique was too difficult and time-consuming. The personal skill of the investigator has to be high, and 20–30% of the intended examinations were lost as a result of the typical US barriers (meteorism, obesity, ribs, massive ascites). Later, there was a lack of important questions for daily work.

The spreading of CDDS imaging equipment led in portal hypertension–the most important clinical question in the area of splanchnic venous vessels–more rapidly to diagnostic results than conventional Doppler sonography did (Seitz and Wermke 1995).

State-of-the-art CDDS equipment with comfortable automatic real-time Doppler calculations led to an increase of scientific work in quantitative blood flow measurements.

7.2 Blood Flow Measurement by CDDS: Principles and Difficulties

The venous blood flow velocities in the splanchnic region are slow to moderately rapid, i.e., on average they are between 0 and 30 cm/s. Extremely slow flow or even reversed flow exists in portal hypertension in the portal vein (POV; Seitz and Kubale 1988). These low flow velocities require a special setting of the CDDS system. The flow velocities fluctuate considerably inter- and intraindividually, so if quantitative flow measurements are to be carried out, multiple measurements have to be done. Three or even better five single measurements have to be averaged to get valid and consistent results. The venous blood flow in the splanchnic vessels shows predominantly respiratory, and only in some cases cardiac modulation. All measurements have to be done under standardized conditions which means: fasting patient (minimum of 6 h, normally fasting overnight), examination after a 15-min rest in mid-inspiration, inflation must be held without Valsalva maneuver (Seitz and Kubale 1988; Teichgräber et al. 1997). Flow profiles have to be stable for at least 4 s or longer (Siringo et al. 1994). Under these conditions and by averaging multiple measurements, intraindividual variance is below 10% (Iwao et al. 1994; Arienti et al. 1996).

K. H. Seitz, MD
Associate Professor of Internal Medicine, Innere Abteilung, Kreiskrankenhaus Sigmaringen, Hohenzollernstrasse 40, 72488 Sigmaringen, Germany
M. Merz, MD
Innere Abteilung, Kreiskrankenhaus Sigmaringen, Hohenzollernstrasse 40, 72488 Sigmaringen, Germany

It is of special importance that an identical examination technique is used within one working group. Only under these circumstances will interobserver variance of measurements go down to 6%, and intraobserver variance to 4%, respectively (Arienti et al. 1996). Using different US systems, equipment-related variance was 32%, while observer-related variance was only 5% (Sabba et al. 1995). Each Doppler laboratory has to have its own standard values, and if quantitative measurements are to be compared, the same equipment has to be used.

There are also methodical conditions that have to be considered to reduce measurement error as far as reasonably possible. The so called 'Doppler angle' (the angle between the ultrasound beam carrying the sample volume and the longitudinal axis of blood flow) should not exceed 60°. At an angle of 60°, an angle measurement error of 5° will lead to a variation in the velocity measurement of 20%; in cases of doubt, underestimation of the Doppler angle leads to a smaller error than overestimation (Table 7.1).

Wall filters (high-pass filters) are necessary to reduce wall motion artifacts. These wall filters should not exceed 100 Hz because otherwise with slow flow there will be a considerable overestimation of blood flow velocity (Seitz and Kubale 1988) (Fig. 7.1). Vice versa, very low flow cannot be detected when the Doppler shift frequency is below the frequency of the wall filter. In this case, an apparent zero flow will be detected (Table 7.2). The sample volume should cover the whole cross-sectional area of the vessel.

Table 7.1. Technical errors in CDDS flow measurements

	Deviation	Error in %
Doppler angle		
10°	±5°	± 1%
60°	±5°	±20%
Vessel diameter		
5 mm	±0.5 mm	±20%
10 mm	±0.5 mm	±10%

Table 7.2. Influence of the Doppler angle and the frequency of the low-pass (wall) filter on the minimal detectable flow velocity (note: data for a transducer frequency of 3.0 MHz)

Doppler angle	Wall filter 100 Hz	200 Hz	400 Hz
0°	2.6 cm/s	5.1 cm/s	10.2 cm/s
60°	5.1 cm/s	10.2 cm/s	20.5 cm/s

In normal cases, the pulse repetition frequency (PRF) is sufficient for the unequivocal detection of venous blood flow even at a depth of 10 cm or more.

Measurement of the blood flow volume involves the determination of the mean blood flow velocity (v_{mean}), whereas the maximum flow velocities (v_{max}) are sufficient for inter- and intraindividual comparisons of blood flow velocity; the measurement of maximum blood flow velocity is normally unaffected by wall filters.

Modern ultrasound systems are able to measure different velocities (v_{mean}, v_{max}) in real time and to actualize the flow parameters in short intervals and to demonstrate the results on a display (Fig. 7.2).

The flow volume (*FV*) is the product of mean flow velocity (v_{mean}) and the cross-sectional area (*F*) of the vessel $FV(\text{ml/min}) = 60 \cdot v_{mean}\ (\text{cm/s}) \cdot F\ (\text{cm}^2)$. The vessels in the venous capacitative system show an oval cross-section, so both different diameters have to be taken into account [$F = a \cdot b \cdot 0.5\pi\ (\text{cm}^2)$]. Errors

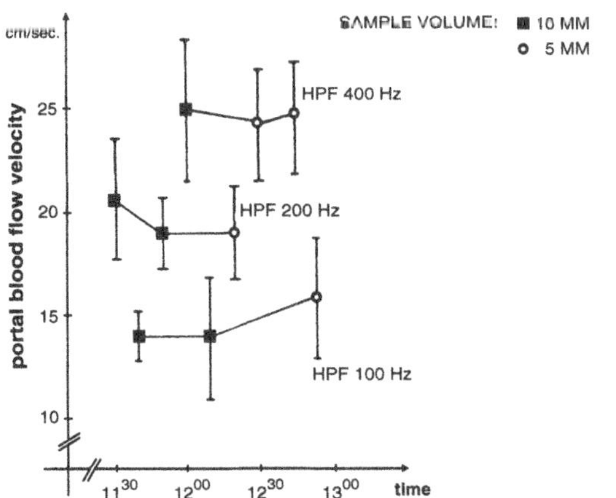

Fig. 7.1. Influence of wall filters on quantitative duplex sonography

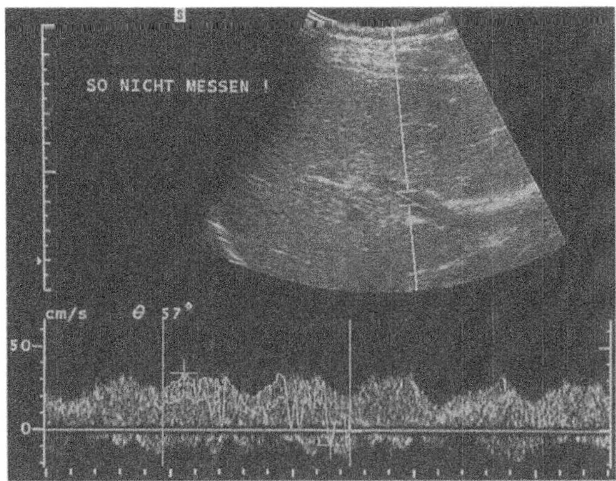

Fig. 7.2. Normal hepatocentric portal venous blood flow (v_{max} 45 cm/s, v_{mean} 23 cm/s)

of 0.5–1 mm in the measurement of vessel diameters below 10 mm will lead to a variation of up to 20% (Table 7.1) (Seitz and Kubale 1988; Delahunt et al. 1996). Blood flow velocity and cross-sectional area have to be measured in two steps at an identical site of the vessel. The ultrasound plane during the diameter measurement is different to the examination plane during Doppler measurement; in the optimum case, they are perpendicular to each other (Doppler angle 0°).

Changes of the vessel diameter due to respiratory modulation cannot be considered quantitatively due to the examination technique. In addition, one has to keep in mind that in unfavorable conditions, the different variabilities can add up to 50%. Therefore, the use of such measurements has to be regarded very critically. Before planning a study, one has to consider whether flow measurements by the Doppler technique are sufficiently accurate to detect the expected effects on blood flow and velocity.

Quantitative blood flow measurements by the Doppler technique are still only used for scientific research; there are only rare clinical questions in daily routine which have to be answered by this method.

Anemia, fever, splenomegaly (without splenic vein thrombosis), and other hyperdynamic states with increased cardiac output lead to an elevation of the splanchnic blood flow volume.

7.3 Blood Flow in Splanchnic Venous Vessels–Qualitative Assessment

7.3.1 Portal Vein

The normal POV has a length of 5–6.5 cm and is best scanned in the supine or right anterior oblique position. CDDS measurements should be performed at its extrahepatic course near the crossing of the hepatic artery at a Doppler angle of 45–60° (Fig. 7.2). The intrahepatic course of the POV can be insonated from an intercostal space with an angle below 15°. In obese or uncooperative persons and patients with massive ascites, measurements of the blood flow velocity may become very difficult or even impossible. The anteroposterior diameter of the POV normally ranges between 10 and 15 mm. There is hepatopetal blood flow with respiratory modulation and, without pathologic significance, variable cardiac modulation.

7.3.2 Splenic Vein

The normal hepatopetal SPV blood flow is also characterized by respiratory and sometimes cardiac modulation. Quantitative blood flow measurement is possible in front of the aorta 2 cm away from the confluence with the SMV (Fig. 7.3a), or left of the aorta, where the Doppler angle can usually be kept small (Fig. 7.3b), but the extremely oval vessel prevents an exact measurement of the corresponding cross-sectional area. Hepatofugal, stop and go, pendulum, or zero flow are findings in portal hypertension. The diagnosis of portal hypertension can be achieved easily by CDDS (Fig. 7.4).

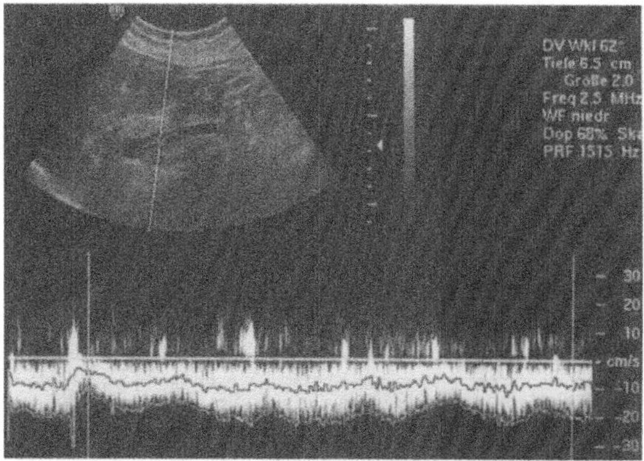

a

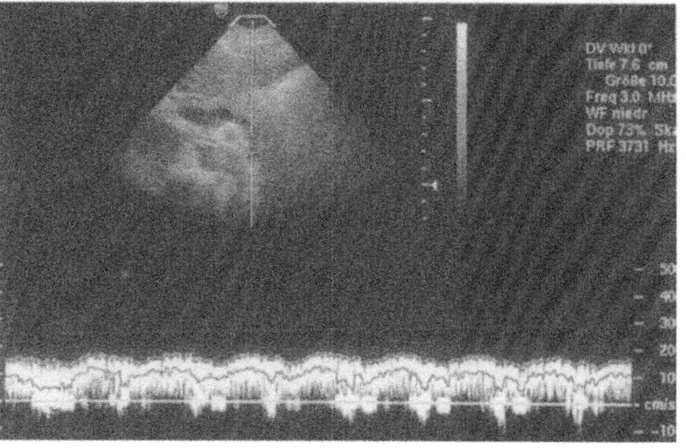

b

Fig. 7.3a, b. Normal blood flow in splenic vein (SPV): typical sites for flow measurements

7.3.3 Superior Mesenteric Vein

The normal blood flow in the SMV is hepatopetal and shows respiratory modulation (Fig. 7.5). During

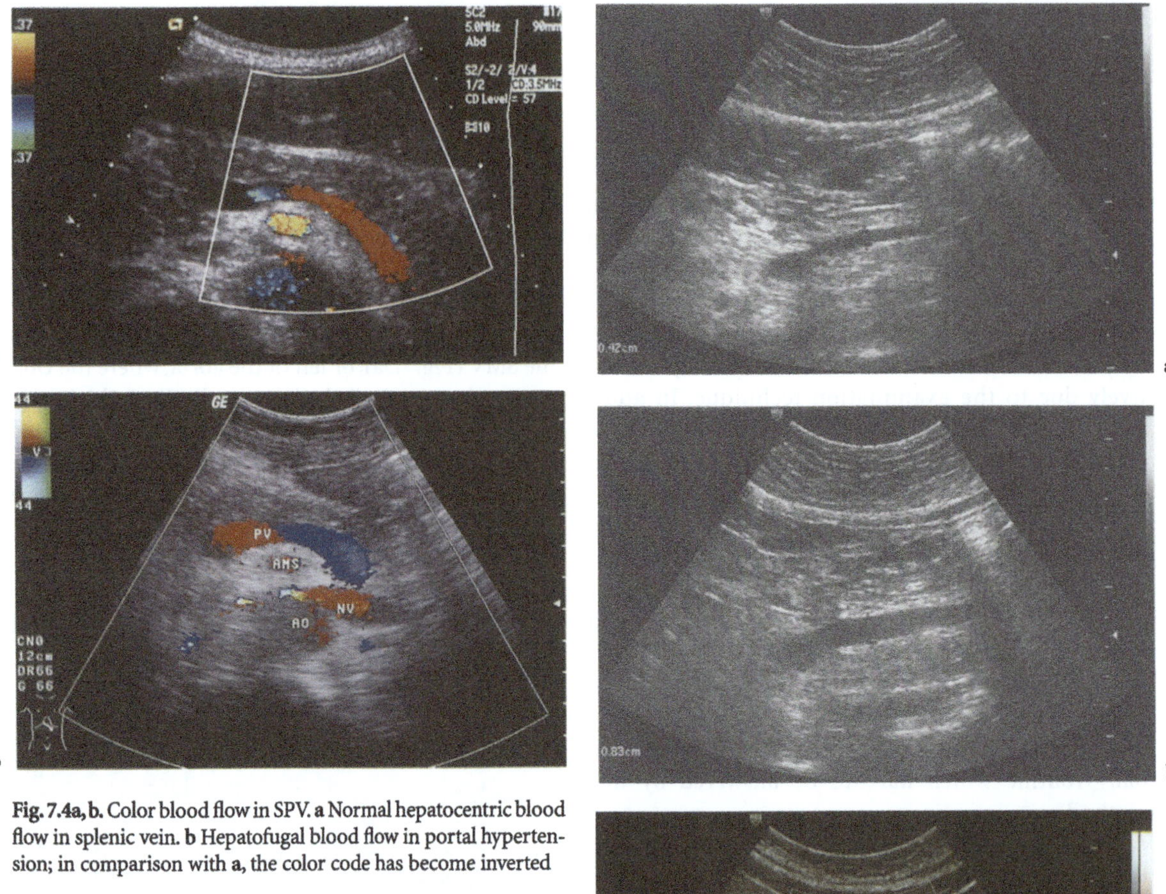

Fig. 7.4a, b. Color blood flow in SPV. **a** Normal hepatocentric blood flow in splenic vein. **b** Hepatofugal blood flow in portal hypertension; in comparison with **a**, the color code has become inverted

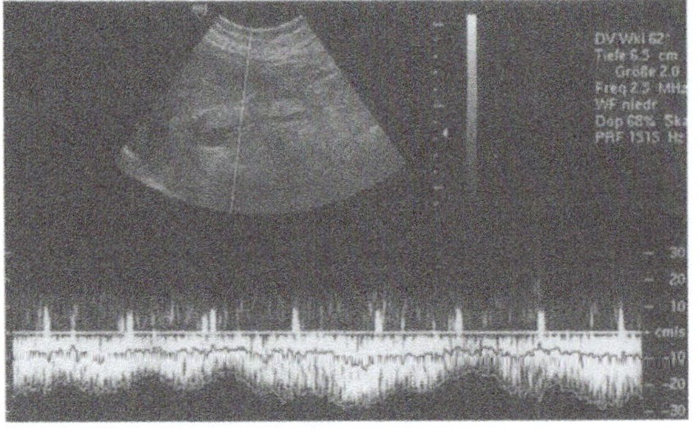

Fig. 7.5. Normal blood flow in superior mesenteric vein (SMV)

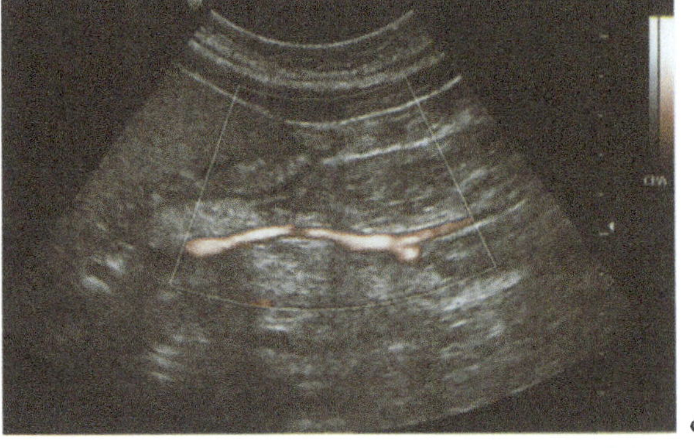

Fig. 7.6a–c. SMV: Alteration of diameter during respiration excludes portal hypertension. **a** End-expiratory diameter: 4 mm. **b** End-inspiratory diameter: 8 mm. **c** Demonstration of normal SMV by power angio mode

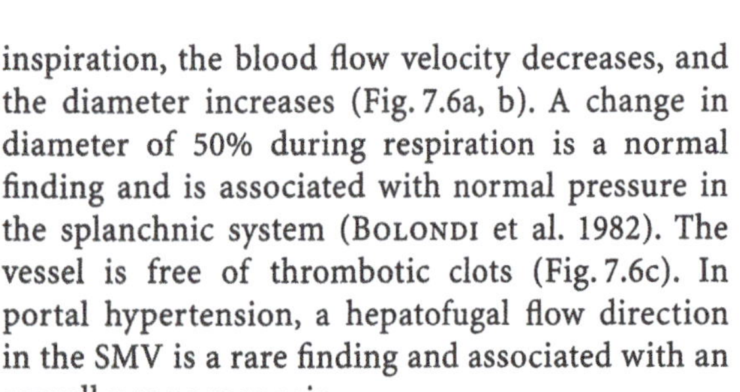

inspiration, the blood flow velocity decreases, and the diameter increases (Fig. 7.6a, b). A change in diameter of 50% during respiration is a normal finding and is associated with normal pressure in the splanchnic system (Bolondi et al. 1982). The vessel is free of thrombotic clots (Fig. 7.6c). In portal hypertension, a hepatofugal flow direction in the SMV is a rare finding and associated with an overall poor prognosis.

7.4 Quantitative Assessment of Blood Flow in Splanchnic Venous Vessels

7.4.1 Splenic and Superior Mesenteric Vein

Quantitative blood flow measurements in the SPV and the SMV have only rare applications in daily clinical practice (Fig. 7.3). Initially, blood flow measurements in these vessels were done to serve as a control for Doppler measurements of blood flow in the POV, because the sum of the blood flow volumes in SMV and SPV must be equivalent to the POV blood flow. Accordingly, blood flow in the superior mesenteric artery (SMA) and SMV should be identical. Blood flow velocities are higher than normal in the SMV in patients with untreated celiac disease and decrease after successful treatment (ARIENTI et al. 1996). Active inflammatory bowel diseases will actually lead to an increase in the mesenteric blood flow and blood flow velocity (MACONI et al. 1996).

7.4.2 Portal Vein

A lot of scientific questions concern POV blood flow. The normal mean POV blood flow velocity has a range between 10 and 25 cm/s, while the maximum velocity may exceed 40 cm/s (Fig. 7.1, Tables 7.3 and 7.4).

In portal hypertension, the mean portal blood flow velocity decreases on average to 6–12 cm/s (Fig. 7.7). In advanced cases, there is stagnant or even hepatofugal blood flow. Due to differences in the study population, there are small differences between the results. The normal blood flow velocity and portal blood flow correlate negatively with age (SEITZ and KUBALE 1988). In portal hypertension, respiratory modulation of POV blood flow may be reduced or absent, and the normally oval cross-sectional area becomes increasingly circular. The normal portal blood flow volume of 600–1300 ml/min may be normal or reduced. In comparison with other measurement techniques, the portal blood flow volume assessed by CDDS is usually underestimated (Table 7.3) (LYCKLAMA et al. 1997).

Portal blood flow volume and velocity do not correlate closely with portal pressure, because the individual hemodynamic condition is influenced by the development of portacaval collaterals (and their blood flow). For example, the portal blood flow velocity will be increased dramatically by a large

Table 7.3. Quantitative Doppler flow measurements in splanchnic veins (POV, portal vein; SMV, superior mesenteric vein; UC, ulcerative colitis; CD, Crohn's disease; CSA, cross-sectional area; FV, flow volume; PCI, portal congestion index)

Reference	n	Diagnosis	POV	Diameter or CSA	v_{mean} (cm/s)	v_{max} (cm/s)	FV (ml/min)	PCI
IWAO et al. 1994	25	Controls	POV	0.72 cm^2	15.7±3.7			
	47	Cirrhosis	POV	0.96 cm^2	11.7±3.5		606±213	
LYCKLAMA et al. 1997	8	Controls/fasting		0.89±0.25 cm^2	12.2±2.2		999±330	
		after meal		1.12±0.23 cm^2	15.5±5.9			
MACONI et al. 1996	10	Controls	POV	10.7±1.4 mm	19.0±2.7		1014±187	
	12	Active UC	POV	11.2±1.4 mm	26.3±4.7		1544±336	
	12	Inactive UC	POV	10.8±1.1 mm	18.8±2.2		1049±243	
	12	Active CD	POV	11.5±1.2 mm	24.3±4.3		1519±350	
	12	Inactive CD	POV	11.6±1.2 mm	23.5±2.7		1513±361	
	12	Irritable bowel syndrome	POV	10.6±1.7 mm	18.7±0.9		1001±225	
	10	Controls	SMV	7.6±1.9 mm	11.3		316±151	
	11	Active UC	SMV	8.2±1.4 mm	20.2±5.7		654±182	
LEEN et al. 1993 (measurement in expiration)	30	Controls	POV				1200±572	0.095±0.051
	20	Cirrhosis	POV				604±507	0.329±0.303
	55	Metastasis	POV				691±344	0.102±0.055
TAI et al. 1996	79	Acute hepatitis			11.1±2.8	20.7±4.0	670±363	
	9	Acute hepatitis fatalities			8.9±2.2	17.6±3.9	422±240	
D'ALIMONTE et al. 1993	52	Cirrhosis	POV			18.6±5.0 (3.5–33.4)		
DE VRIES et al. 1994	55	Controls	POV	10.1±1.4 mm	13.9±4.1		652±203	
	59	Cirrhosis	POV	11.2±2.0 mm	11.0±4.2		672±291	
IWAO et al. 1996	10	Controls	POV	0.82±0.04 cm^2	14.9±0.7		733±46	
	10	Cirrhosis	POV	1.17±0.04 cm^2	10.2±0.8		720±63	
MRI								
LYCKLAMA et al. 1997	8	Controls		1.9±1.4 cm^2	11.0	11.42		
		After meal		2.4±2.0 cm^2	15.5	19.45		

Table 7.4. Average flow velocities in the portal trunk in subjects with normal liver function and patients with cirrhosis of the liver, determined by Doppler sonography

References	Healthy subjects		Cirrhosis	
	n	v_{mean} (cm/s)	n	v_{mean} (cm/s)
Saito et al. (1983)	41	16.5±4.9		
Moriyasu et al. (1984)	88	15.3±4.0	65	9.7±2.6
Zoli et al. (1986)	75	16.0±0.5		10.6±0.6
Ohnishi et al. (1985)	26	14.8±5.6	27	10.1±2.4
Mildenberger et al. (1987)	50	15.2±2.6		
Ozaki et al. (1988)	22	19.0±0.9	29	6.2±1.6
Mostbeck et al. (1989)			11	11.2±6.2
Seitz (1988)	29	15.2±2.9	27	7.6±2.8
Wruck (1990)	18	13.0±1.7	30	7.0±1.9
Wermke (1989)	5	15.1±1.6	144	8.1±2.4

paraumbilical venous portacaval collateral, which, in the authors' experience, can drain up to 2 l of portal blood per minute. In this case, the portal blood volume may exceed 2 l/min, but the portal liver perfusion may be near zero. On the other hand, massive prehepatic collateral vessels reduce the POV blood flow and may lead to hepatofugal flow direction.

Due to these facts, it is important to know that the portal flow does not correlate closely with the POV pressure or with the extent or severity of esophageal varices or with the flow volume in the portacaval collaterals.

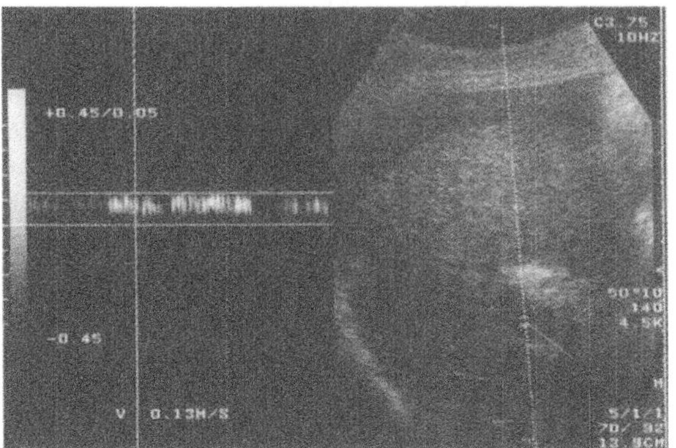

a

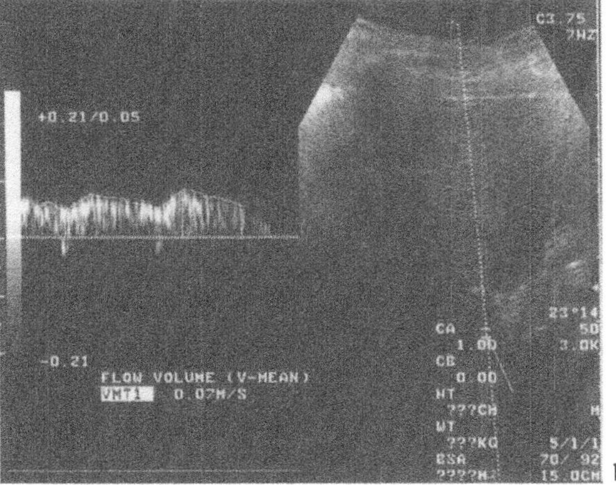

b

Fig. 7.7a, b. Reduced portal blood flow velocity in portal hypertension. **a** Blood flow measurement under difficult conditions (ascites, meteorism), v_{max} 13 cm/s. **b** Portal mean flow velocity v_{mean} 7 cm/s

7.4.2.1
Respiratory Modulation of POV Flow Velocity

During early inspiration, there is an acceleration of the blood flow velocity in the IVC and a collapse of the lumen. The sections of the hepatic veins next to the IVC show identical changes in blood flow. The diaphragm compresses the liver during inspiration, and there is a consecutive decrease of portal blood flow velocity and a dilation of the POV (compare blood flow in SMV, see above). The blood flow volume in the POV remains nearly constant or will be slightly diminished. Vice versa, the blood flow velocity increases upon expiration.

7.4.2.2
Postprandial POV Blood Flow

Due to the postprandial hyperemia in the splanchnic vessels, the flow volume in the POV increases significantly. Comparisons of Doppler measurements with indocyanine green clearance showed similar results (Burggraaf et al. 1996). Normally, both the POV flow velocity and the POV diameter increase. The flow volumes increase by nearly 100% in healthy persons but by only 30–50% in patients with liver cirrhosis (Iwao et al. 1996). Similar results were shown by Kawamura et al. (1983) and Limberg (1991). In our own experience, POV flow velocity and diameter may not always show the previously mentioned changes after food intake in individual cases. The portal blood flow increment was examined after a standardized meal: After fatty meals, it was more pronounced than after meals which contained less fat or different proportions of proteins and carbohydrates (Hoost et al. 1996).

7.4.2.3
Effects of Posture Change and Exercise

In healthy persons and patients with chronic hepatitis or cirrhosis, the POV blood flow and velocity are significantly higher in the supine than the sitting position. Additionally, there is a further decrease of POV blood flow immediately after exercise when measured in the sitting position (Ohnishi et al. 1985).

7.4.2.4
POV Blood Flow in Acute Hepatitis

In severe acute hepatitis, the POV blood flow and prothrombin time were found to be the only two independent risk factors. During hospital care, transient reduced portal blood flow was followed by a hyperdynamic stage (Tai et al. 1996).

7.4.2.5
POV Blood Flow in Portal Hypertension

CDDS POV blood flow measurements in portal hypertension are statistically valid concerning inter- and intraobserver variation (Lomas et al. 1993).

Several studies demonstrate a significant decrease in portal blood flow velocity in patients with cirrhosis compared with normal controls (Fig. 7.8), whereas POV blood flow is not significantly reduced (Tables 7.3 and 7.4) (Seitz and Kubale 1988; de Vries et al. 1994; Iwao et al. 1994; Iwao et al. 1996). The overall decrease in POV blood flow velocity depends on the number of patients within the study population presenting with spontaneous splenorenal shunts and reverse blood flow in the SPV. To a substantial extent, the results of portal blood flow volume measurement are influenced by the number of patients included with zero, pendulum, stop and go, or reverse portal flow. Without considerable portacaval collaterals, there is no or only a small difference between normal subjects and patients with portal hypertension.

Generally, the results of the measurements are less than the actual flow velocity because there is a slight, systematic underestimation when measuring during inspiration. One has to keep in mind that the error in velocity measurement can reach 20%, and the measurement of the portal cross-sectional area may cause a second error, around 20% as well (in extreme cases 30%). Thus, in individual cases, the error can add up to 40%, which is rather unacceptable for a quantitative method. So the results are complex, and the POV flow volume is not identical to portal hepatic perfusion. POV blood flow volume or velocity tells us nothing about the portacaval, umbilical, and portovenous shunt volumes, which are of clinical importance. So interpretation of the POV blood flow volume is very difficult.

Measurement of POV blood flow velocities (v_{mean}) separates 80% of normal subjects and patients with cirrhosis and portal hypertension with overlapping values in 20%, whereas the simple measurement of the diameter of the POV overlaps in 80% between the two groups (Fig. 7.9) (Seitz and Kubale 1988). The problem is not the diagnostic differentiation between normal subjects and patients with portal hypertension, the main problem is that changes of POV blood flow develop gradually from normal to definitely abnormal. There is a broad overlap of measurements between patients suffering from chronic hepatitis and other liver diseases progressing to cirrhosis (Saito et al. 1983).

Similar results were found when the maximum POV blood flow velocity (v_{max}) was measured. Of patients with portal hypertension, 70% presented with a v_{max}<20 cm/s (velocity range in normal subjects in this study: 20–33 cm/s), resulting in a sensitivity of 0.76 and a specificity of 1.0 (D'Alimonte et al. 1993).

The portal congestion index, calculated by dividing the mean POV flow velocity by the POV cross-sectional area, is referred to as the best index for the diagnosis of portal hypertension (Moriyasu et al. 1986). The hemodynamic changes with portal hypertension are demonstrated more clearly. With this 'mathematical trick', the congestion index sepa-

a
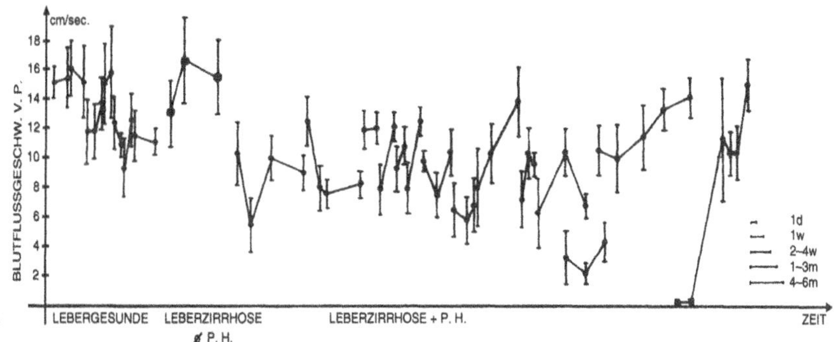

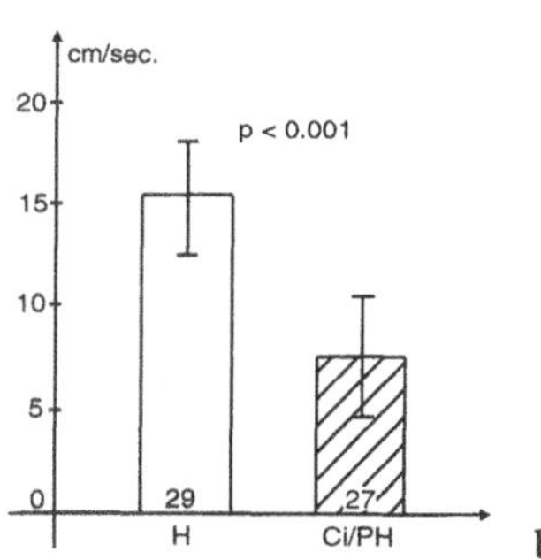

b

Fig. 7.8a, b. Mean portal blood flow velocities in healthy volunteers and cirrhotic patients with portal hypertension. **a** Repeated averaged mean flow velocity measurements within different time intervals (*d* day, *w* week, *m* month). **b** Portal mean flow velocity differs significantly in both groups

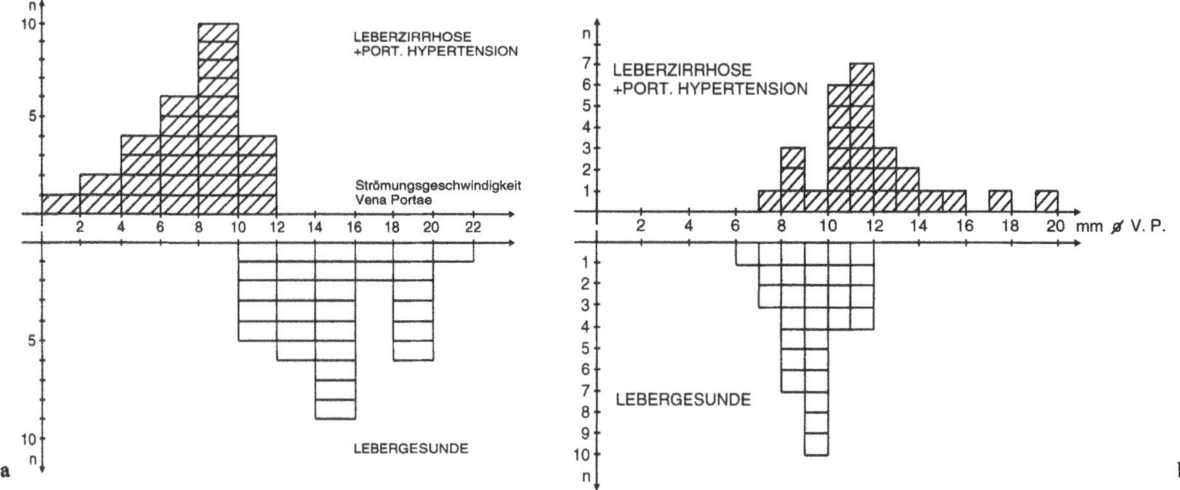

Fig. 7.9a, b. Mean portal blood flow velocity (**a**) and vessel diameter (**b**) in normal subjects and portal hypertensive patients. Compare the different overlaps

rates these groups. This relation explains why portal flow volume cannot be used as a diagnostic tool, as it only plays a role in hemodynamic studies (Iwao et al. 1994).

Additionally, the error in POV flow measurements may be related to the shunt flow, which can be ruled out by special measurements to some extent. An estimation of the prehepatic portacaval shunt flow can be obtained by the Doppler technique by comparing the difference between the POV flow volume and the sum of the flow volumes obtained in the splenic and superior mesenteric arteries (Iwao et al. 1996).

Interestingly, hemodynamic alterations of POV blood flow can be observed when big portacaval collaterals appear or when in advanced alcoholic liver disease alcohol abuse is stopped and the fatty infiltration diminishes very fast (Fig. 7.8, last patient on the right).

Another reliable way to diagnose portal hypertension is the demonstration of a significant reduction in the normal postprandial increase of POV blood flow velocity. The difference between normal subjects and patients with portal hypertension evidently increases because both the blood flow velocity and the POV diameter have increased (Kawamura et al. 1983; Limberg 1991). However, this approach is very time-consuming and limited by the fact that up to 20% of measurements are impossible after postprandial conditions, as US visibility of the POV worsens.

Regional hepatic blood flow is difficult to assess. Compared with indocyanine green extraction, sinusoidal perfusion was significantly predicted by changes in the main POV. Intrahepatic shunting was correlated with flow changes in the main and right POVs (Gibson et al. 1996). These results require further investigation and confirmation.

POV blood flow measurements obtained in patients with either liver cirrhosis or metastatic disease to the liver showed similar POV blood flow volumes but differences in the POV congestive index. Further differences between patients with cirrhosis and liver metastasis could be demonstrated in the hepatic arterial blood flow and Doppler perfusion index (Di Giulio et al. 1997; Leen et al. 1993). POV blood flow velocities in cirrhotic patients with a history of variceal bleeding are lower than in patients without a bleeding history, but the POV blood flow velocity or volume cannot be used as a predictor of variceal bleeding (Seitz and Kubale 1988). However, the POV congestion index was found to be an independent predictor of variceal bleeding, like red cherry spots, variceal size, or serum bilirubin. The congestion index in nonbleeders was 1.3±0.7, 1.8±0.9 in early bleeders (within 6 months), and 1.5±0.4 in late bleeders (after 6 months). However, prediction of variceal bleeding with clinical and endoscopic parameters and the congestive index remains quite poor (Siringo et al. 1994). Portal hypertensive gastropathy does not affect the portal blood flow (Iwao et al. 1994).

7.4.2.6
Drug-Induced Flow Changes in the POV

Various drugs influence the POV flow velocity and/or blood flow as measured by the CDDS technique. The decrease of POV blood flow velocity after the administration of β-blocking agents (propanolol) is less in cirrhotic patients than in controls (Fig. 7.10). Nadolol decreases the POV flow velocity and POV flow volume in cirrhotic patients as well (Table 7.5). With chronic oral administration of β-blocking agents, therapeutic nonresponders could be evaluated using this technique (Bolognesi et al. 1997). In a study performed in our laboratory, the i.v. administration of 2 mg of glucagon led within 2–10 min to an increase of the POV blood flow velocity of about 20% in healthy controls, whereas patients with portal hypertension did not show any response (Fig. 7.11). Similar results in healthy persons were found by Renda et al. (1994). In contrast to studies with pre- and postprandial POV hemodynamic assessment, these examinations can be done during one single CDDS investigation, which is less time-consuming.

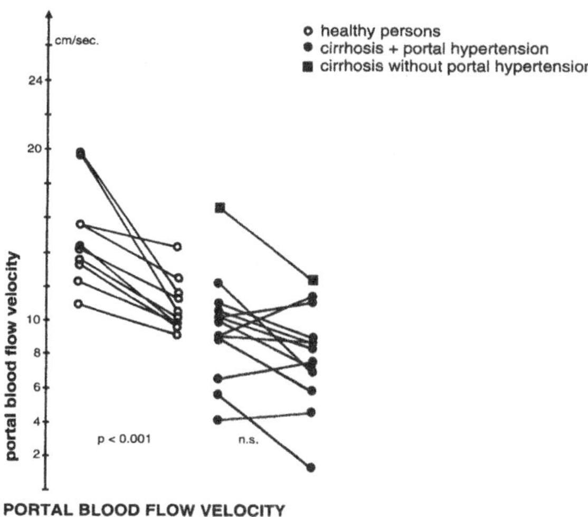

Fig. 7.10. Propanolol and portal blood flow velocity. In most cases, the portal blood flow velocity drops after propanolol (40 mg orally)

In daily clinical routine, quantitative blood flow measurements in the POV system are of little importance except for controls after transjugular intrahepatic portosystemic shunt (see Chapter 8). The examination is technically rather complicated and time-consuming, and in individual cases, the results are not reliable enough, due to intraindividual, interobserver, and technical (different CDDS systems) variability. However, CDDS plays a big role in the diagnosis of portal hypertension because the blood flow direction in the POV can be detected quickly and reliably. Qualitative criteria like hepatofugal, stagnant, stop and go, or pendulum flow support the diagnosis as well as the detection of portacaval collateral veins. Qualitative registration of the intrahepatic portal blood flow is highly interesting in some cases. The flow direction in the right and left intrahepatic POV can vary, and arterioportal shunts produce a typical flow profile which can be easily identified.

The therapy of portal hypertension with β-blocking agents led to a number of Doppler investigations. Propanolol, nadolol, nitrates, and glycilpressin induce a decrease of portal blood flow in both

Table 7.5. Duplex sonographic examinations of the drug-induced effects in portal venous flow (*PBF* portal blood flow)

Reference	n	Diagnosis	Drug/dose	Effect
Zoli et al. 1996	9	Cirrhosis	Nitroglycerin transdermal 15 mg	18–22% decrease of v_{mean}
Seitz and Kubale 1988	10	Controls	Glucagon (iv) 2 mg	21% increase of v_{mean}
	10	Cirrhosis	Glucagon (iv) 2 mg	No effect
Renda et al. 1994	30	Normal	Glucagon (iv) 1 mg	15.6% increase of v_{mean}
Seitz and Kubale 1988	10	Controls	Propranolol 40 mg (60 min)	v_{mean} before 15.0, after 11.0 cm/s
	10	Cirrhosis	Propranolol 40 mg (60 min)	v_{mean} before: 9.0 after 7.5 cm/s
Bolognesi et al. 1997	30	Portal hypertension cirrhosis	Nadolol dose: 25% heart rate reduction	v_{mean} reduction from 11.7 to 9.1 cm/s PBF before: 917±368 ml/min after: 666±276 ml/min
	16		Nadolol 80 mg acute	v_{mean} reduction from 11.8 to 10.4 cm/s PBF before: 905±387 ml/min after: 774±320 ml/min
Dinç et al. 1996	14	Cirrhosis	Verapamil (orally) 80 mg	Portal vein diameter before: 11.6, after: 12.6 mm v_{mean} before: 11.6, after: 10.9 cm/s PBF before: 654, after: 788 ml/min
Ljubicic and Bilic 1992	12	Cirrhosis	Verapamil (orally) 80 mg (measured after 30 min)	Portal vein diameter before: 1.52, after: 1.51 cm/s v_{mean} before: 13.2, after: 13.4 cm/s PBF before: 931, after: 954 ml → no change

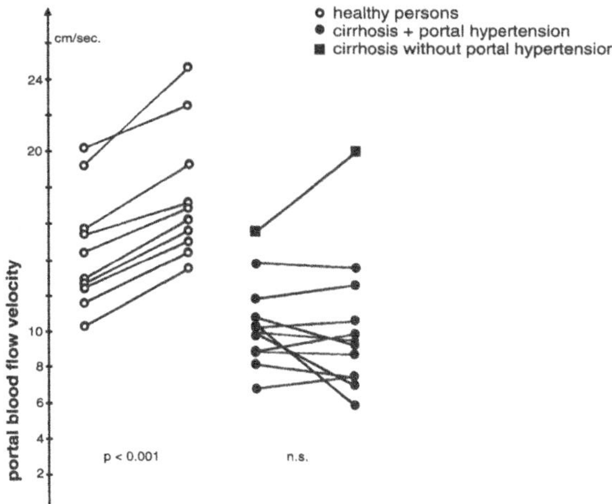

Fig. 7.11. Glucagon and portal blood flow velocity. After i.v. administration of 2 mg of glucagon, the portal flow velocity rises in normal persons and stays constant in patients with portal hypertension

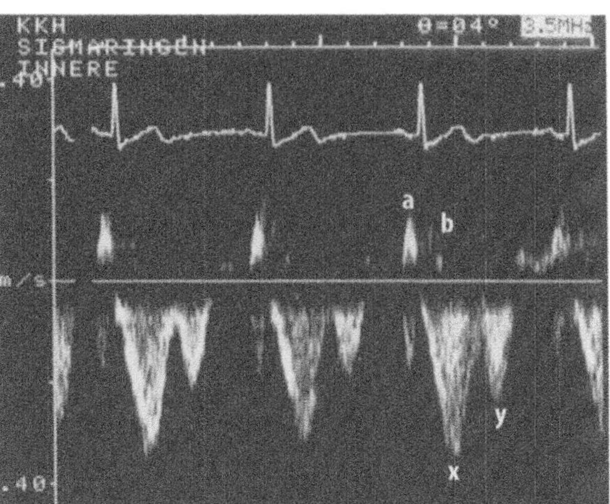

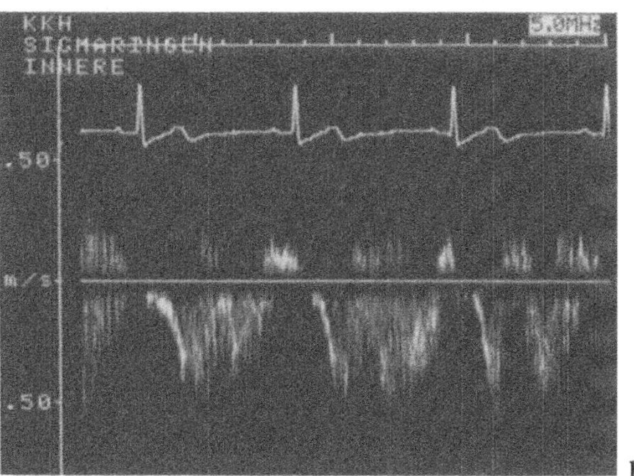

Fig. 7.12a, b. Cardial modulation of the hepatic venous flow. **a** Hepatic vein: *x*=phase I, *y*=phase II, *a*=phase III. **b** Jugular vein: compare the identical flow pattern

cirrhotic patients and controls (Zoli et al. 1996). Cigarette smoking and Ranitidine do not alter the POV blood flow parameters as assessed by CDDS (Rapaccini et al. 1996). Verapamil and glucagon were without effect in portal hypertensive patients (Dinç et al. 1996; Seitz and Kubale 1988; Ljubicic and Bilic 1992).

Our own results of CDDS POV flow parameters obtained 2–5 min after sublingual administration of nitroglycerine in patients with heart failure were somewhat different between two groups. In patients with prevailing left heart failure, there was a tremendous decrease in the mean POV flow velocity. In contrast, patients with right heart failure presented without changes in POV flow velocity, probably because further venous pooling could not take place in the congested portal vessels (Seitz and Kubale 1988).

7.5 Hepatic Veins

The normal blood flow in the right, middle, and left hepatic vein (HV) shows cardiac and respiratory modulation (Figs. 7.12 and 7.13a). HV Doppler curves are similar to flow curves obtained in the IJV. The physiological flow in the HVs is triphasic. Teichgräber et al. described the normal hepatic flow systematically in 1997 (Table 7.3). The HV blood flow velocity increases from the periphery of the liver towards the IVC. Standardized flow profiles and flow velocities can be obtained very reliably 1–2 cm distant from the HV–IVC junction (Table 7.6). The flow velocities in the middle and right HV are similar, while the flow velocity in the left HV is higher. The triphasic flow pattern can best be described by the quotient between the maximum flow velocities in phase 1 and phase 2. The quotient increases during inspiration and decreases during expiration, corresponding to the alteration in blood flow velocities (Table 7.6).

In heart failure, especially with tricuspid insufficiency, a typical augmentation of the back stream component is visible, and the flow curve becomes biphasic (Fig. 7.13b). All phasic modulations derive from the caval flow pattern, whereas monophasic flows exclude cardiac or caval modulation. Alterations of the liver parenchyma due to cirrhosis, sometimes even due to high-grade fatty infiltration, but also diminished tissue compliance in the neigh-

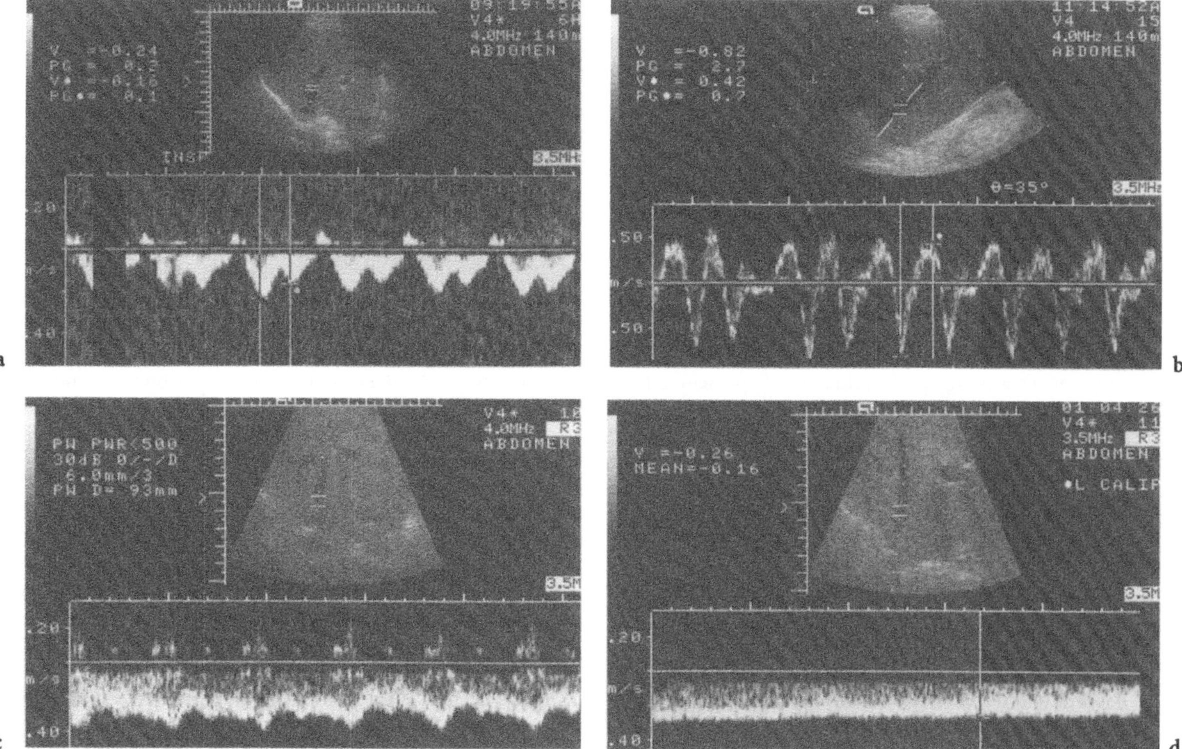

Fig. 7.13a–d. Flow profiles in hepatic veins: normal (**a**), heart failure (**b**), reduced modulation in diffuse hepatopathy (**c**), flat flow profile in 'severe' hepatopathy (**d**)

Table 7.6. Flow velocity in the middle hepatic vein (MLV) and right hepatic vein (RLV) (mid-inspiratory) (Teichgräber et al. 1997)

Phase	Hepatic vein	*v* (±SD)
I	MLV	–0.21±0.019 m/s
	RLV	–0.25±0.013 m/s
II	MLV	–0.16±0.016 m/s
	RLV	–0.16±0.016 m/s
III	MLV	0.08±0.011 m/s
	RLV	0.09±0.006 m/s

borhood of tumors lead to a damping of the blood flow profiles (Fig. 7.13c,d). The flow profile in the HVs becomes mono- or aphasic, and the cardiac or respiratory modulation is lost. According to these rather complex alterations, in portal hypertension at least six different flow profiles in the HV have been described. The typical decreased flow velocity or flat flow profile was found in 29 of 100 patients (Ohta et al. 1994; Lycklama et al. 1997).

In Budd-Chiari syndrome or any other obstruction of the HVs, the flow profile is very flat and aphasic or completely absent.

Until now, there has been no distinct relation between the different HV flow patterns and a specific liver disease. However, an aphasic blood flow pattern in Doppler curves of HVs is a sign of severe liver disease like frank cirrhosis or HV obstruction.

7.6 Summary

Despite the fact that CDDS flow measurements, especially those obtained in the POV, are reliable and reproducible under specific conditions as described previously, these measurements are of little clinical importance. A good correlation has been obtained between CDDS flow measurements and those obtained by MRI (Lycklama et al. 1997) or indocyanine green (Burggraaf et al. 1996; Zentner and Zoller 1992). So far, the noninvasive nature of CDDS measurements has prompted many investigators to look for physiologic hemodynamic alterations in the blood flow or the influence of pharmacological interventions. The new generation of CDDS equipment enables real-time Doppler calculations and will perhaps lead to a new wave of publications. However, currently there are hardly any new results which exceed those obtained over the past 15 years. Accordingly, quantitative blood flow measurement in the splanchnic circulation will probably remain a domain of scientific questions, especially in portal hypertension and liver transplantation.

References

Arienti V, Califano C, Brusco G, Boriani L, Biagi F, Giulia Sama M, Sottoili S, Domanico A, Corazza GR, Gasbarrini G (1996) Doppler ultrasonographic evaluation of splanchnic blood flow in coeliac disease. Gut 39:369–373

Bolognesi M, Sacerdoti SD, Merkel C, Bombonato G, Enzo E, Gatta A (1997) Effects of chronic therapy with nadolol on portal hemodynamics and on splanchnic impedance indices using Doppler sonography: comparison between acute and chronic effects. J Hepatol (Denmark) 26:305–311

Bolondi L, Gandolfi L, Arienti V, Caletti GC, Corioni E, Gasbarrini G, Labo G (1982) Ultrasonography in the diagnosis of portal hypertension: diminished response of portal vessels to respiration. Radiology 142:167–172

Bru C, Bosch J, Mastai R, Kravetz D, Fabregas I, Bianchi L, Rodes J (1983) Noninvasive measurement of portal venous blood flow in man by combined Doppler real time ultrasonography. Effects of propanolol [abstract]. Hepatology 3:855

Burggraaf J, Schoemaker HC, Cohen AF (1996) Assessment of changes in liver blood flow after food intake–comparison of ICG clearance and echo-Doppler. Br J Clin Pharmacol 42:499–502

D'Alimonte P, Cioni G, Cristani A, Ferrari A, Ventura E, Romagnoli R (1993) Duplex-Doppler ultrasonography in the assessment of portal hypertension. Utility of the measurement of maximum portal flow velocity. Eur J Radiol 17: 126–129

Dauzat M, Layrargues GP (1989) Portal vein blood flow measurements using pulsed doppler and electromagnetic flowmetry in dog: a comparative study. Gastroenterology 96:913–919

Delahunt TA, Geelkerken RH, Hermans J, van Baalen JM, Vaughan AJ, van Bockel JH (1996) Comparison of trans- and intra abdominal duplex examinations of the splanchnic circulation. Ultrasound Med Biol 22:165–171

De Vries PJ, Hoekstra BL, de Hooge P, van Hattum J (1994) Portal venous flow and follow-up in patients with liver disease and healthy subjects. Scand J Gastroenterol 29:172–177

Di Giulio G, Lupo L, Tirelli A, Vinci R, Rotondo A, Angelelli G (1997) Valutazioni flussimetriche con eco color Doppler nei tumori epatici primitivi e secondari Radiol Med (Torino) 93:225–229

Dinç H, Kapicioglu S, Cihanyurdu N, Can G, Ünal M, Topkaya L, Gümele HR (1996) Effects of verapamil on portal and splanchnic hemodynamics in patients with advanced posthepatic cirrhosis using duplex Doppler ultrasound. Eur J Radiol 23:97–101

Gibson PR, Gibson RN, Donlan JD, Jones PA, Colman JC, Dudley FJ (1996) A comparison of Doppler flowmetry with conventional assessment of acute changes in hepatic blood flow. J Gastroenterol Hepatol 11:14–20

Hoost U, Kelbaek H, Rasmusen H, Court-Payen M, Christensen NJ, Pedersen-Bjergaard U, Lorenzen T (1996) Haemodynamic effects of eating: the role of meal composition. Clin Sci 90:269–276

Iwao T, Toyonaga A, Ikegami M, Sumino M, Oho K, Shigemori H, Sakaki M, Nakayama M, Tanikawa K, Iwao J (1994) Portal vein hemodynamics in cirrhotic patients with portal hypertensive gastropathy: an echo-Doppler study. Hepatogastroenterology 41:230–234

Iwao T, Toyonaga A, Oho K, Sakai T, Tayama C, Masumoto H, Sato M, Nakahara K, Tanikawa K (1996) Postprandial splanchnic hemodynamic response in patients with cirrhosis of the liver: evaluation with "triple-vessel" duplex US. Radiology 201:711–715

Kawamura S, Miyatake K, Okamoto K, Beppu S, Kinoshita N, Sakakibara H, Nimura Y (1983) Analysis of the portal vein flow with two-dimensional echo-Doppler-method. In: Lerski RA, Morley P (eds) Ultrasound '82. Pergamon, Oxford, pp 511–515

Kurz CS, Klosa W, Graf HP, Schillinger H (1985) Ultraschall-Doppler-Verfahren zur nicht invasiven Bestimmung fetaler Blutflußvolumina. Ultraschall 6:90–96

Leen E, Goldberg JA, Anderson JR, Robertson J, Moule B, Cooke TG, McArdle CS (1993) Hepatic perfusion changes in patients with liver metastases: comparison with those patients with cirrhosis. Gut 34:554–557

Limberg B (1991) [The duplexsonographic diagnosis of portal hypertension in liver cirrhosis. The effect of a standardized test meal on portal hemodynamics] (in German). Dtsch Med Wochenschr 116:1384–1387

Ljubicic N, Bilic A (1992) Effect of verapamil on portal blood flow in patients with liver cirrhosis. J Ultrasound Med 11: 517–520

Lomas DJ, Britton PD, Summerton CB, Seymour CA (1993) Duplex Doppler measurements of the portal vein in portal hypertension. Clin Radiol 48:311–315

Lycklama A, Nijeholt GJ, Burggraaf K, Wasser MNJ, Schultze Kool LJ, Schoemaker RC, Cohen AF, de Roos A (1997) Variability of splanchnic blood flow measurements using MR velocity mapping under fasting and post-prandial conditions–comparison with echo-Doppler. J Hepatol 26: 298–304

Maconi G, Imbesi V, Bianchi Porro G (1996) Doppler ultrasound measurement of intestinal blood flow in inflammatory bowel disease. Scand J Gastroenterol 31:590–593

Mildenberger P, Lotz R, Kreitner K (1987) Duplexsonographie der normalen Pfortader. Dtsch Med Wochenschr 112: 1936–1939

Moriyasu F, Ban N, Nishida O et al (1984) Quantitative measurement of portal blood flow in patients with chronic liver disease using an ultrasonic duplex system consisting of a pulsed Doppler flowmeter and B-mode electroscanner. Gastroenterol Jpn 19:529–536

Moriyasu F, Ban N, Nishida O, Nakamura T, Miyake T, Uchino H, Kanematsu Y, Koizumi S (1986a) Clinical application of an ultrasonic duplex system in the quantitative measurement of portal blood flow. J Clin Ultrasound 14:579–588

Moriyasu F, Nishida O, Bar N (1986b) Congestion index of the portal vein. Am J Gastroenterol 146:735–739

Mostbeck GH, Wittich GR, Herold C et al (1989) Hemodynamic significance of the paraumbilical vein in portal hypertension: assessment with Doppler US. Radiology 170:339–342

Nakayama T, Ohnishi K, Saito M, Hatano H, Nomura F, Kono K, Okuda K (1983) Effects of propranolol on portal vein pressure, portal blood flow and cardiac output in patients with chronic liver disease. Hepatology 3:812

Ohta M, Hashizume M, Tomikawa M, Ueno K, Tanoue K, Sugimachi K (1994) Analysis of hepatic vein waveform by Doppler ultrasonography in 100 patients with portal hypertension. Am J Gastroenterol 89:170–175

Ohnishi K, Saito M, Koen H, Nakayama T, Nomura F, Okuda K (1985) Pulsed Doppler flow as a criterion of portal venous velocity: comparisons with cineangiographic measurements. Radiology 154:495–498

Ohnishi K, Terabayashi H, Tsunoda T (1990) Budd-Chiari-syndrome: diagnosis with duplex sonography. Am J Gastroenterol 85:165–169

Ozaki CF, Anderson JC, Liebermann RP et al (1988) Duplex ultrasonography as a non-invasive technique for assessing portal hemodynamics. Am J Surg 155:70–75

Rapaccini Gl, Pompili M, Marzano MA, Grattagliano A, Cedrone A, Aliotta A, Pignataro F, Caturelli E, Cellerino C (1996) Comment. J Gastroenterol Hepatol 11:995–996

Renda F, Olivieri A, Migliorato L, Sanita di Toppi G, Colagrande C (1994) Valutazione con eco-Doppler degli effetti del glucagone sul flusso portale nei soggetti normali. Radiol Med (Torino) 87:447–451

Sabba C, Merkel C, Zoli M, Ferraioli G, Gaiani S, Sacerdo D, Bolondi L (1995) Interobserver and interequipment variability of echo-Doppler examination of the portal vein: effect of a cooperative training program. Hepatology 21: 428–433

Saito M, Ohnishi K, Nakayama T, Nomura F, Kono K, Koen H, Okuda K (1983) Ultrasonic measurements of portal and splenic vein blood flows and their velocities in normal subjects and patients with chronic liver disease. Hepatology 3:812–817

Seitz K (1988) Duplexsonographische Befunde am Portalsystem. Klin Wochenschr 66 [Suppl 13]:172–173

Seitz K, Kubale R (1988) Duplex sonography of the abdominal and retroperitoneal vessels. VCH, Weinheim

Seitz K, Wermke W (1995) Portale Hypertension–derzeitiger Stand der sonographischen Diagnostik. Z Gastroenterol 33:349–361

Siringo S, Bolondi L, Gaiani S, Sofia S, Zironi G, Rigamonti A, di Febo G, Miglioli M, Cavalli G, Barbara L (1994) Timing of the first variceal hemorrhage in cirrhotic patients: prospective evaluation of Doppler flowmetry, endoscopy and clinical parameters. Hepatology 20:66–73

Tai D, Changchien C, Chen C, Chiou S, Lee C, Kuo C, Chen J, Chiu K, Chuah S, Hu T, Hsiaw C (1996) Sequential evaluation of portal venous hemodynamics by Doppler ultrasound in patients with severe acute hepatitis. Am J Gastroenterol 91:545–550

Walter JP, Mcgahan JP, Lantz PM (1986) Absolute flow measurements using pulsed Doppler US. Radiol 159:545–548

Wermke W (1989) Sonomorphometrische und dopplersonographische Untersuchungen bei chronischen Leberkrankheiten. Habilitationsschrift, Humboldt-Universität, Berlin

Wruck U (1990) Sonomorphometrische und dopplersonographische Untersuchungen bei Leberzirrhose unter besonderer Berücksichtigung des Akuteffektes von Propanolol. Habilitationsschrift, Humboldt-Universität, Berlin

Zentner J, Zoller WC (1992) Indocyanine green clearance and duplex sonography in hepatic blood flow. Clin Invest 70:620

Zoli M, Marchesini G, Brunori A et al (1986) Portal venous flow in response to acute _-blocker and vasodilatory treatment in patients with liver cirrhosis. Hepatology 6:1248–1251

Zoli M, Magalotti D, Ghigi G, Marchesini G, Pisi E (1996) Transdermal nitroglycerin in cirrhosis. A 24-hour echo-Doppler study of splanchnic hemodynamics. J Hepatol 25:498–503

8 Doppler Imaging of TIPS

G. Nics and F. Karnel

CONTENTS

8.1 Introduction

The transjugular intrahepatic portosystemic shunt (TIPS) is a nonsurgical method of decompressing the portal venous system. TIPS involves the creation of a portosystemic shunt by forming an intrahepatic tract between the hepatic and portal veins using angiographic techniques. From a hemodynamic point of view, TIPS is a small caliper H-shunt with partial decompression of portal hypertension. In 1989, Richter et al. described the first clinical use of a metallic stent for TIPS. During the past few years, TIPS has been shown to be an effective treatment alternative in patients suffering from complications due to portal hypertension.

CDDS plays a major role in the evaluation of patients before the TIPS procedure and in the postinterventional follow-up (Koslin and Mizutani 1995). Thorough patient selection is one of the keys to successful intervention. Shunt dysfunction is a common problem especially in the first year after the procedure. Early detection of malfunctioning stents allows prompt reintervention to achieve improved long-term patency (Haskal et al. 1997).

The goal of this chapter is to demonstrate hemodynamic changes after the TIPS procedure and CDDS characteristics of patent and malfunctioning stents.

8.2 Preinterventional Sonographic Evaluation

As patient selection is one of the keys for a successful TIPS procedure, a standardized preinterventional examination program is necessary. Table 8.1 gives the evaluation program used in the KFJ Hospital, Vienna. CDDS plays a key role in the assessment of patients prior to TIPS placement. Several points have to be mentioned. Besides checking the indication and ruling out contraindications, the preinterventional examination has to alert the interventionalist to the vascular anatomy and any possible vascular abnormality and to serve as a baseline study for CDDS evaluation of portal hypertension as there is wide variation in the individual expression of portal hypertension (Koslin and Mizutani 1995).

8.2.1 Indications and Contraindications

Indications. Major indications for TIPS are active, refractory variceal bleeding and recurrent variceal bleeding, Budd-Chiari syndrome, and acute POV thrombosis in combination with thrombolysis. TIPS is probably effective in patients with intractable ascites, hydrothorax, or severe hepatorenal syndrome (Lakin et al. 1995; Flora and Benner 1995; Saxon and Keller 1997).

Contraindications. Severe hepatic failure is a contraindication for TIPS. In 1995, Flora and Benner reported that patients with a Child-Pugh score greater than 12 have a 30 day survival after TIPS insertion of

G. Nics, MD; F. Karnel, MD
Röntgeninstitut, Kaiser-Franz-Josef-Spital, Kundratstrasse 3, 1100 Vienna, Austria

Table 8.1. Evaluation of TIPS patients

Gray-scale US	Liver (morphology, focal lesions), spleen, ascites
CCDS	Anatomy, patency, flow direction, peak velocity of POV (main, right, left), SPV, SMV and HVs Presence of and flow within collateral veins: – Intrahepatic: paraumbilical, posterior portal branches – Extrahepatic: esophageal, coronary gastric collaterals, splenorenal, gastrorenal, retrocaval, mesocaval shunts
S-CT, MR, biopsy	Focal liver lesions or etiology of cirrhosis
Indirect splenoportography or S-CT-A or MR-A of the portal venous system	If CDDS inconclusive

S-CT = spiral CT, S-CT-A = spiral-CT angiography, MR-A = MR angiography

only 60% versus 90% in patients with Child-Pugh scores less than 12. In cases of severe right heart failure, the increase in blood flow to the right heart may lead to acute decompensation after successful TIPS insertion. TIPS should be avoided in patients with active cholangitis, hepatic abscesses, or systemic sepsis (Flora and Benner 1995).

Relative contraindications are hepatic neoplasms, polycystic liver disease, hepatic encephalopathy, and POV thrombosis. Thorough sonographic evaluation of the liver for the presence of possible masses is necessary, as patients with liver cirrhosis are known to have an increased risk for hepatocellular carcinoma. Only large central neoplasms are absolute contraindications for TIPS, as the tumor may be traversed by TIPS insertion, and therefore there will be an increased risk of seeding of neoplastic cells (Flora and Benner 1995).

As there is some risk of intraperitoneal bleeding if liver cysts are punctured, US has to show a safe access route for the intervention in case of multiple cysts in the liver or polycystic liver disease. As there have been published cases of recanalization of a thrombosed portal vein in addition to a TIPS procedure, CDDS has to show the extent of the thrombosis and to rule out extensive and chronic forms, or cases of portal venous cavernomas. TIPS implanted in patients with POV thrombosis show an increased risk for shunt thrombosis, but these patients might become eligible for liver transplantation after a successful TIPS procedure (Saxon and Keller 1997).

Table 8.2 lists indications and contraindications for the TIPS procedure.

Table 8.2. Indications and contraindications for TIPS (modified according to LAKIN et al. 1995)

Indications
- TIPS is effective for:
  - uncontrolled acute variceal bleeding
  - recurrent variceal bleeding
- TIPS is probably effective for:
  - Budd–Chiari syndrome
  - refractory ascites
  - cirrhotic hydrothorax
  - hepatorenal syndrome
- TIPS may be useful:
  - in patients waiting for a liver transplant
  - as preoperative intervention in patients with esophageal varices before gastric or esophageal surgery

Contraindications
- Absolute:
  - severe hepatic failure
  - severe right heart failure
- Relative:
  - hepatic neoplasm
  - polycystic liver disease
  - hepatic encephalopathy
  - portal vein thrombosis

8.2.2 Anatomical Considerations

There are some anatomical variants of liver size and shape, in particular, the size of the left lobe varies widely. A well-known variant is Riedel's lobe, a right lobe extending far caudally. Usually, cirrhotic livers are small, with a shrunken right and a larger, often hypertrophic left lobe. If there is a large amount of ascites, the liver is shifted medially and caudally (La Berge et al. 1995).

Outflow Tract. The patency of the outflow tract of the shunt is of great importance for a well-functioning TIPS. Occlusion or atresia of the IVC is rare but can be demonstrated by CDDS. Dilatation and loss of respiratory modulation of the IVC or the hepatic veins are signs of right heart failure, which is a relative contraindication for TIPS. Occlusion of all or some hepatic veins or variant anatomy may influence the selection of the puncture site. There are commonly three hepatic veins. Usually, the right hepatic vein is the largest and therefore the first choice for puncture. There are some anatomical variants, the most common is an inferior right hepatic vein. If the inferior right hepatic vein becomes large, sometimes draining most of the right lobe, the superior right hepatic vein may be small or even absent. In severe cirrhosis, the liver is small and shrunken, and the hepatic veins may be small and tortuous (La Berge 1995). Using CDDS, a large and patent hepatic vein has to be found for access.

Portal Venous System. A patent POV is mandatory for a functioning TIPS. The puncture site into the POV must be intrahepatic to avoid intra-abdominal hemorrhage. Shultz et al. (1994) found the bifurcation of the portal vein to be outside the liver capsule in nearly 50% of patients. As the right hepatic vein is commonly chosen for access, the entry site into the portal venous system is usually the right portal venous branch. In up to 20%, there are variations of the portal venous branching such as a trifurcation of the POV or segmental branches to segments of the right lobe coming from the left portal venous branch (La Berge 1995). Patency of the SPV and the SMV is important to provide good shunt flow. Three-dimensional US can be helpful to determine if the POV entry site is functionally intrahepatic (Rose et al. 2002).

The aim of the TIPS procedure is to decompress portal hypertension. Preinterventional sonography is important as a baseline study for comparison to evaluate shunt function in the follow-up. Various signs of portal hypertension at CDDS have been published, varying widely from patient to patient (Table 8.3). Maximum velocity in the POV and direction of flow in the main POV and in the intrahepatic branches should be recorded. The amount of ascites should be quantified as regression of ascites is a good sign for shunt function. Portosystemic shunts and collaterals should be identified (Koslin and Mizutani 1995). Especially a recanalized paraumbilical vein can become very large in diameter and may reduce flow through the TIPS significantly, possibly leading to shunt thrombosis. An accurate CDDS examination with exact documentation of pathologic findings is necessary for a useful baseline study.

Hepatic Artery. A patent hepatic artery is mandatory as the TIPS procedure leads to a decrease of portal venous liver perfusion. Hepatic artery occlusion may therefore result in hepatic insufficiency.

8.3 Sonographic Follow-up of TIPS

Follow-up CDDS examination should focus on the question of whether the TIPS remains patent or is in danger of malfunction. Diagnosis of shunt dysfunction is achieved by CDDS by demonstrating stenosis or occlusion and by assessing signs of an increased pressure in the portal venous system (Table 8.4). Post-TIPS follow-up should begin the day after the intervention as early occlusion of the stent is a rare, but well-known complication. The evaluation after 1 month allows assessment of postinterventional hemodynamic changes compared with the baseline study to obtain an individual glance at shunt function, as there is great interindividual variation in the expression of portal hypertension. Afterwards, a 3 month follow-up interval will be sufficient.

Table 8.3. US and CDDS criteria and findings associated with portal hypertension (modified according to Hennerici and Neuerburg-Heusler 1998)

Portal vein
Extrahepatic dilatation of the POV (>13–15 mm)
Round cross-sectional area
Decreased or absent respiratory modulation of flow velocity
Splenic vein
Dilated SPV (>10 mm)
Decreased or absent respiratory modulation of flow velocity
Hepatofugal flow in the SPV
Splenomegaly
Additional findings
Dilated SMV (>15 mm)
Dilated veins in the round ligament of the liver (>2.5 mm)
Hepatofugal flow in these veins (with or without dilatation)
Portocaval collateral veins
Ascites

Table 8.4. CDDS signs of normal functioning and dysfunctioning TIPS

	Normal function	Dysfunction
Peak velocity POV	30–60 cm/s	<25 cm/s
Peak velocity TIPS	100–200 cm/s	<60 cm/s
Flow within intrahepatic POV branches	Hepatofugal	Hepatopedal
Extrahepatic portosystemic collaterals	Not visible	Visible
Ascites volume	Small/absent	Increasing in
Draining liver vein	Large, hepatofugal monophasic flow	Small, cardiac variability of flow

8.3.1
Examination Technique

Using real-time gray-scale US of the upper abdomen, the position of the stent, the amount of ascites, and the morphology of the liver and spleen can be evaluated. CDDS shows the shunt from the POV up to the IVC. Peak flow velocities should be measured in the stent, most usefully in its central part, and in the POV. However, positioning of the Doppler sample volume to obtain Doppler angles less than 60° may be difficult. Use of intercostal windows for insonation, different positioning maneuvers, and the patient's cooperation are necessary. A good overview of the stent from the POV to the draining hepatic vein is found with an intercostal position of the scan head in the supine position, as shown in Fig. 8.1. Most often, the POV with real-time US and the peak velocity in the POV by CDDS near the TIPS and in the stent entrance can best be evaluated in the left decubitus position using a subcostal view. The central part of the stent may be evaluated best in the left decubitus position with an intercostal position of the scan head. This position allows a Doppler angle of less than 60° in most patients. The outflow tract is best evaluated in the supine position with a subxiphoidal CDDS approach (Fig. 8.2).

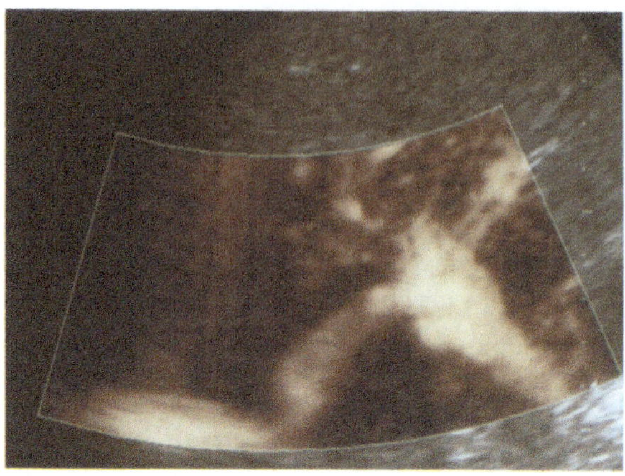

Fig. 8.1. CDDS (amplitude-encoded) image of a patent TIPS, transcostal view, supine position. The shunt is shown from the portal vein down to the IVC

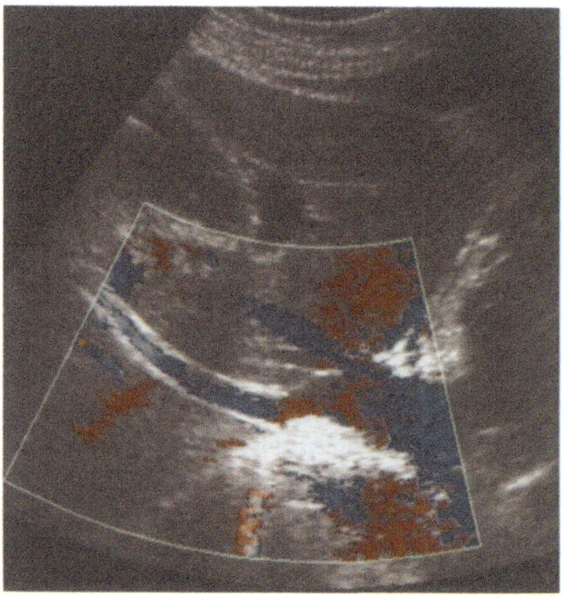

Fig. 8.2. CDDS of a patent shunt, subxiphoidal view, left lateral decubitus position. The caval aspect of the stent, the draining hepatic vein, and the IVC (forming the outflow tract) are nicely demonstrated

8.3.2
Hemodynamic Changes After TIPS Insertion

The aim of the TIPS procedure is the reduction of pressure in the portal venous system to maintain a portosystemic gradient of less than 12–15 mmHg, a level reported in the literature to be necessary to prevent recurrent hemorrhage (Saxon et al. 1995). After successful TIPS insertion, most of the portal venous blood will flow from the portal vein via the stent to the draining hepatic vein, and thus flow in and the size of portosystemic shunts and varices will decrease. Blood flow velocity in the SPV, the SMV, and the POV will increase significantly by the reduction of hemodynamic resistance, and flow will be directed hepatopedally towards the stent entrance (Sanyal et al. 1997). Maximum velocities measured in the main POV after TIPS insertion vary from 30 to 60 cm/s in patients with patent stents (Foshager et al. 1995). Flow in the intrahepatic portal venous branches will slow down and often turn hepatofugally (Wachsberg et al. 2002); in some cases, even thrombosis of intrahepatic portal venous branches will occur.

In CDDS imaging, the stent should be filled with color pixels. Within a TIPS, there is fast flow with slight undulation, and peak velocities up to 100–200 cm/s are considered normal. A normal shunt flow is shown in Fig. 8.3. There may be some variation in peak velocity measured in different parts of the stent. Usually, the fastest flow velocity will be measured in the central part of the stent and next to the draining hepatic vein, whereas flow is slowest near the portal venous side of the stent. In a recent study of 72 patients with a normally functioning TIPS, a

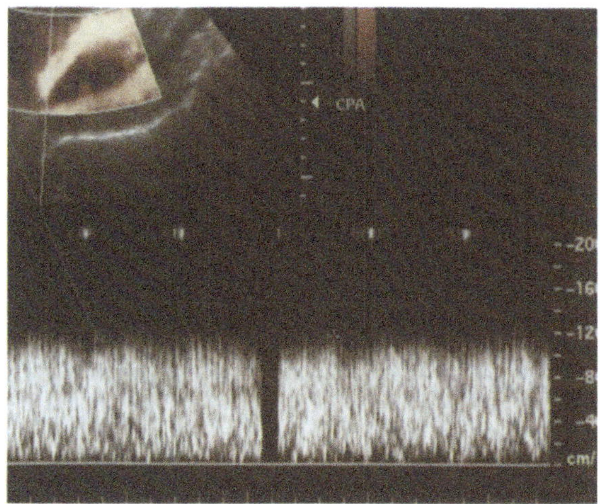

Fig. 8.3. CDDS (amplitude-encoded) image of a patent shunt, transcostal view in left lateral decubitus position. Doppler sample volume in the central part of the stent. Peak velocity about 120 cm/s

velocity gradient between the portal (range of velocities: 40–109 cm/s) and the venous side (range of velocities: 88–220 cm/s) of the TIPS was a normal finding (Bodner et al. 2000). The draining liver vein usually has a wide diameter, and the blood flow is monophasic towards the right atrium (Koslin and Mizutani 1995). In case of a weak duplex Doppler signal, the application of an attenuation-enhancing US contrast agent can be used for troubleshooting (Fürst et al. 1998).

8.3.3 TIPS Occlusion

Occlusion may be the consequence of stenosis but can also occur during the first days after the procedure, caused by procedure-related problems (Saxon et al. 1995). CDDS has a nearly 100% sensitivity and specificity for the diagnosis of shunt occlusion (Haskal et al. 1997). With frequency-encoded color Doppler, occlusion is demonstrated by the absence of color flow, a sign which may be unclear in some patients, as a weak Doppler signal may be a problem in TIPS in large patients. With amplitude-encoded Doppler, an occluded stent can be demonstrated as two parallel lines with no flow in between. Figure 8.4 shows a patent stent and an occluded stent in the same patient. These parallel lines are motion artifacts of the metallic stent caused by heartbeat or breathing motion. Besides these direct CDDS signs of occlusion, all US signs of portal hypertension may reappear. The peak flow velocity in the POV decreases, with a threshold of less than 20 cm/s proving TIPS dysfunction. The direction of flow in the intrahepatic portal venous branches turns hepatopedal again, and portosystemic shunt vessels may become visible on US again (Koslin and Mizutani 1995). In a recent study of 1192 CDDS examinations in 216 patients with TIPS during a follow-up period of 5 years, shunt occlusion was shown by CDDS in 25 of 26 angiographically proven cases (Zizka et al. 2000). Another indicator for shunt occlusion is an increasing amount of ascites. However, attention has to be paid to other causes of ascites like cardiac insufficiency or worsening liver or renal function. In patients with long-time TIPS occlusion, dislocation of the stent may occur by retraction and growth of regeneration nodules.

8.3.4 TIPS Stenosis

As reintervention is usually easier to perform in stenosed than in occluded stents, detection of stenosis as a precursor of occlusion is mandatory. As there are differences both in the diagnosis and in the reintervention procedure of stenosis of the stent itself and of the outflow tract, these entities should be differentiated. Stenosis of the POV itself is very rare. Table 8.5 summarizes CDDS criteria to differentiate occlusion, stent stenosis, and outflow tract stenosis (Dodd et al. 1995)

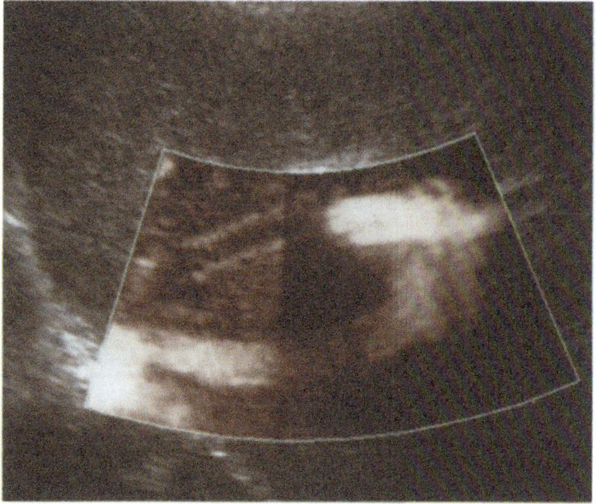

Fig. 8.4. CDDS (amplitude-encoded) image, transcostal view. Patent (color flow between 'tramlines') and occluded stent ('tramlines' without color flow more anteriorly) in the same patient

Table 8.5. CDDS differential diagnosis of shunt dysfunction

	TIPS occlusion	TIPS stenosis	Outflow tract stenosis
Stent CDDS flow	No flow, tramlines	Turbulence, narrowing	Laminar flow
Stent velocity	0	Decreased prestenotic velocity (<60 cm/s) and/or focal site of high velocity (>50 cm/s difference to prestenotic velocity)	Decreased flow velocity (<60 cm/s)
Draining liver vein	Small	Small	Severe narrowing

8.3.4.1
Outflow Tract Stenosis

The outflow tract consists of the IVC and the draining HV. As known from dialysis fistulas, the turbulent and fast flow from the stent induces intimal hyperplasia in the draining liver vein. Intimal hyperplasia reduces the diameter of the draining HV. Additionally, there can be some mechanical injury of the stent in the HV (SAXON et al. 1995). The caval aspect of the stent and the draining HV may be difficult to evaluate by CDDS because of motion artifacts (heart, respiration) and normal high velocity. In our experience, amplitude-encoded color Doppler may be superior to conventional color Doppler in identifying stenosis, as frequency-encoded Doppler relies on the detection of high velocity and focal turbulence, which may be obscured by artifacts. Figure 8.5 shows a severe stenosis of the caval aspect of the stent and the HV. Severe HV stenosis reduces the flow in the stent, and peak velocity in the stent decreases. A decrease of the peak velocity in the TIPS to less than 60 cm/s and a decrease of flow velocity in the POV to less than 20 cm/s are recommended thresholds to diagnose shunt dysfunction. However, one has to consider that there is great interindividual variation in peak velocities (besides interobserver variation), leading to high specificity (0.86) but low sensitivity (0.57) of these thresholds (HASKAL et al. 1997). Comparison with baseline studies is very important for accurate interpretation of the velocity parameters. In addition, there are some other causes for a decrease in peak velocities within the TIPS and POV like right heart insufficiency or hypovolemia.

8.3.4.2
Stent Stenosis

Stenosis of the stent itself is caused by pseudointimal hyperplasia. Bile duct injury during the TIPS procedure might be a causative factor (SAXON et al. 1995). Using CDDS, stent stenosis can be proven by showing focal acceleration and turbulence of flow within the stenotic segment or by demonstrating the peripheral

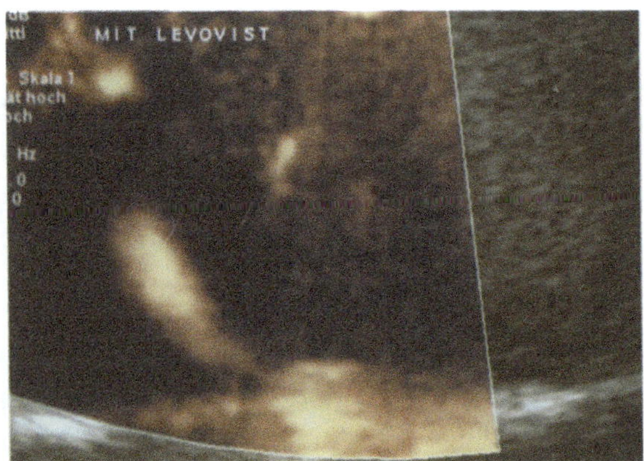

a

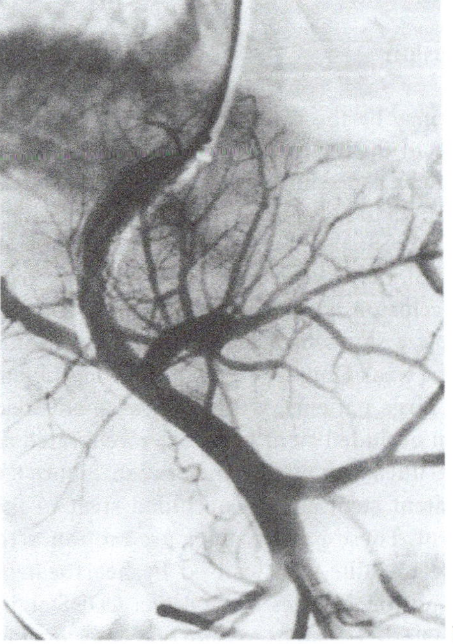

b

Fig. 8.5a,b. Severe stenosis of the hepatic vein. **a** CDDS (amplitude-encoded) image, subxiphoidal view, supine position. **b** Corresponding shunt angiogram

decrease of flow. There is some increase in flow velocity from the portal aspect towards the caval aspect of the stent, but focal turbulence and an increase of flow velocity of more than 50 cm/s above baseline are considered evident signs for stenosis. In a recent study, the combination of velocity criteria (peak intrashunt velocity ≥250 cm/s, maximum velocity in the portal third of the shunt ≤50 cm/s, or maximum POV velocity less than or equal to two-thirds of the baseline value) revealed shunt stenosis in 103 of 110 cases (sensitivity 0.94) (Zizka et al. 2000). Another parameter influenced by shunt malfunction is the number of cardiac pulsations in the Doppler spectral waveforms within the stent and in the POV and HV (Sheiman et al. 2002).

In our experience, a short stenosis is easier to diagnose with frequency-encoded color Doppler, as artifacts may obscure these stenoses when using amplitude-encoded color Doppler. Figure 8.6 shows a short but significant stenosis in the central part of a stent. Extensive stenosis may be difficult to detect, as sometimes the whole length of the stent appears concentrically narrowed. In this situation, the peak flow velocity in the whole stent is increased, simulating normal flow within a patent stent. In this situation, one has to rely on the reduced peak velocity in the POV and other signs of shunt dysfunction. Most helpful is the comparison with a previous CDDS examination under identical technical circumstances. The stenosis itself may be demonstrated with amplitude-encoded color Doppler as shown in Fig. 8.7 by demonstrating the narrowed lumen and the stent mesh. A large dilated paraumbilical vein in a patient with a TIPS may impede the diagnosis

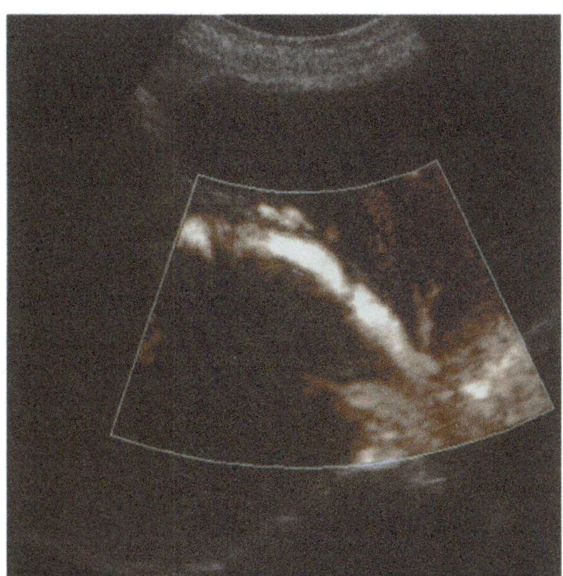

a

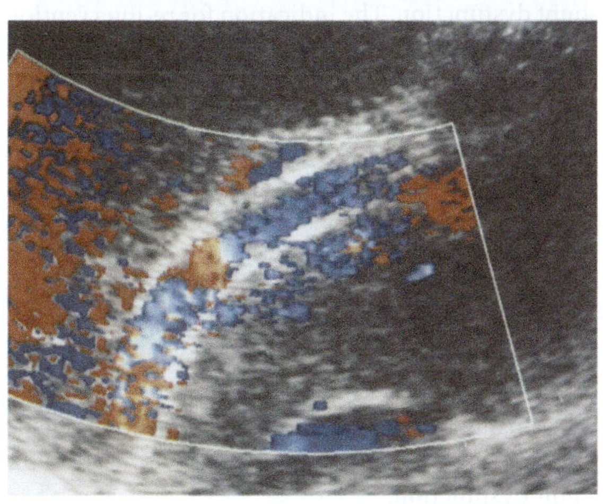

b

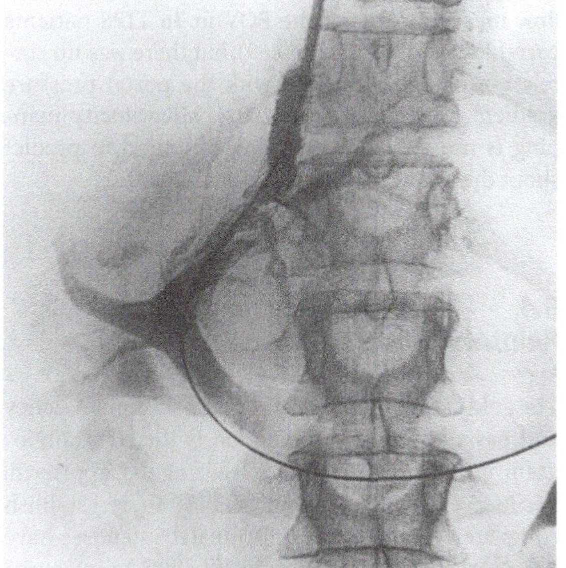

c

Fig. 8.6a–c. Severe stenosis in the center of the stent proven by shunt angiography. **a** CDDS (amplitude-encoded image, subxiphoidal view, left lateral decubitus position) shows short narrowing of the stent. **b** CDDS (frequency-encoded) shows focal increase in shunt flow velocity (aliasing, red color). **c** Corresponding shunt angiogram demonstrating severe narrowing in the center of the shunt

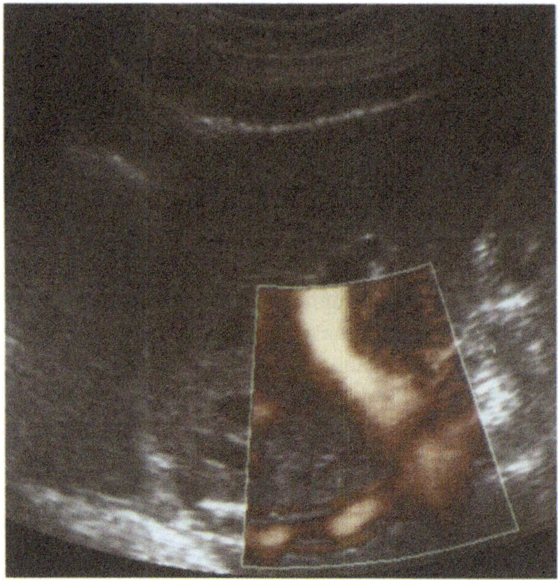

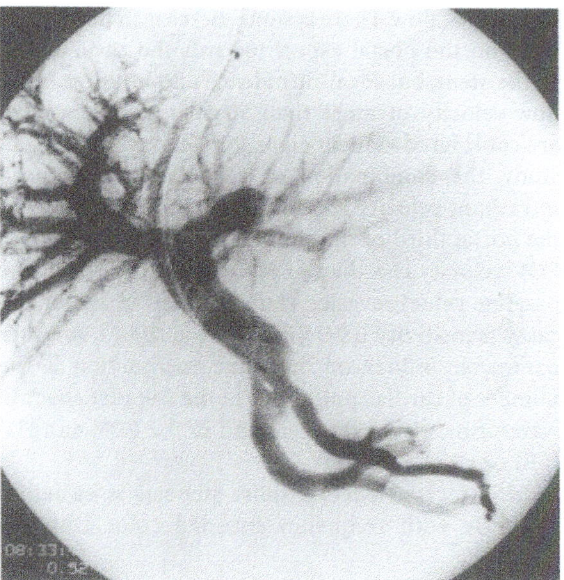

Fig. 8.7a,b. Severe stenosis of the shunt and the outflow tract. **a** CDDS (amplitude-encoded image, subxiphoidal view, supine position) shows significant stenosis of the outflow tract. The stent mesh can be delineated as motion artifacts, indicating severe stenosis. **b** Stent angiogram proves significant stenosis

of shunt dysfunction. One of our patients presented with severe stenosis of the stent in combination with a widely dilated paraumbilical vein serving as a portosystemic collateral. In this patient, both the peak velocity in the stent (150 cm/s) and the peak velocity in the POV (70 cm/s) suggested a patent shunt, as POV blood flow bypassed the liver and the stenosed TIPS via the paraumbilical vein.

Recently, MR flow quantification in the POV has been used for the follow-up of patients with TIPS instead of CDDS (Schlegel et al. 2002). MR-derived flow measurements of the POV in 36 TIPS patients correlated with CDDS (r=0.69), but there was no correlation of either method with the portal pressure gradient (Schlegel et al. 2002). MR velocity mapping is not adequate as a single method to predict shunt dysfunction (Schlegel et al. 2002).

8.4 Reintervention

The gold standard for the evaluation of shunt patency and basis of any re-intervention is the stent angiogram usually obtained via a transjugular approach. Re-intervention has a 90% chance to re-establish complete TIPS patency. Unfortunately, stenoses have a tendency to reoccur, and thus further re-interventions will be necessary to achieve continued optimal shunt function (Saxon et al. 1995). As every re-intervention is an invasive procedure requiring sedation or general anesthesia of the patient, a careful indication is mandatory. Indications for re-intervention may be clinical signs of shunt dysfunction or significant stenosis or stent occlusion suggested by CDDS. Clinical signs of shunt dysfunction are rebleeding or growing amounts of ascites. Saxon et al. reported in 1995 that all patients with endoscopically documented variceal re-bleeding had shunt stenosis or occlusion proven by stent angiography. On the other hand, about two-thirds of patients with shunts found to be stenosed or occluded by CDDS or venogram lack symptoms of shunt dysfunction. The indication for re-intervention therefore has to consider both clinical symptoms and the results of CDDS. In patients undergoing regular CDDS follow-up, without re-bleeding, shunt angiograms should only be performed if signs of occlusion or severe stenosis are found. In patients with a recurrent episode of upper gastrointestinal bleeding, a shunt angiogram is necessary if there are any CDDS signs of shunt dysfunction. If CDDS demonstrates a patent shunt in these patients, gastroscopy will be performed to find any another source of bleeding. In patients with fast growing amounts of ascites, right heart insufficiency or deteriorating hepatic or renal function have to be ruled out if CDDS is negative for shunt dysfunction.

References

Bodner G, Peer S, Kreczy A, Waldenberger P, Fries D (2000) Results of Doppler sonography in normally functioning transjugular portosystemic shunts. Ultraschall Med 2: 160–164

Dodd GD, Zajko AB et al (1995) Detection of transjugular intrahepatic portosystemic shunt dysfunction: value of duplex Doppler sonography. Am J Roentgenol 164: 1119–1124

Flora KD, Benner KG (1995) TIPS: a hepatologist's view. Semin Interv Radiol 12:389–395

Foshager MC, Ferral H et al (1995) Duplex sonography after transjugular intrahepatic portosystemic shunts (TIPS): normal hemodynamic findings and efficacy in predicting shunt patency and stenosis. Am J Roentgenol 165:1–7

Fürst G, Malms J et al (1998) Transjugular intrahepatic portosystemic shunts: improved evaluation with echo enhanced color Doppler sonography, power Doppler sonography and spectral duplex sonography. Am J Roentgenol 170: 1047–1054

Haskal ZJ, Carroll JW et al (1997) Sonography of transjugular intrahepatic potosystemic shunts: detection of elevated portosystemic gradients and loss of shunt function. J Vasc Interv Radiol 8:849–856

Hennerici M, Neuerburg-Heusler D (1998) Vascular diagnosis with ultrasound. Springer, Stuttgart Berlin Heidelberg New York

Koslin DB, Mizutani PA (1995) Noninvasive evaluation of TIPS. Semin Interv Radiol 12:368–374

LaBerge JM (1995) Anatomy relevant to the transjugular intrahepatic portosystemic shunt procedure. Semin Interv Radiol 12:337–346

LaBerge JM, Somberg KA et al (1995) Two-year outcome following transjugular intrahepatic portosystemic shunt for variceal bleeding: results in 90 patients. Gastroenterology 108:1143–1151

Lakin PC, Saxon RR et al (1995) TIPS: indications and techniques. Semin Interv Radiol 12:347–354

Richter GM, Palmaz JC et al (1989) Der transjuguläre intrahepatische portosystemische Stentshunt (TIPSS). Radiologe 29:406–411

Rose SC, Behling C, Roberts AC, Pretorius DH, Nelson TR, Kinney TB, Masliah E, Hassanein TI (2002) Main portal vein access in transjugular portosystemic shunt procedures: use of three-dimensional ultrasound to ensure safety. J Vasc Interv Radiol 13:267–273

Sanyal AJ, Freedman AM et al (1997) The natural history of portal hypertension after transjugular intrahepatic portosystemic shunts. Gastroenterology 112:889–898

Saxon RR, Keller FS (1997) Technical aspects of accessing the portal vein during the TIPS procedure. J Vasc Interv Radiol 8:733–744

Saxon RR, Barton RE et al (1995) Prevention, detection, and treatment of TIPS stenosis and occlusion. Semin Interv Radiol 12:375–383

Schlegel PM, Tombach B, Reimer P, Vestring T, Menzel J, Moller HE, Heindel W (2002) The value of magnetic resonance imaging (MRI) for the follow-up of patients with transjugular intrahepatic portosystemic shunts (TIPS). Fortschr Geb Röntgenstr Neuen Bildgeb Verfahr 174:224–230

Sheiman RG, Vrachliotis T, Brophy DP, Ransil BJ (2002) Transmitted cardiac pulsations as an indicator of transjugular intrahepatic portosystemic shunt function: initial observation. Radiology 224:225–230

Shultz SR, La Berge JM et al (1994) Anatomy of the portal vein bifurcation: intra- versus extrahepatic location—implications for transjugular intrahepatic portosystemic shunts. J Vasc Interv Radiol 5:457–459

Wachsberg RH, Bahramipour P, Sofocleous CT, Barone A (2002) Hepatofugal flow in the portal venous system: pathophysiology, imaging findings, and diagnostic pitfalls. Radiographics 22:123–140

Zizka J, Elias P, Krajina A, Michl A, Lojik M, Ryska P, Maskova J, Hulek P, Safka V, Vanasek T, Bukaz J (2000) Value of Doppler sonography in revealing transjugular intrahepatic portosystemic shunt malfunction: a 5-year experience in 216 patients. Am J Roentgenol 175:141–148

9 Doppler Imaging of Lower Extremity Deep Venous Thrombosis

M. M. Baldt, T. Zontsich, G. H. Mostbeck

CONTENTS

9.1 Introduction

Acute deep venous thrombosis (DVT) is a common and serious clinical entity that requires early and accurate diagnosis and therapy before life-threatening complications, e.g., pulmonary thromboembolism (PE), occur. It is estimated that over 90% of pulmonary emboli originate from the area of the lower extremity and the pelvis, demonstrating the intimate relationship between PE and DVT as a pathophysiological entity (venous thromboembolism, VTE) (Weinmann and Salzman 1994).

Furthermore, a significant number of patients develop a postphlebitic syndrome following DVT, leading to severe edema and inability to work (Gaitini et al. 1990; Monreal et al. 1993). Early diagnosis can lead to immediate treatment, possibly reducing the incidence and the severity of postphlebitic syndrome.

During the last 20 years, a significant number of published articles have described the different ultrasound techniques such as real-time B-mode ultrasound, duplex scanning (DS), and color-coded duplex Doppler sonography (CDDS) in the diagnosis of DVT and compared these results to other tests.

Today, US is an established and widely available technique for the diagnosis of DVT. However, several critical issues remain unsolved, such as the accuracy in the detection of free-floating thrombi and of isolated calf vein thromboses, the usefulness of bilateral examinations in the asymptomatic patient, and the role of CDDS in the diagnostic algorithm of VTE in times of increasing clinical application of spiral computed tomography (CT) and magnetic resonance imaging (MR) for the detection of PE and DVT.

This article will review the assessment of venous clot by US techniques compared with other imaging modalities such as contrast venography (CV), CT and MR, the relationship of DVT to PE, and the long-term-consequences of DVT.

9.2 Clinical Epidemiology

DVT and PE generally are common disorders. In 1985, a total of 187,000 patients was treated in the USA for DVT, PE contributed to more than 30,000 deaths and was diagnosed 120,000 times in inpatients (Gillum 1987). These figures have not improved over the intervening years. The risk of DVT after a knee or hip operation is high, with estimated frequencies of 40–70%, and a 2–5% risk for symptomatic PE (Gallus et al. 1973).

Most venous thrombi are clinically silent when they are first detected by imaging methods (Wein-

M. M. Baldt, MD
Associate Professor of Radiology, Bilddiagnostik Wolfsberg, Rossmarkt 14, 9400 Wolfsberg, Austria
T. Zontsich, MD
Ambulatorium für Computertomographie, Ultraschall und moderne Schnittbilddiagnostik, Ferdinand Porsche Ring 10, 2700 Wiener Neustadt, Austria
G. H. Mostbeck, MD
Professor of Radiology, Sozialmedizinisches Zentrum, Baumgartner Höhe mit Pflegezentrum, Otto Wagner Spital, Sanatoriumstrasse 2, 1140 Vienna, Austria

mann and Salzman 1994), probably because they do not totally obstruct the vein or there is sufficient collateral circulation. Therefore, the clinical diagnosis is unreliable, and less than one-third of patients present with classic symptoms (pain, discomfort, edema, positive Homans's sign, etc.) (Haeger 1969). In fewer than 50% of patients with a clinical suspicion of DVT is this diagnosis confirmed by imaging tests (Weinmann and Salzman 1994).

The most important risk factors for venous thromboembolism are immobilization (after trauma or operation, bus or air travel: 'economy class syndrome'), hypercoagulability, obesity, and neoplasm. There is a significantly higher incidence of cancer in patients with DVT in follow-up periods (Baron et al. 1998).

9.3 Ultrasound Assessment of DVT of the Lower Extremity

9.3.1 Real-time B-mode US

The compression technique of the deep veins is usually performed from the level of the inguinal ligament to the confluens of the peroneal and tibial veins below the knee (Cronan 1993). Adequate gain settings require that normal vessels be free of internal echoes. This can be managed by comparing the US signal within the vein to that of the accompanying artery (or vein of the opposite side, where appropriate). The examination is performed in the longitudinal and transverse planes with respect to the vessel's course. The longitudinal plane is used for primary orientation and localization of the vein, whereas the optimal plane for the compression technique is transverse, since the transducer cannot 'roll off' the vein.

The compression should be sufficient to dimple the overlying skin. The pressure is excessive when the arterial vessel is compressed, too. Compression of a normal vein completely collapses the venous lumen, while DVT prevents venous wall collapse (Fig. 9.1). In some patients, complete compression of the vein in the adductor canal region may be difficult or even impossible (Cronan 1993). Some authors report a very low specificity of vein incompressibility for this part of the thigh (Killewich et al. 1989). The amount of compression required in these areas may be significant.

Comparison with CV has demonstrated that US may sometimes underestimate the extent of the clot. Clot echogenicity is very variable, depending on the age, localization, and extent of the clot and transducer frequency (Fobbe et al. 1991). Fresh thrombi may demonstrate no internal echoes and can be missed by US (Murphy and Cronan 1990). Therefore, clot echogenicity is an unreliable parameter for determining the age of a clot. Further confusion may arise because slow-flowing blood can appear highly echogenic, mimicking a clot (Fig. 9.2). The only parameter which allows us to estimate the age of a clot is the diameter of the occluded vein. If the diameter of the vein exceeds twice the diameter of the accompanying artery, the age of the thrombus can be estimated to be less than 10 days (Fobbe et al. 1991).

The normal response of veins of the lower extremity to the Valsalva maneuver is an increase in diameter, while an occluded vein does not do this. While

a 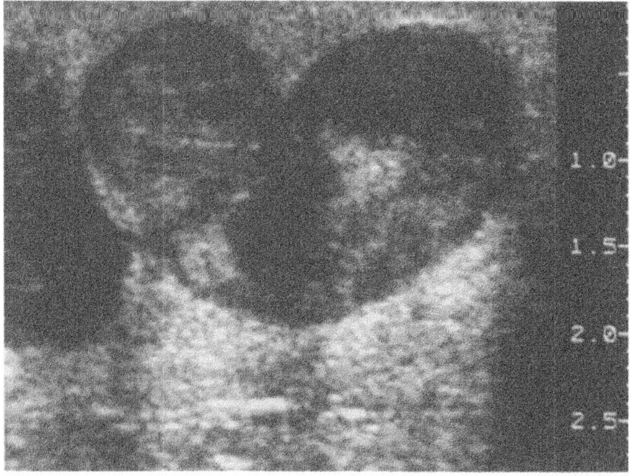

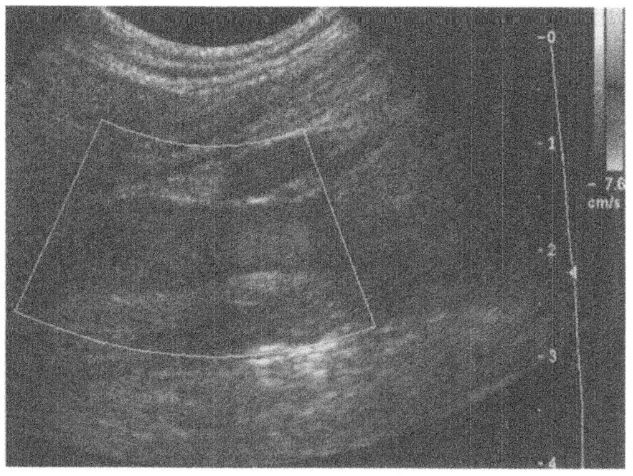 b

Fig. 9.1. a Thrombosis of the GSV. Echogenic material (clot) in the vein, the GSV cannot be compressed by the scan head. **b** Thrombosis of the POPV. Lack of color coding and echogenic material in the POPV

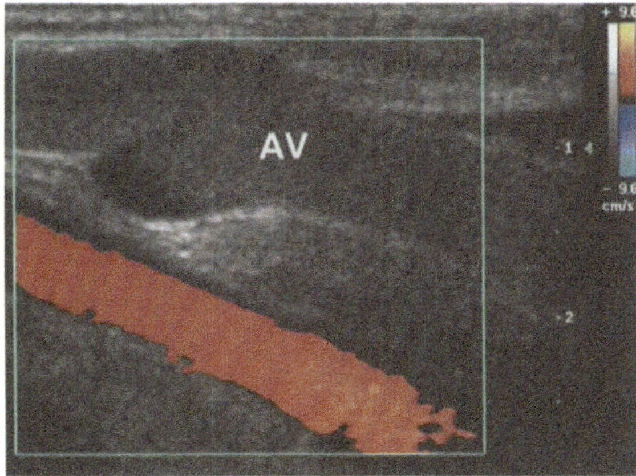

Fig. 9.2. Longitudinal CDDS of the left AV and axillary artery (encoded in *red*) in a patient with compression of the SV and AV by massive lymph node enlargement due to B-cell lymphoma (not shown). Note high echogenicity of stagnant blood in the AV

this finding is very efficient in the inguinal and upper femoral region, its significance diminishes down to the knee or calf region. Excellent patient cooperation is essential for the usefulness of this finding (Effeney et al. 1984).

Numerous articles indicate that B-mode US is an excellent tool for the diagnosis of above-the-knee clots. However, others argue that vein incompressibility as the major criterion for DVT should be used with caution (Killewich et al. 1989). Nevertheless, among the diagnostic criteria for DVT (Table 9.1), the most reliable sign is the detection of a filling defect during compression (Appelman et al. 1987). The abnormal response to the Valsalva maneuver is less reliable, with a reported sensitivity of 82% and specificity of 80% (Effeney et al. 1984).

Table 9.1. B-mode criteria for the detection of DVT

Filling defect during compression
Increase of venous diameter
Abnormal or missing response to Valsalva maneuver
Direct visualization of thrombus

Direct visualization of the thrombus is unreliable. Cronan et al. (1987) detected 14 of 25 true-positive DVTs (56%) only by abnormal compressibility. Direct visualization of the clot was not possible in these cases (Cronan et al. 1987). However, as US techniques have improved over the years, this might not hold true to that extent for state-of-the-art US today, but compression still remains the diagnostic key using B-mode US.

Table 9.2 demonstrates an overview of published articles comparing real-time B-mode sonography to CV. For the thigh region, most authors report high sensitivities and specificities (up to 98% and 100%, respectively). In contrast, Ginsberg et al. (1991) reported a low sensitivity of 65% for the detection of DVT in postoperative asymptomatic patients, compared with a sensitivity of 92% in symptomatic patients. This points to the fact that in this cohort of patients, isolated, nonoccluding, proximal thrombi are at present easily missed by US. A recent article (Screaton et al. 1998) reports a higher number of false-negative US findings in patients with duplicated femoral veins (6%) compared with patients with single femoral veins (2%).

US data for the detection of calf vein thrombosis are very inhomogeneous (Dauzat et al. 1986; Ginsberg et al. 1991; Habscheid and Landwehr 1990; Herzog et al. 1991; Pedersen et al. 1991). The reported sensitivities range from 14% to 90%. These differences can only be explained in part by different criteria for thrombosis (e.g., occluding vs nonoccluding thrombi) and different inclusion criteria (e.g., symptomatic vs asymptomatic patients).

Table 9.2. Comparison of real-time B-mode US to CV for the diagnosis of DVT

Reference	Patients	Extremities	Total (%)	Thigh (%)	Calf (%)
			Sens/Spec	Sens/Spec	Sens/Spec
Habscheid and Landwehr (1990)	238	301	91/99	97/99	90/99
Pedersen et al. (1991)	215	218	-/-	89/97	50/-
Vogel et al. (1987)	54	54	-/-	91–94	-/-
Cronan et al. (1987)	51	51	89/100	-/-	-/-
Ginsberg et al. (1991)	130 (asympt.)	247	-/-	65/99	52/97
	65 (sympt.)	98	-/-	92/95	-/-
Appelman et al. (1987)	112	112	-/-	96/97	-/-
Dauzat et al. (1986)	145	145	-/-	94/100	62/-
Herzog et al. (1991)	101	113	-/-	98/98	60/97

9.3.2 Duplex Scanning

The combination of real-time B-mode US with pulsed Doppler technique allows us to evaluate blood flow noninvasively. Although Duplex without color Doppler is technically outdated, evaluation of blood flow by pulsed Doppler remains an integral part of a comprehensive CDDS examination. Normal and augmented duplex Doppler findings of the lower leg and pelvic veins are discussed in Chapter 3. All these parameters are impaired or not detectable with DVT. In addition, valvular competency can be assessed by DS using the Valsalva maneuver or manual compression of a more proximal part of the vein. If retrograde flow is observed in deep lower leg veins, this indicates valvular incompetence resulting from valve damage due to either prior DVT (postthrombotic syndrome) or massive recirculation in extensive varicosis.

Duplex Doppler criteria of DVT are demonstrated in Table 9.3. Killewich et al. (1989) evaluated different duplex Doppler criteria for the diagnosis of DVT and concluded that a single criterion is insufficient. The best results are obtained with a combination of direct clot visualization, absence of spontaneous flow, and absence of respiration-modulated phasicity.

Table 9.4 reviews the results of DS compared with CV in the diagnosis of DVT. In general, the results of DS in the diagnosis of above-the-knee DVT are excellent (sensitivity 90–100% and specificity 83–100%) (De Valois et al. 1990; Killewich et al. 1989; Krings et al. 1990; Mitchell et al. 1991; Quintavalla et al. 1992; Rosner and Doris 1988; Wichert et al. 1993). Again, inhomogeneous results are given for the calf. Here, the best result is a reported sensitivity of 93% and a specificity of 96% (Krings et al. 1990), in contrast to a study which was false-negative in all 20 cases (Mitchell et al. 1991).

Table 9.3. Duplex Doppler criteria for the detection of DVT

No flow signal at the DVT
Proximal to thrombus:
Impaired flow velocity
No flow augmentation following distal compression
Distal to thrombus:
No cardiac or respiratory phasicity of flow
Impaired or missing response to Valsalva maneuver
Increased flow velocity in GSV compared to other (normal) limb

9.3.3 CDDS

CDDS adds an additional criterion to the diagnosis of DVT: the lack of color coding. Nearly all authors recommend the use of color imaging, if available (Baxter et al. 1992; Becker et al. 1997; Cronan 1992, 1993; Davidson et al. 1992; Dorfman and Cronan 1992; Fernandez-Canton et al. 1994; Fobbe et al. 1989; Fürst et al. 1990; Grosser et al. 1991; Lausen et al. 1995; Lewis et al. 1994; Mattos et al. 1992; Mostbeck et al. 1993; Rose et al. 1990; Vanninen et al. 1993). Another advantage using CDDS is that the vein can be localized very quickly, thus shortening the examination time (Cronan 1992, 1993; Mostbeck et al. 1993) and allowing the detection of flow in small calf veins by using the color signal of adjacent arteries as a useful landmark. The color signal can be augmented by distal manual compression of the vein (Cronan 1992, 1993). This is especially helpful in regions where compression B-mode US is limited, such as the pelvic veins, the SFV in the adductor channel or the calf veins, or when there is severe edema. Another advantage of CDDS is the unequivocal differentiation between floating and wall-adherent thrombus (Dorfman and Cronan 1992; Mostbeck et al. 1993) (Fig. 9.3). Free-floating thrombi represent a greater risk for PE (Mostbeck et al. 1993; Voet and Afschrift 1991).

Table 9.5 summarizes the literature comparing CDDS with CV. Again, excellent results are reported

Table 9.4. Comparison of DS to CV for the diagnosis of DVT

Authors	Patients	Extremities	Total (%)	Thigh (%)	Calf (%)
			Sens/Spec	Sens/Spec	Sens/Spec
Wichert et al. (1993)	98	113	88/88	94/97	91/95
Rosner and Doris (1988)	32	32		90/100	
Krings et al	182	235		98/97	93/96
Quintavalla et al. (1992)	157	157	77/98	97/98	0/0
De Valois et al. (1990)	180	101		92/90	
Mitchell et al. (1991)	65	64	96/85	93/92	81/89
Killewich et al. (1989)	47	50	95/83		

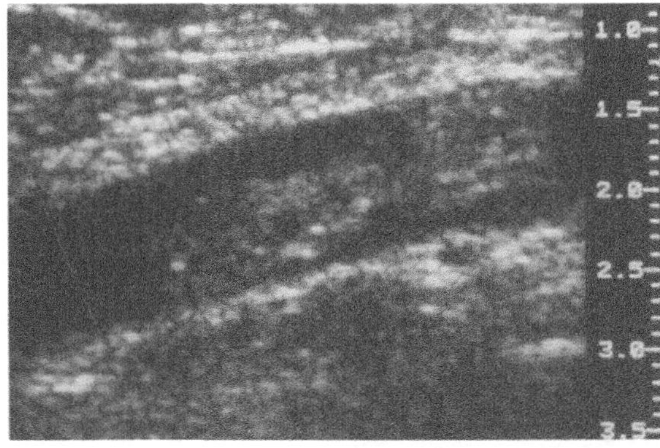

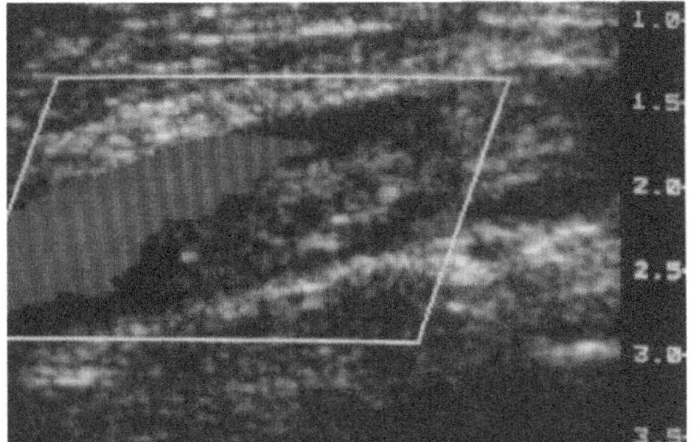

Fig. 9.3a,b. B-mode (**a**) and CDDS image (**b**) of floating thrombus within POPV

for proximal DVT in symptomatic patients. Results in asymptomatic patients and below-the-knee results are more inhomogeneous.

9.4 Regions of the Lower Limb

9.4.1 Calf Veins

The clinical importance of calf vein DVT is a matter of debate. Demers et al. (1998) found calf DVT in 24 of 184 asymptomatic patients (13%) after knee arthroscopy, other authors report calf DVT in 15% after hip or knee surgery and more than 45% after coronary artery surgery (Demers et al. 1998; Ginsberg et al. 1991; Reis et al. 1991). In symptomatic patients, the incidence of calf DVT is even higher (De Valois et al. 1990).

Over the last few years, many clinicians considered the benefits of treating isolated calf DVT worth the risk of anticoagulation, thus pointing to the need for an early and accurate diagnosis (Weinmann and Salzman 1994). Some 20–30% of primary isolated calf thrombi may propagate to the femoropopliteal veins with increasing risk for PE (Weinmann and Salzman 1994). Even without propagation, calf thrombi can cause PE. The risk of isolated calf vein DVT causing PE is discussed controversially. Some authors think that PE predominantly originates from proximal extension (Dorfman and Cronan 1992), others found PE in 29–50% of patients with isolated calf DVT (De Valois et al. 1990, Mostbeck et al. 1979; Stiegler et al. 1991). Different methods of diagnosing DVT and PE as well as different scintigraphic definitions of PE only partly explain these differences.

Table 9.5. Comparison of CDDS to CV for the diagnosis of DVT

References	Patients	Extremities	Total (%)	Thigh (%)	Calf (%)	Comments[a]
			Sens/Spec	Sens/Spec	Sens/Spec	
Baxter et al. (1992)	50	40		100/100	95/100	sy
Grosser et al. (1991)	325	325		98/98	96/96	sy
Fürst et al. (1990)	75	102		90–95/ 97–99	72/100	sy
Fobbe et al. (1989)	103	129		96/97		sy
Lewis et al. (1994)	97	99		95/99		sy
Becker et al. (1997)	268	526	98/96			sy
Rose et al. (1990)	69	75	79/88	92/100	73/86	sy
Mattos et al. (1992)	75	77		100/99	94/75	sy
	99	190		67/100	56/98	asy
Fernandez-Canton et al. (1994)	30	60	53/100	83/100	40/100	asy
Davidson et al. (1992)	319	319		38/92	20/-	asy
Vanninen et al. (1993)	51	102	77/96			asy
Lausen et al. (1995)	82	164			43/99	asy

[a] *sy*, symptomatic patients; *asy*, asymptomatic patients

Direct US evaluation of the calf veins is successful in approximately 60–80% of patients (Cronan 1993; Rose et al. 1990). Calf vein US requires a commitment of an additional 10–20 min examination time and is much easier using CDDS. Some authors prefer the patient in the sitting position, as it causes passive distention of the calf veins, permitting them to be visualized more easily (Cronan 1993).

Nevertheless, the diagnostic accuracy of B-mode and compression US to detect calf thrombi is discussed controversially. Reported sensitivities range from 14% to 90% (see Table 9.4) in comparison with the 'gold standard' CV, and one has to be aware that CV is subject to a high interobserver variability (McLachlan et al. 1979) and that up to 6.6% of calf venograms may be inadequate (Baldt et al. 1993). This prompted some investigators to recommend a repeated sonographic study between 1 and 14 days later when the first sonographic study is negative for DVT (Birdwell et al. 1998). However, a recent study demonstrated that this strategy can be avoided in patients classified with intermediate or high clinical risk for DVT, as a second examination 1 week later detected only an additional 1% of DVTs (Friera et al. 2002).

When technically adequate, US may identify DVT in muscle veins like the soleus veins, which are not visualized by CV (Simons et al. 1995). Hollerweger et al. (2000) investigated 357 consecutive patients with a suspicion of DVT by CDDS. A total of 85 patients (47% of all patients with DVT) showed isolated calf vein thrombosis, in 45 patients (25%) the gastrocnemial and/or soleal veins were the only site of thrombosis. Interestingly, the embolic frequency for isolated calf vein thrombosis and muscular calf vein thrombosis was 48% and 50%, respectively (Hollerweger et al. 2000).

Thus, in daily clinical practice, calf veins should not be disregarded during examination for DVT as is done by some authors, for the sake of saving examination time. The examination of the whole leg is recommended to prevent some loss of diagnostic efficacy (Frederick et al. 1996). The whole leg should be systemically examined with the useful addition of CCDS, if available. In addition, an excellent knowledge of venous anatomy and variant anatomy and enough time for the examination are factors leading to good results in the diagnosis of calf vein DVT (Mostbeck et al. 1993).

In a review of 1231 patients with DVT, 96% had one or more predisposing risk factors (Anderson and Wheeler 1992). Therefore, patients with clinical risk factors and negative US as well as patients with ambiguous or inconclusive US results should undergo other tests like CV, which seems to remain the accepted 'standard' in the detection of calf vein DVT (Fig. 9.4) (Becker et al. 1997; Laissy et al. 1996; Redman 1988; Vanninen et al. 1993).

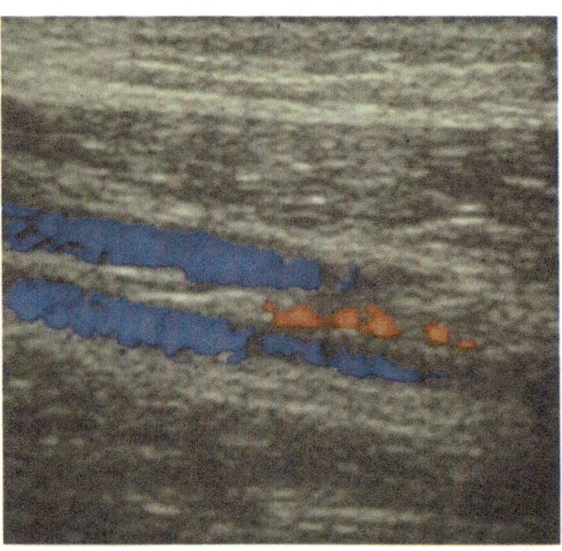

a

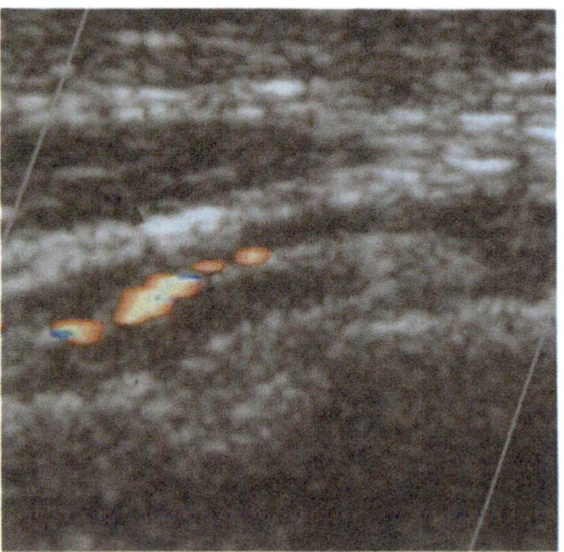

b

Fig. 9.4a,b. DVT of the PTV. **a** CDDS in a normal volunteer. Posterior tibial artery (*red*) accompanied by the paired PTVs (*blue*). **b** CDDS in DVT of the PTVs. Artery (*red*) accompanied by hypoechoic, thrombosed veins without color-encoded blood flow

9.4.2 Femoropopliteal Veins

In general, there are excellent results for US in the diagnosis of femoropopliteal DVT in symptomatic patients (see Tables 9.2, 9.4, 9.5) due to the good US visibility of these veins and ease of compression

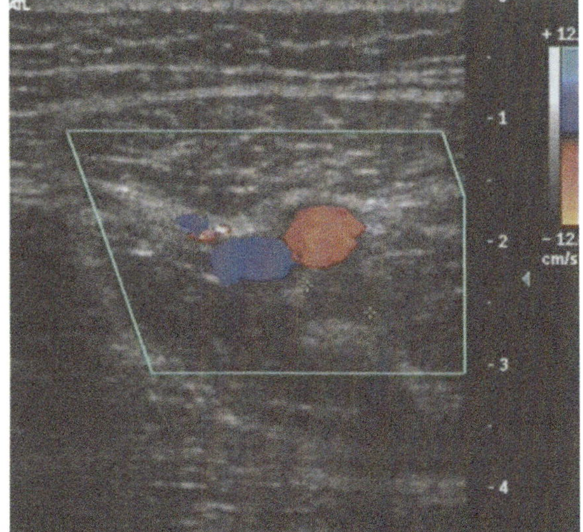

a

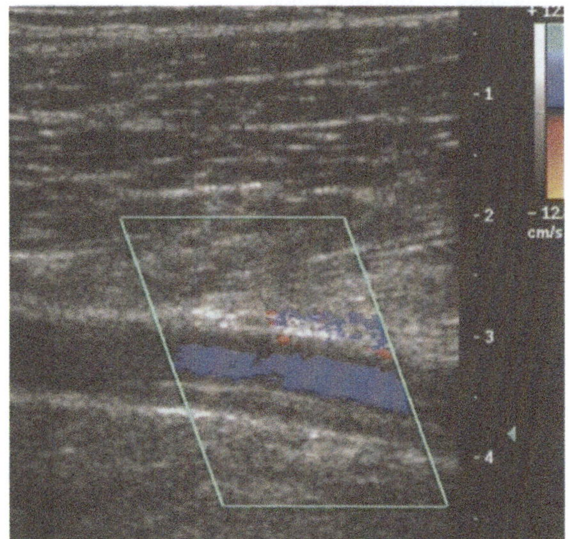

b

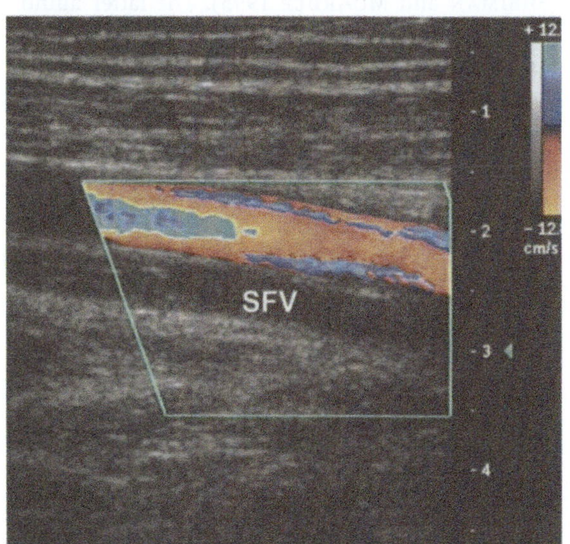

c

Fig. 9.5a–c. DVT of one branch of a doubled SFV. **a** Transverse CDDS image of the right thigh. Superficial femoral artery (*red*), patent lateral (*blue*) and thrombosed (between *crosses*) medial branch of the doubled SFV. Longitudinal CDDS images of the patent (*blue*) (**b**) and thrombosed (**c**) branch of the SFV. SF artery encoded in *red*

applied to them (Fig. 9.5). An exception to this rule is SFV within the adductor's channel, where it may be difficult to examine due to severe adipositas, edema, or hematoma (Zwiebel and Priest 1990). Isolated or free-floating thrombi are better evaluated by CDDS than by compression US alone (Mostbeck et al. 1993; Voet and Afschrift 1991).

However, a meta-analysis of 30 studies of asymptomatic patients after orthopedic surgery showed only a moderate overall sensitivity of 62% and a positive predictive value (PPV) of 66% for US detection (including CDDS) of proximal DVT (Wells et al. 1995). Articles were only included if they fulfilled three criteria. These were: established, objective criteria for CV and US, independent blinded comparison of US and CV, and prospective study design. The same authors analyzed another group of papers not fulfilling all three criteria: Sensitivity and PPV in this group were 100%. The authors concluded that US has only a moderate sensitivity when used to screen for DVT after surgery in asymptomatic patients (Wells et al. 1995).

9.4.3 Iliac Veins

Isolated iliac vein thrombosis is a rare event (Zwiebel and Priest 1990), but frequently associated with PE (Figs. 9.6, 9.7) (Stiegler et al. 1991). CIV and in part EIV are not visible in some patients due to overlying bowel gas and/or adipositas (Zwiebel and Priest 1990). In addition, these veins cannot be compressed adequately (Herzog et al. 1991; Mostbeck et al. 1993; Zwiebel and Priest 1990).

Many studies comparing US and CV for the diagnosis of DVT did not evaluate the pelvic veins, and vice versa, other authors found difficulties in the delineation of the proximal extent of DVT in the iliac veins or IVC (Cronan et al. 1987; Habscheid and Landwehr 1990). Using duplex Doppler, the reported sensitivity is 78% for the detection of DVT (Herzog et al. 1991). CDDS may further improve US results (Mostbeck et al. 1993). Even if the iliac veins are not completely visible, duplex and color

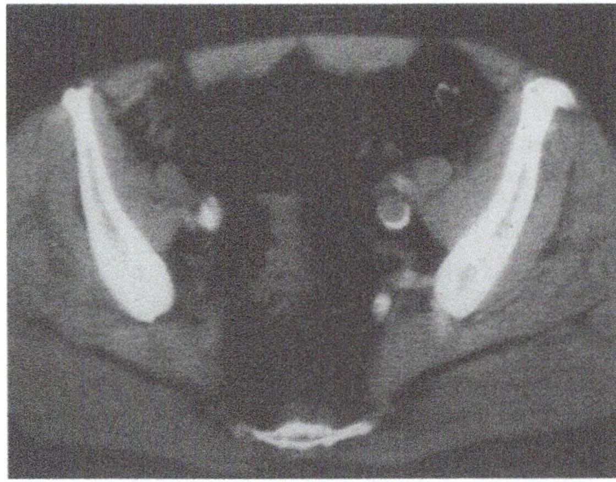

Fig. 9.6. **a** DVT of the left iliac vein. Note hypoechoic clot surrounded by some blood flow encoded in blue. **b** Corresponding S-CT venography demonstrating hypodense clot surrounded by contrasted blood

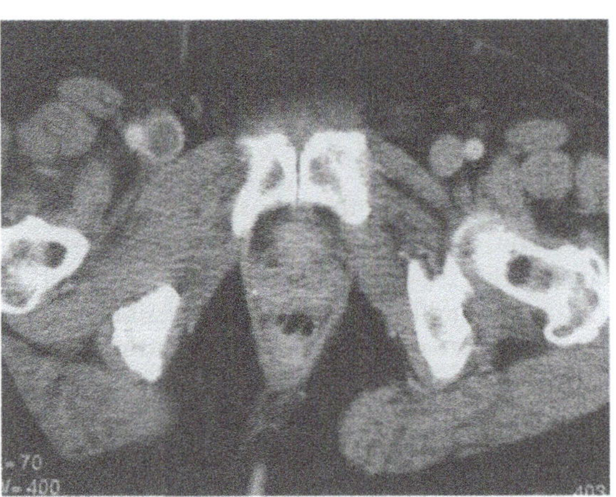

Fig. 9.7. S-CT of right CFV thrombosis. Note hypodense clot within enlarged right CFV compared with the normal left CFV

Doppler may show indirect hemodynamic changes in the femoral vein suggesting pelvic DVT (Dorfman and Cronan 1992). As CV also may be limited in the pelvic region (Baldt et al. 1993; McLachlan et al. 1979), some authors recommend CT or MRI for evaluation of the iliac veins and IVC (Baldt et al. 1997; Laissy et al. 1996; Mostbeck et al. 1993). Using MR and CV, Laissy et al. (1996) detected thrombi in the pelvic and lumbar veins which were missed by CDDS. MR may become the noninvasive method of choice to clarify ambiguous US or CV results (Carpenter et al. 1993; Evans et al. 1993; Laissy et al. 1996).

9.5 Bilateral vs Unilateral Imaging in DVT

There is some controversy about the need for bilateral diagnostic imaging in the patient with unilateral symptoms of DVT (Cronan 1996; Keogan et al. 1994; Lohr et al. 1994; Naidich et al. 1996; Sheiman and McArdle 1995). In three publications, DVT was detected by US in the asymptomatic limb of 5–27% patients with unilateral symptomatic DVT (Keogan et al. 1994; Lohr et al. 1994; Naidich et al. 1996). In contrast, another US study of 206 patients with symptoms suspicious for DVT on one side found no DVT in any contralateral asymptomatic extremity (Sheiman and McArdle 1995). The latter authors concluded that bilateral examination is not necessary in patients with unilateral symptoms. In another series, DVT was detected in 4 asymptomatic limbs among 47 patients (9%), 2 of them with a history of PE (Baldt et al. 1997).

Thus, a bilateral US examination seems to be justified in patients with both bilateral and unilateral symptoms and in suspected PE, if there are clinical risk factors for DVT (Cronan 1996).

9.6 Recurrent DVT

Late changes after DVT include not only incompetent, damaged valves but also persistent organized clot and venous occlusion with echogenic material. There may be partial recanalization of the clot with thickening of the walls and the presence of collateral veins (Fig. 9.8) (GAITINI et al. 1990). Thus, compression US may not be reliable for making a diagnosis (CRONAN 1993). The high incidence of postphlebitic changes (40–80% of patients) and the high risk of recurrent acute DVT in postphlebitic veins may create a diagnostic dilemma: Are the patient's symptoms due to 'old' DVT, or is there acute, recurrent DVT (GAITINI et al. 1990; MONREAL et al. 1993)?

The size of the vein may help in determining the age of the thrombus. In acute DVT, the vein can enlarge to twice the size of the accompanying artery (FOBBE et al. 1991). In chronic disease, the vein is nearly similar to the size of the artery or even smaller. CDDS seems to be helpful in assessing the thickness of the wall by contrasting the flowing blood (CRONAN 1993; FOBBE et al. 1991). However, neither the normal size of the vein nor accompanying collateral veins can rule out acute DVT (CRONAN 1993). Therefore, some authors recommend serial US examinations after DVT or a baseline US after 12 months to look for changes suggesting recurrent disease (CRONAN 1993; GAITINI et al. 1990). If these examinations are not available, patients should undergo other tests like CV.

Recent studies have demonstrated the usefulness of CT and MRI in recurrent DVT, resulting in a better accuracy compared with CV and surgery (BERGIN et al. 1997; SPRITZER et al. 1998). MR can demonstrate changes of the signal intensity of a thrombus over a period of at least 1.5 years, thus helping to distinguish acute DVT from residual changes (SPRITZER et al. 1998).

9.7 Postphlebitic Syndrome

The anatomic and pathophysiologic changes after DVT are known as postphlebitic or postthrombotic syndrome. Damage to the valves following DVT leads to permanent venous valve incompetence. Increased pressure develops in the venous system, especially when the patient is standing or sitting. Fluid extrav-

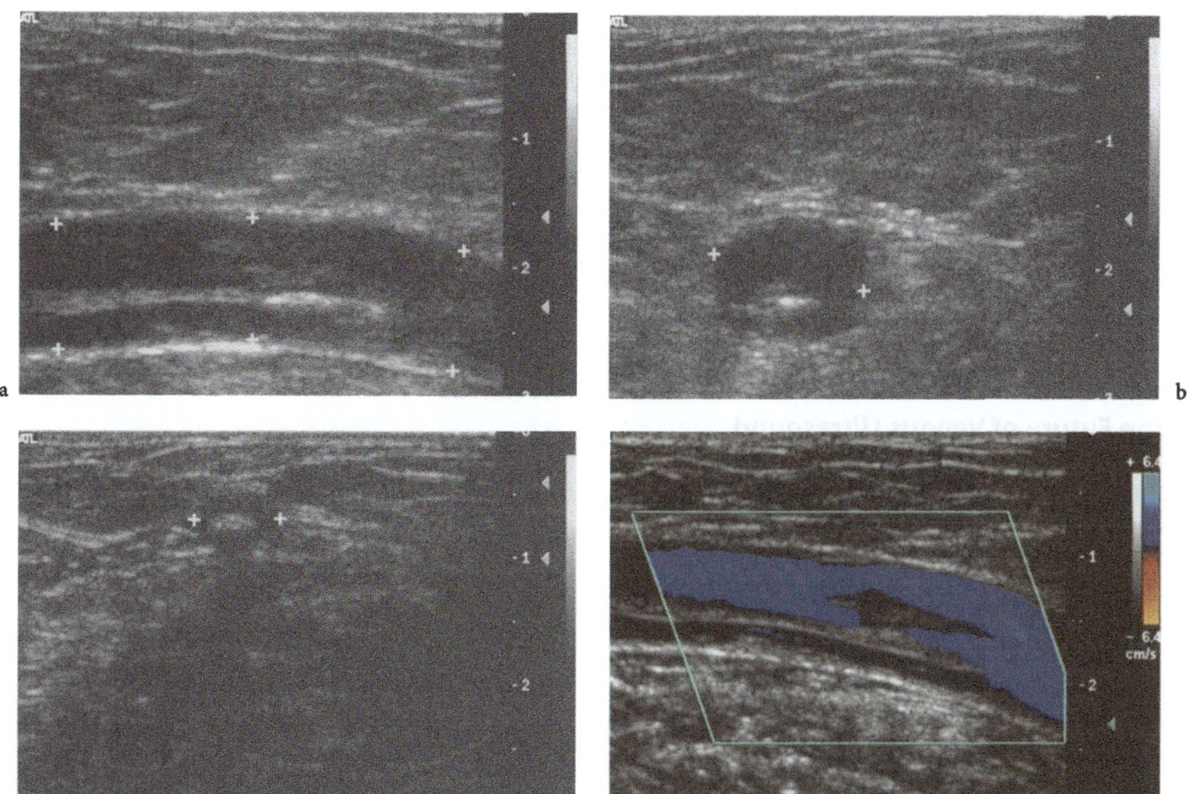

Fig. 9.8a–d. Old (>1.5 years) DVT of the GSV. **a** Longitudinal scan demonstrates echogenic material within GSV (GSV between *crosses*). Transverse scan (**b**) also demonstrating old clot within GSV, which is not completely compressible (**c**). **d** CDDS demonstrating old clot and partial recanalization

asates out of the vein into the soft tissues, leading to edema, pain, cell death, and ulceration (Cronan 1993). Venous backflow shifts from the intrafascial to the extrafascial venous system, resulting in extensive collateral veins.

US evaluation of chronic venous insufficiency should be performed in the supine and erect positions using CDDS (Baldt et al. 1995). Reversal of flow following the Valsalva maneuver or manual compression should last not longer than 0.5 s if the valves are competent. Pathological reflux is mostly detected in the GSV or in the CFV (Cronan 1993).

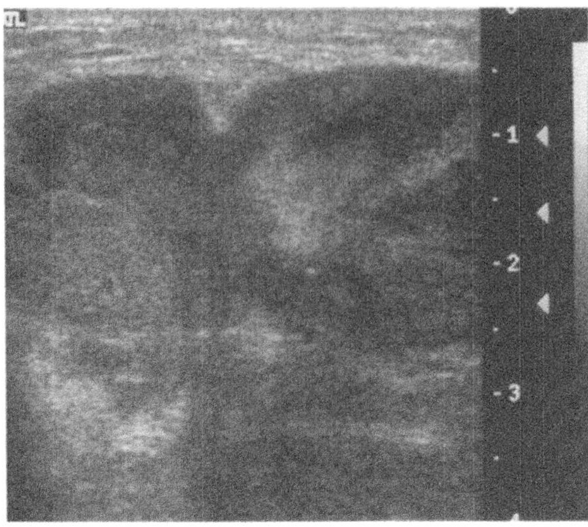

Fig. 9.9. Enlarged, pathologic lymph node in the left inguinal region in a patient with B-cell lymphoma and lower extremity edema without DVT

9.8 Ancillary Findings

One major advantage of US compared with CV is that other possible reasons for the patient's symptoms beside DVT, such as enlarged lymph nodes, Baker cysts, or muscle injury, are easily depicted (Fig. 9.9). Using CDDS, arterial disease (pseudoaneurysms, etc.) can be evaluated. In addition, superficial thrombophlebitis can be detected (see Fig. 9.1a), which may have an underestimated role in the development of VTE. A review of this topic found a 35% rate of superficial clot extension into the deep venous system, accompanied by episodes of PE (Lutter et al. 1991). Thus, in patients with superficial clot, follow-up examinations to determine clot extension are strongly recommended (Cronan 1993).

9.9 The Future of Venous Ultrasound

Many authors indicate an expanded use of lower limb venous US for the future, with US probably becoming the primary imaging technique used in the detection of DVT in symptomatic patients, as already done in many centers. Even the refinement of the CT and MR technique with 'one-stop shopping' for PE and DVT by multislice-spiral CT angiography and venography or MR-venography has not displaced US from its role as the first-choice study in VTE.

The use of contrast media in combination with harmonic imaging and new transducer technologies are possible recommendations for the future for clot detection (Coley et al. 1994; Rizzatto 1998; Whittingham 1997). However, some of the above-mentioned limitations and difficulties for the diagnosis of DVT will remain.

State-of-the-art CDDS of the lower limb veins has dramatically increased in importance for the diagnosis of DVT during the last few years. Today, US in experienced hands offers high sensitivity and specificity in symptomatic patients. In asymptomatic patients with risk factors for DVT and in recurrent DVT, the accuracy is lower, but US is still the primary imaging technique, leaving other invasive or expensive modalities to patients with inconclusive US results.

References

Anderson FA, Wheeler HB (1992) Physician practices the management of venous thromboembolism: a community-wide survey. J Vasc Surg 15:707–714

Appelman PT, de Jong TE, Lampmann LE (1987) Deep venous thrombosis of the leg: US findings. Radiology 163: 743–746

Baldt MM, Zontsich T, Wiesmayr M et al (1993) Phlebographie der Beinvenen. Radiologe 33:491–497

Baldt MM, Böhler K, Zontsich T et al (1995) Preoperative imaging of lower extremitiy varicose veins. J Ultrasound Med 15:143–154

Baldt MM, Zontsich T, Kainberger F et al (1997) Spiral CT evaluation of deep venous thrombosis. Semin Ultrasound CT MRI 18:369–375

Baron JA, Gridley G, Weiderpass E et al (1998) Deep venous thromboembolism and cancer. Lancet 351:1077–1080

Baxter GM, Duffy P, Partridge E (1992) Color flow imaging of calf vein thrombosis. Clin Radiol 46:198–201

Becker D, Günter E, Strauss R et al (1997) Color Doppler imaging versus phlebography in the diagnosis of deep leg and pelvic vein thrombosis. J Ultrasound Med 16:31–37

Bergin CJ, Sirlin CB, Hauschildt JP et al (1997) Chronic thromboembolism: diagnosis with helical CT and MR imaging with angiographic and surgical correlation. Radiology 204: 695–702

Birdwell BG, Raskob GE, Whitsett TL et al (1998) The clinical validity of normal compression ultrasonography in outpatients suspected of having deep venous thrombosis. Ann Intern Med 128:1–7

Carpenter JP, Holland GA, Baum RA et al (1993) Magnetic resonance venography for the detection of deep venous thrombosis: comparison with contrast venography and duplex Doppler ultrasonography. J Vasc Surg 18:734–741

Coley BD, Trambert MA, Mattrey RF (1994) Perfluorocarbon-enhanced sonography value in the detection of acute venous thrombosis in rabbits. Am J Roentgenol 163:961–967

Cronan JJ (1992) Ultrasound evaluation of deep venous thrombosis. Semin Roentgenol 27:39–52

Cronan JJ (1993) Venous thromboembolic disease: the role of US. Radiology 186:619–630

Cronan JJ (1996) Deep venous thrombosis: one leg or both legs? Radiology 200:323–324

Cronan JJ, Dorfman GS, Scola FH, Schepps B, Alexander J (1987) Deep venous thrombosis: US assessment using vein compression. Radiology 162:191–194

Dauzat MM, Laroche JP, Charras C et al (1986) Real-time B-mode ultrasonography for better specificity in the noninvasive diagnosis of deep venous thrombosis. J Ultrasound Med 5:625–631

Davidson BL, Elliott CG, Lensing AW (1992) Low accuracy of color Doppler ultrasound in the detection of proximal leg vein thrombosis in asymptomatic high-risk patients. Ann Intern Med 117:735–738

Demers C, Marcoux S, Ginsberg JS et al (1998) Incidence of venographically proved deep venous thrombosis after knee arthroscopy. Arch Intern Med 158:47–50

De Valois JC, van Schaik CC, Verzijlbergen F et al (1990) Contrast venography: from gold standard to „golden backup" in clinically suspected deep vein thrombosis. Eur J Radiol 11:131–137

Dorfman GS, Cronan JJ (1992) Venous ultrasonography. Radiol Clin North Am 30:879–894

Effeney DJ, Friedman MB, Gooding GAW (1984) Ileofemoral thrombosis: real time ultrasound diagnosis, normal criteria and clinical application. Radiology 150:787–792

Evans AJ, Sostman HD, Knelson MH et al (1993) Detection of deep venous thrombosis: prospective comparison of MR imaging with contrast venography. Am J Roentgenol 161: 131–139

Fernandez-Canton G, Vidaur IL, Munoz F et al (1994) Diagnostic utility of color Doppler ultrasound in lower limb deep vein thrombosis in patients with clinical suspicion of pulmonary thromboembolism. Eur J Radiol 19:50–55

Fobbe F, Koennecke HC, El Bedewi M et al (1989) Diagnostik der tiefen Beinvenenthrombose mit der farbkodierten Duplexsonographie. Rofo Fortschr Geb Röntgenstr Neuen Bildgeb Verfahr 151:569–573

Fobbe F, Ruhnke-Trautmann M, Gemmeren D et al (1991) Age determination of venous thrombosis by ultrasound. Fortschr Röntgenstr 155:344–348

Frederick MG, Hertzberg BS, Kliewer MA et al (1996) Can the US examination for lower extremity deep venous thrombosis be abbreviated? A prospective study of 755 examinations. Radiology 199:45–47

Friera A, Gimenez NR, Caballero P, Molini PS, Suarez C (2002) Deep vein thrombosis: can a second sonographic examination be avoided? Am J Roentgenol 178:1001–1005

Fürst G, Kuhn FP, Trappe RP et al (1990) Diagnostik der tiefen Beinvenenthrombose. Farbdopplersonographie versus Phlebographie. Rofo Fortschr Geb Röntgenstr Neuen Bildgeb Verfahr 152:151–158

Gaitini D, Kaftori JK, Pery M et al (1990) Late changes in veins after deep venous thrombosis: ultrasonographic findings. Fortschr Röntgenstr 153:68–72

Gallus AS, Hirsh H, Tuttle RJ et al (1973) Small subcutaneous doses of heparin in prevention of venous thrombosis. N Engl J Med 288:545–551

Gillum RF (1987) Pulmonary embolism thrombophlebitis in the United States 1970–1985. Am Heart J 114:1261–1264

Ginsberg JS, Caco CC, Brill-Edwards PA et al (1991) Venous thrombosis in patients who have undergone major hip or knee surgery: detection with compression US and impedance plethysmography. Radiology 181:651–654

Grosser S, Kreymann G, Kühns A (1991) Stellenwert der farbkodierten Duplexsonographie bei der Diagnostik von akuten und chronischen venösen Erkrankungen der unteren Extremität. Ultraschall Med 12:222–227

Habscheid W, Landwehr P (1990) Diagnostik der akuten tiefen Beinvenenthrombose mit der Kompressionssonographie. Ultraschall Med 11:268–273

Haeger K (1969) Problems of acute deep venous thrombosis. The interpretation of signs and symptoms. Angiology 20: 219–230

Herzog P, Anastasiu M, Wollbrink W et al (1991) Real-time Sonographie bei tiefer Becken- und Beinvenenthrombose. Ein prospektiver Vergleich zur Phlebographie. Med Klin 86:132–137

Hollerweger A, Macheiner P, Rettenbacher T, Gritzmann N (2000) Sonographic diagnosis of thrombosis of the calf muscle veins and the risk of pulmonary embolism. Ultraschall Med 21:66–72

Keogan MT, Paulson EK, Paine SS et al (1994) Bilateral lower extremity evaluation of deep venous thrombosis with color flow and compression sonography. J Ultrasound Med 13: 115–118

Killewich LA, Bedford GR, Beach KW (1989) Diagnosis of deep venous thrombosis. A prospective study comparing duplex scanning to contrast venography. Circulation 79:810–814

Krings W, Adolph J, Diederich S et al (1990) Diagnostik der tiefen Becken- und Beinvenenthrombose mit der hochaiflösenden real-time und CW-Doppler-Sonographie. Treffsicherheit und Grenzen. Radiologe 30:525–531

Laissy JP, Cinqualbre A, Loshkajian A et al (1996) Assessment of deep venous thrombosis in the lower limbs and pelvis: MR venography versus duplex Doppler sonography. Am J Roentgenol 167:971–975

Lausen I, Jensen R, Wille-Jorgensen P et al (1995) Colour Doppler flow imaging ultrasonography versus venography as screening method for asymptomatic postoperative deep venous thrombosis. Eur J Radiol 20:200–204

Lewis BD, James EM, Welch TJ et al (1994) Diagnosis of acute deep venous thrombosis of the lower extremities: prospective evaluation of color Doppler flow imaging versus venography. Radiology 192:651–655

Lohr JM, Hasselfeld KA, Byrne MP et al (1994) Does the asymptomatic limb harbor deep venous thrombosis? Am J Surg 168:184–187

Lutter KS, Kerr TM, Roedersheimer LR et al (1991) Superficial thrombophlebitis diagnosed by duplex scanning. Surgery 110:42–46

Mattos MA, Londrey GL, Leutz DW et al (1992) Color flow duplex scanning for the surveillance and diagnosis of acute deep venous thrombosis. J Vasc Surg 15:366–375

McLachlan MSF, Thomson JG, Taylor DW et al (1979) Observer variation in the interpretation of lower limb venograms. Am J Roentgenol 132:227–229

Mitchell DC, Grasty MS, Stebbings WS et al (1991) Comparison of duplex sonography and venography in the diagnosis of deep venous thrombosis. Br J Surg 78:611–613

Monreal M, Martorelli A, Callejas JM et al (1993) Venographic assessment of deep venous thrombosis and risk of developing postthrombotic syndrome: a prospective study. J Intern Med 233:233–238

Mostbeck A, Partsch H, Lofferer O (1975) Untersuchungen zur Häufigkeit von Lungenembolien bei tiefer Bein- und Beckenvenenthrombose. Folia Angiol 23:243–249

Mostbeck GH, Kettenbach J, Henk C (1993) Comparison of sonography and venography in the diagnosis of lower extremity deep venous thrombosis. Radiologe 33:498–507

Murphy TP, Cronan JJ (1990) Evolution of deep venous thrombosis: a prospective evaluation with US. Radiology 177: 543–548

Naidich JB, Torre JR, Pellerito JS et al (1996) Supected deep venous thrombosis: is US of both legs necessary? Radiology 200:429–431

Pedersen OM, Aslaksen A, Vik MH, Bassoe AM (1991) Compression ultrasonography in hospitalized patients with suspected deep venous thrombosis. Arch Intern Med 151: 2217–2220

Quintavalla R, Larini P, Miselli A et al (1992) Duplex ultrasound diagnosis of symptomatic proximal deep venous thrombosis of lower limbs. Eur J Radiol 15:32–36

Redman HC (1988) Deep venous thrombosis: is contrast venography still the diagnostic «gold standard»? Radiology 168:277–278

Reis SE, Polak JF, Hirsch DR et al (1991) Frequency of deep venous thrombosis in asymptomatic patients with coronary artery bypass grafts. Am Heart J 122:475–481

Rizzatto G (1998) Ultrasound transducers. Eur J Radiol 27 [Suppl 2]:188–195

Rose SC, Zwiebel WJ, Nelson BD et al (1990) Symptomatic lower extremity deep venous thrombosis: accuracy, limitations, and role of color duplex flow imaging in diagnosis. Radiology 175:639–644

Rosner NH, Doris PE (1988) Diagnosis of femoropopliteal venous thrombosis: comparison of duplex sonography and plethysmography. Am J Roentgenol 150:623–627

Screaton JS, Gillard JH, Berman LH, Kemp PM (1998) Duplicated superficial femoral veins: a source of error in the sonographic investigation of deep vein thrombosis. Radiology 206:397–401

Sheiman RG, McArdle CR (1995) Bilateral lower extremity US in the patient with unilateral symptoms of deep venous thrombosis: assessment of need. Radiology 194:171–173

Simons GR, Skibo LK, Polak JF et al (1995) Utility of leg ultrasonography in suspected isolated calf deep venous thrombosis. Am J Med 99:43–50

Spritzer CE, Trotter P, Sostman HD (1998) Deep venous thrombosis: gradient-recalled-echo MR imaging changes over time—experience in 10 patients. Radiology 208: 631–639

Stiegler H, Weichenhain B, Chatzopulos D et al (1991) Incidence and symptomatology of lung embolism in relation to the site of deep venous thrombosis. Vasa 20:119–124

Vanninen R, Manninen H, Soimakallio S et al (1993) Asymptomatic deep venous thrombosis in the calf: accuracy and limitations of ultrasonography as a screening test after total knee arthroplasty. Br J Radiol 66:199–202

Voet D, Afschrift M (1991) Floating thrombi: diagnosis and follow-up by duplex ultrasound. Br J Radiol 64:1010–1014

Vogel P, Laing FC, Jeffrey RJ, Wing VW (1987) Deep venous thrombosis of the lower extremity: US evaluation. Radiology 163:747–751

Weinmann EE, EW Salzman (1994) Deep-vein thrombosis. N Engl J Med 331:1630–1641

Wells PS, Lensing AWA, Davidson BL (1995) Accuracy of ultrasound for the diagnosis of deep venous thrombosis in asymptomatic patients after orthopedic surgery: a meta-analysis. Ann Intern Med 122:47–53

Whittingham TA (1997) New and future developments in ultrasonic imaging. Br J Radiol 70:119–132

Wichert C, Gmelin E, Jansen O (1993) Diagnostik der Beinvenenthrombose mit der Duplexsonographie. Aktuel Radiol 3:37–42

Zwiebel WJ, Priest DL (1990) Color duplex sonography of extremity veins. Semin Ultrasound CT MR 11:136–167

10 Preoperative Assessment of Varicosis of the Lower Extremity by Doppler Techniques

T. Zontsich and M. Baldt

CONTENTS

10.1 Introduction

Varicose veins affect an estimated 57% of men and 68% of women in the middle-aged population of the Western world. Approximately 13% of patients with varicosis ultimately develop venous ulceration. In addition to conservative treatment, complete stripping of the GSV has been recommended as the surgical procedure of choice for patients with varicose veins. This approach has been questioned in recent years because normal veins could be required as graft material for bypass procedures. Thus, preservation of normal segments of the GSV with more sophisticated surgical approaches is justified. These more complex and less invasive or even endoscopic surgical techniques also require detailed preoperative information about normal and variant venous anatomy, incompetent venous segments, and incompetent perforators.

T. Zontsich, MD
Ambulatorium für Computertomographie, Ultraschall und moderne Schnittbilddiagnostik, Ferdinand Porsche Ring 10, 2700 Wiener Neustadt, Austria
M. Baldt, MD
Associate Professor of Radiology, Bilddiagnostik Wolfsberg, Rossmarkt 14, 9400 Wolfsberg, Austria

10.2 Etiology

10.2.1 Primary Varicosis

The most important predisposing factors for the development of primary varicosis are genetic disposition and sex. In addition, hormonal factors, age, and lifetime habits influence the probability for the development of primary varicosis. Because of these predisposing factors, a primary dilatation of the superficial venous system develops, which leads to primary insufficiency of the venous valves in the saphenofemoral or saphenopopliteal junction. In some cases, an isolated valvular insufficiency develops in perforating veins. Because of this insufficiency of the transfascial communications and reflux into the superficial venous system, an overload of blood volume evolves in the GSV or SSV, leading to progressive dilatation and to insufficiency of more distal valves (Fig. 10.1).

There are different forms of primary varicosis depending on the location of the incompetent superficial venous valves.

Complete truncal varicosis of the GSV is the most common manifestation, which is characterized by reflux in the saphenofemoral junction (Fig. 10.2). Depending on the degree of insufficiency, the reflux may be seen down to the proximal thigh, defined as grade 1 insufficiency (Fig. 10.3). If there is reflux down to the distal thigh, grade 2 is present (Fig. 10.4). Grade 3 is defined as reflux down to the proximal calf, and in patients with grade 4 insufficiency, dilatation

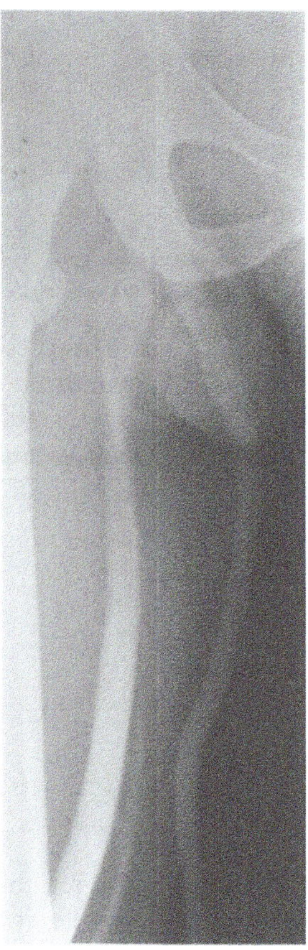

Fig. 10.1. Ascending venogram demonstrating a dilatation of the proximal GSV in a patient with primary varicosis

of and reflux within the GSV down to the ankle is demonstrated (Fig. 10.5).

Complete truncal insufficiency of the SSV results from incompetence of the saphenopopliteal junction (Fig. 10.6). The location of the saphenopopliteal junction varies greatly. Because of this wide variance, knowledge of the site of the saphenopopliteal junction is very important information for the surgeon prior to ligation and stripping of the SSV. A reflux down to the first valves of the SSV is defined as grade 1 insufficiency (Fig. 10.7), whereas grade 2 is defined as reflux down to the middle of the calf (the area where the SSV penetrates through the superficial fascia). In grade 3 varicosis of the SSV, the reflux is seen down to the ankle (Fig. 10.8).

The second group of primary varicosis is incomplete truncal varicosis of the GSV or SSV. Incomplete truncal varicosis develops when the insufficient junction between the superficial and the deep venous system is located more distally. In most cases, this is caused by incompetence of perforating veins, while the saphenofemoral or saphenopopliteal junction is sufficient. In these cases, the identification of this proximal incompetent perforator is crucial prior to surgery.

A third group of primary varicose veins involves isolated varicosis of branches of the GSV. In these cases, the location of the site of the junction with regard to the deep venous system is the most important task of

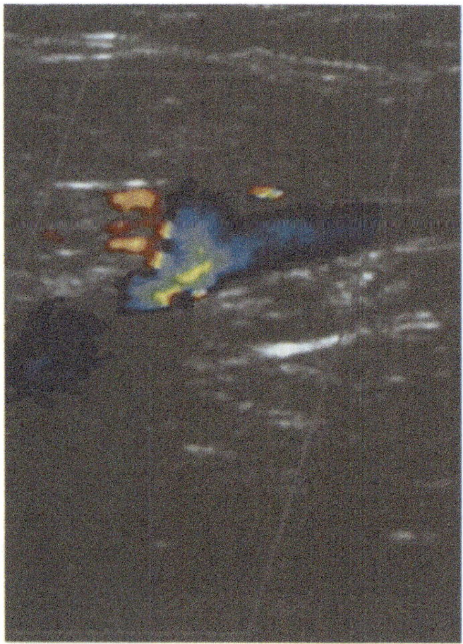

a

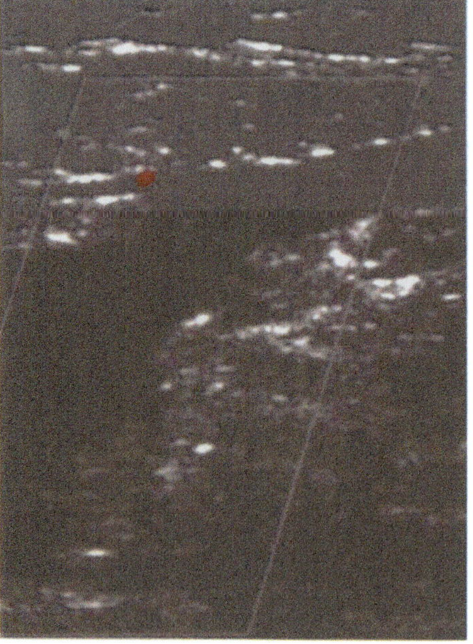

b

Fig. 10.2a, b. Sufficient saphenofemoral junction. CDDS before (a) and during (b) the Valsalva maneuver. Antegrade flow in a, no reflux in b

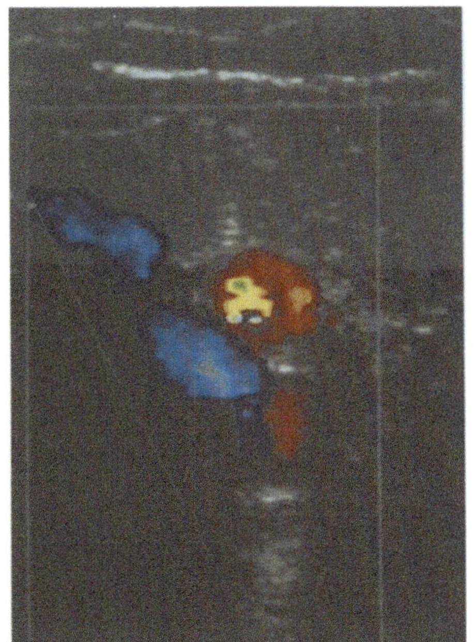

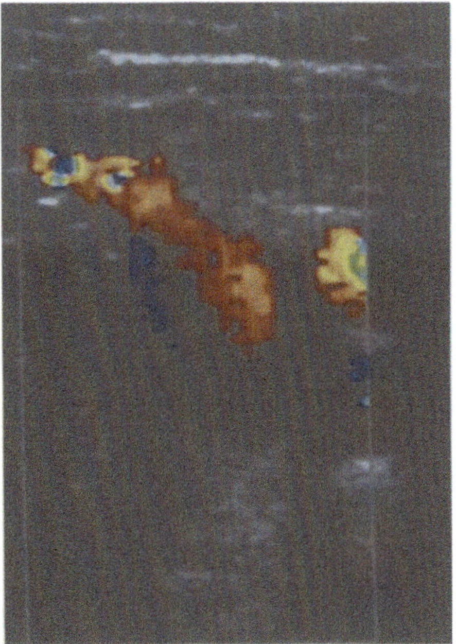

Fig. 10.3a, b. Incompetent saphenofemoral junction. CDDS before (a) and during (b) the Valsalva maneuver. There is reversed blood flow in b indicating valve incompetence

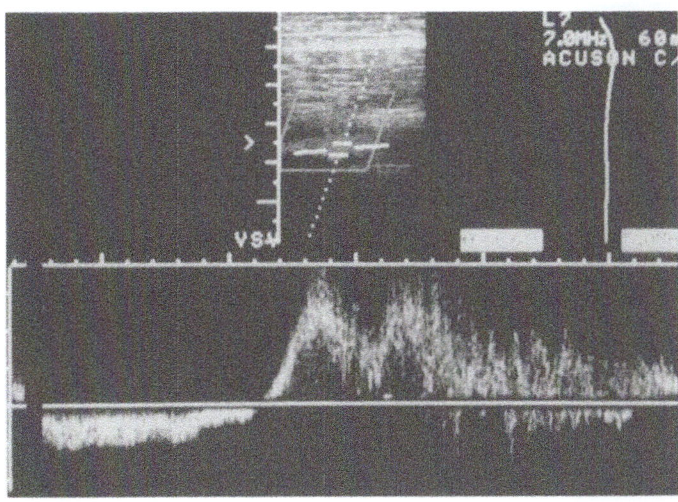

Fig. 10.4. Longitudinal CDDS scan of the saphenofemoral junction during the Valsalva maneuver. There is reflux in the GSV lasting more than 2 s. Reflux in Doppler curve indicated as a change in signal from below to above the zero line

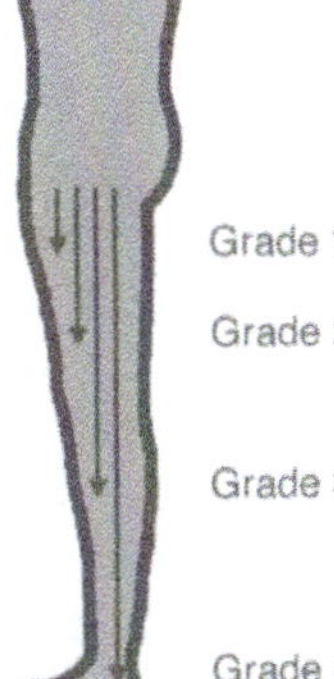

Fig. 10.5. Grading of saphenofemoral reflux

imaging prior to varicose surgery. For example, the medial or lateral branch of the GSV in the thigh may end in the GSV itself or directly in the SFV.

10.2.2 Secondary Varicosis

With DVT, the superficial venous system has to serve as a collateral vascular system. Due to the increased circulating blood volume and raised venous blood pressure, there is dilatation of the superficial veins,

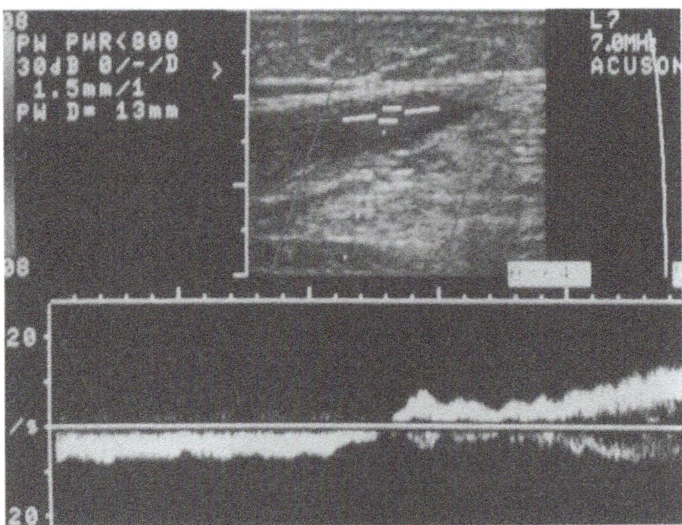

Fig. 10.6. Longitudinal CDDS image of the saphenopopliteal junction during manual compression of the popliteal vein. There is reflux in the SSV lasting more than 2 s. Reflux in Doppler curve indicated as a change in signal from below to above the zero line

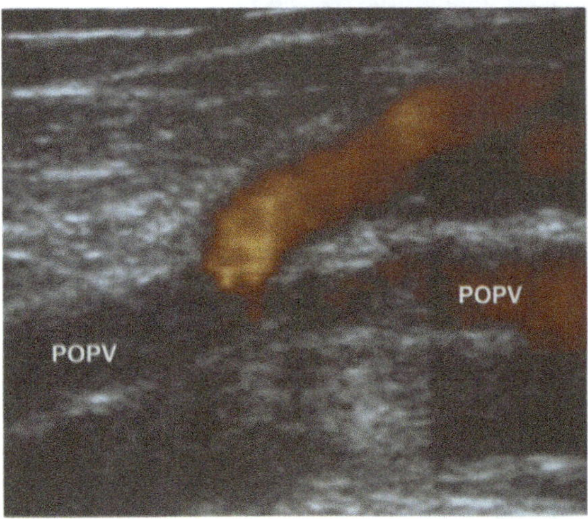

Fig. 10.7. Longitudinal CDDS image of the saphenopopliteal junction. There is dilatation and reversal of blood flow (from *blue* to *red*) in the saphenopopliteal junction indicating valve incompetence

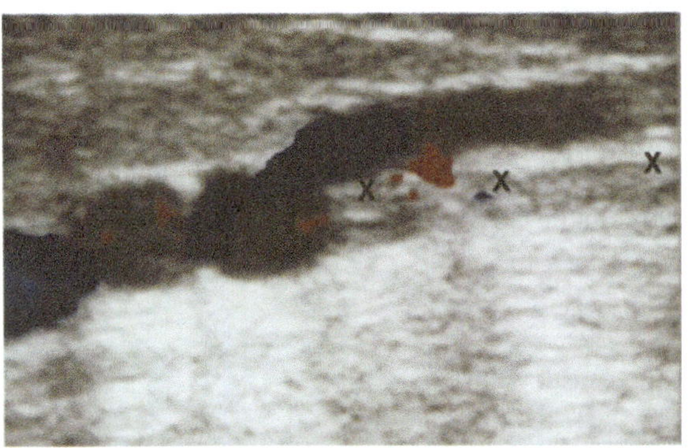

Fig. 10.8. Longitudinal CDDS image of the SSV in the middle of the calf. The SSV perforates the superficial fascia (*crosses*) and is dilated in a patient with grade 3 insufficiency

leading to incompetence of the valvular system. The location of the secondary varicosis depends on the location of the DVT or the deep veins that are involved due to postphlebitic changes.

10.3 Doppler Techniques

10.3.1 CDDS of the Venous System

CDDS should be performed using 3 MHz to 12 MHz transducers, depending on the region and vein of interest. For the superficial veins, high spatial resolution transducers are considered most suitable. CDDS allows exact placement of the pulsed Doppler sample volume within the center of a vein to obtain Doppler spectra. The most important advantage of CDDS is the direct visualization of the blood flow direction.. For more details, see Chapters 2 and 3.

10.3.2 Effect of Patient Position

For venous CDDS examinations or the detection of DVT, a supine or 10 deg reverse Trendelenburg position is appropriate. This patient position is clearly inadequate for studying valve function. It has been shown that valves which show reflux while the patient is in the erect position may appear competent when the patient is in the supine position. Thus, in mobile patients, the standing position is recommended for examination of the thigh and either sitting or standing position for the examination of the calf.

10.3.3 Evaluation of Valve Incompetence

There are three techniques used to provoke reflux in the venous system of the lower extremities (Table 10.1).

Manual limb compression is usually performed at the level of the thigh to assess the competence of the popliteal vein valves. It also may be useful for the assessment of the proximal valves of the SSV or to test the competence of perforating veins (Fig. 10.9). A study by van Bemmelen et al. (1990) demonstrated that in healthy volunteers in the supine position, valve closure only occurs when reverse blood flow velocities exceed 30 cm/s. These authors also showed that the maximum reverse velocity generated by using manual compression was less than 20 cm/s. Thus, manual compression on a patient in the supine position may lead to false-negative results concerning valvular competence.

Table 10.1. Evaluation of valve incompetence

Valsalva maneuver
Common femoral vein and saphenofemoral junction
Manual compression
Popliteal vein and saphenopopliteal junction, perforators
Cuff compression
Superficial femoral vein, popliteal vein, saphenopopliteal junction

With the Valsalva maneuver, the obtained reverse velocities exceed 30 cm/s in 90% of healthy volunteers in the CFV. However, reverse flow velocities obtained in response to a Valsalva maneuver become progressively lower in more distal venous segments. Average reverse velocities of 15 cm/s in the DFV, of 12 cm/s in the SFV, and of 7 cm/s in the POPV have been found. Thus, the Valsalva maneuver leads to a sufficient reverse velocity only in the CFV. These results indicate that the Valsalva maneuver is also an adequate method for the assessment of valve function in the proximal GSV.

The third technique for the creation of reverse blood flow is cuff compression. It has been demonstrated that reverse velocities of more than 30 cm/s can be obtained with a cuff pressure of 80 mmHg or more. Cuff compression is helpful for the assessment of the saphenopopliteal junction if the venous segments between the cuff around the thigh and the saphenopopliteal junction have no valves.

10.4 CDDS Findings in Patients with Varicose Veins of the Lower Extremity

Most studies using CDDS in the imaging work-up prior to varicose surgery describe a broad distribution of valvular incompetence. There is dilatation of incompetent venous segments in most cases, particularly in cases of primary varicosis. Masuda and Kistner (1992) evaluated the time of reflux duration

a 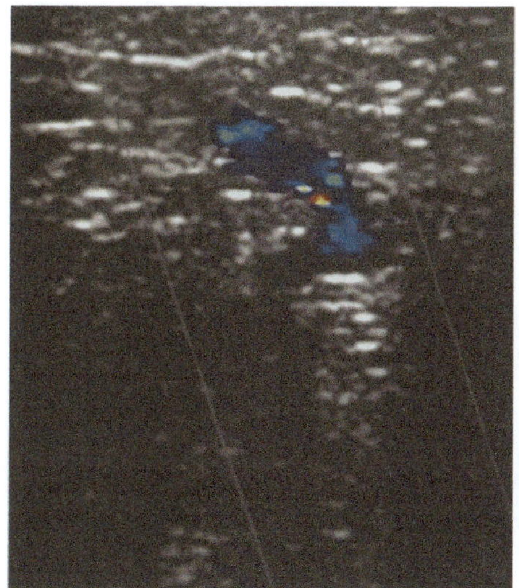

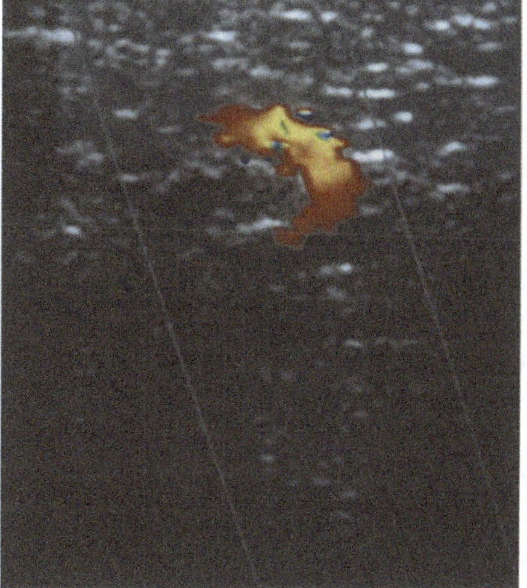 b

Fig. 10.9a, b. CDDS images of an insufficient perforating vein in the distal calf at rest (**a**) and with manual compression proximal of the vessel (**b**). Without compression, normal flow from the superficial to the deep vein is indicated by *blue* color coding. During compression, the color coding changes to *red*, indicating flow from the deep to the superficial vein

and the flow velocity of reverse blood flow by duplex Doppler US and compared these results to findings from descending venography (MASUDA and KISTNER 1992). Their results demonstrated that a reflux duration of >0.5 s measured by duplex Doppler correlated with venographic reflux with a sensitivity of 0.9, a specificity of 0.84, and an accuracy of 0.88. On the other hand, when the duration of reflux exceeded 2.0 s, the specificity was 1, but the sensitivity was only 0.72. In the patient population with duration of reflux between 0.5 and 2.0 s, there were significant discrepancies between the venographic and Doppler findings. These authors therefore concluded that reflux duration between 0.5 and 2.0 s should be interpreted with caution.

10.5 Distribution of Incompetent Valves

Appropriate treatment of varicose veins requires adequate ligation or eradication of all incompetent connections between the superficial and deep venous system. These connections can be the saphenofemoral junction, saphenopopliteal junction, and the perforating veins (Table 10.2).

There are a few studies dealing with the distribution of valvular incompetence in patients with varicose veins. HANRAHAN et al. (1991a, b) demonstrated severe heterogeneity of venous disease in these patients and that saphenofemoral junction incompetence is a common but rarely an isolated finding. They also demonstrated that valvular incompetence is much more frequent in the branches of the GSV or SSV than in the main trunks, and that normal GSV trunks were often present, even with widespread incompetence of branches. Specifically, there was a 28% rate of trunk incompetence in the GSV, a 2% rate in the SSV, and a 96% rate of branch disease in one or both of these veins.

GOREN and YELLIN (1990), in a study of 163 patients with primary varicosis, found that 71% of this group had typical saphenous varicosities with incompetence of the escape points. In this study population, the authors described incompetence of the saphenofemoral junction in 90% and incompetence of the saphenopopliteal junction in 10%. Atypical saphenous varicosities with nonjunctional escape points were present in 22%. In 10% of these patients, the Doppler examination failed to detect the presence or site of an escape point, whereas 43% presented primarily with calf tributary varicosities with reflux originating in the main perforators.

Table 10.2. Distribution of venous incompetence

Complete truncal insufficiency of great saphenous vein
without branch incompetence
with branch incompetence
Incomplete truncal insufficiency of great saphenous vein
Complete truncal incompetence of short saphenous vein
Incomplete truncal incompetence of short saphenous vein

In the study by HANRAHAN et al. (1991b), incompetent perforating veins were identified in almost 50% of the study population, and these were almost always located below the knee. Using Doppler sonography, these authors detected 63 incompetent perforating veins in 54 extremities with varicose veins. In another study, published by our group, 254 incompetent perforators in 37 limbs were diagnosed by CDDS and ascending venography. There were 219 incompetent perforators in the calf (Fig. 10.10), whereas the remaining 35 incompetent perforators were located in the thigh (BALDT et al. 1996). In this group of incompetent calf perforators, 78 (36%) connected the medial gastrocnemius vein with the GSV or SSV.

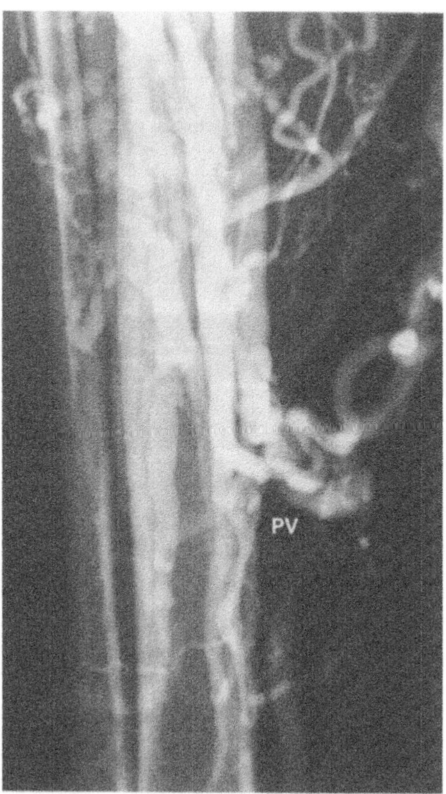

Fig. 10.10. Ascending venogram demonstrating perforating veins (*PV*) from the posterior tibial veins. The perforators are dilated, and no valves are seen, indicating perforator incompetence

10.6 CDDS Comparison with Physical Examination and Hand-Held CW-Doppler

DePalma et al. (1993) compared physical and hand-held CW-Doppler examination to CDDS in 80 limbs with mild to moderate symptoms related to GSV varicosis. The sensitivity and negative predictive value for physical examination and hand-held Doppler were low, while the specificity and positive predictive values were higher. Accordingly, these authors recommended a CDDS examination prior to surgical intervention for primary saphenous varicosis. Another study, published by Grunewald (1995), assessed the value of a clinical examination and hand-held Doppler compared with CDDS. False-positive clinical findings concerning incompetent perforators were found in 67%. The rate of false-positive hand-held Doppler findings was 40%. In this study, 45% of all incompetent perforating veins were found only using CDDS.

According to these studies, we conclude that CDDS is more accurate than physical examination and hand-held Doppler in the preoperative assessment of varicose veins of the lower limb.

10.7 CDDS Comparison with Venography

10.7.1 CDDS Comparison with Ascending Venography

Comparing CDDS to ascending venography in patients with varicose veins, Phillips et al. (1995) showed that CDDS is an accurate method for the assessment of primary and recurrent saphenofemoral and saphenopopliteal incompetence. On the other hand, in this study, CDDS was of limited value in assessing perforator incompetence. Our own results comparing CDDS to venography showed excellent agreement between CDDS and ascending venography in the grading of superficial venous reflux in the GSV and SSV. More incompetent perforating veins were detected by ascending venography than by CDDS. However, 15 of 254 incompetent perforators were detected only by CDDS and were not evident on ascending venography (Baldt et al. 1996). Thus, CDDS is a very useful tool for the detection and grading of reflux in the GSV and SSV but has some limitations in the detection of incompetent perforators.

10.7.2 CDDS Comparison with Descending Venography

Baker et al. (1993) compared descending venography to CDDS in 98 limbs with healed venous ulcers. They found good agreement between these methods in the detection of reflux in the GSV and concluded that CDDS is an ideal method to assess reflux in the GSV and SSV. In this study, CDDS was more sensitive in detecting superficial venous reflux below the knee than descending venography. This is particularly true for reflux in the SSV and in patients with incomplete truncal varicosis that cannot be assessed by descending venography. Accordingly, CDDS is a very valuable tool for preoperative imaging in patients with varicose veins. The combination of CDDS with ascending venography may lead to a higher detection rate of incompetent perforating veins. In cases with inconclusive results with regard to valvular competence in the saphenofemoral junction, descending venography may be helpful to avoid overestimation of reflux disease.

References

Araki CT, Back TL, Padberg FT, Thompson PN, Duran WN, Hobson RW (1993) Refinements in the ultrasonic detection of popliteal vein reflux. J Vasc Surg 18:742–748

Baker SR, Burnand KG, Sommerville KM, Thomas LM, Wilson NM, Browse NL (1993) Comparison of venous reflux assessed by duplex scanning and descending phlebography in chronic venous disease. Lancet 341:400–403

Baldt MM, Böhler K, Zontsich T, Bankier AA, Breitenseher M, Schneider B, Mostbeck G (1996) Preoperative imaging of lower extremity varicose veins: color coded duplex sonography or venography? J Ultrasound Med 15:143–154

Barnes RW (1985) Noninvasive techniques in chronic venous insufficiency. In: Bernstein ER (ed) Noninvasive diagnostic techniques in vascular disease. Mosby, St. Louis, MO, p 724

Bradbury A, Evans CJ, Allan P, Lee AJ, Ruchley CV, Fowkes FG (2000) The relationship between lower limb symptoms and superficial and deep venous reflux on duplex ultrasonography: the Edinburgh Vein Study. J Vasc Surg 32:921–931

Butie A (1995) Clinical evaluation of varicose veins. Dermatol Surg 21:52–56

Campanello M, Hammarsten J, Forsberg C, Bernland P, Henrikson O, Jensen J (1996) Standard stripping versus long saphenous vein saving surgery for primary varicose veins: a prospective, randomized study with patients as their own controls. Phlebology 11:45–49

De Cossart L (2001) Varicose veins and pregnancy. Br J Surg 88:323–324

DePalma RG, Hart MT, Zanin L, Massarin EH (1993) Physical examination, Doppler ultrasound and colour flow duplex scanning: guides to therapy for primary varicose veins. Phlebology 8:7–11

Fischer H (1981) Venenleiden – eine repräsentative Untersuchung in der Bevölkerung der BRD (Tübinger Studie). Urban and Schwarzenberg, Baltimore

Goldman MP, Fronek A (1989) Anatomy and pathophysiology of varicose veins. J Dermatol Surg Oncol 15:138–145

Goren G, Yellin AE (1990) Primary varicose veins: topographic and hemodynamic correlations. J Cardiovasc Surg 31: 672–677

Gottlob R, May R (1989) Venous valves. Springer, Vienna Berlin Heidelberg New York

Grunewald AM (1995) Gegenüberstellung von klinischem Untersuchungsbefund und Doppler- sowie Duplexsonographie bei der Perforantendiagnostik. Phlebologie 24: 15–19

Hach W, Hach-Wunderle V (1996) Phlebographie der Bein- und Beckenvenen Schnetztor, Konstanz

Hanrahan LM, Araki CT, Rodriguez AA, Kechejian GJ, LaMorte WW, Menzoian JO (1991a) Distribution of valvular incompetence in patients with venous stasis ulceration. J Vasc Surg 13:805–812

Hanrahan LM, Kechejian GJ, Cordts PR, Rodriguez AA, Araki CA, LaMorte WW, Menzoian JO (1991b) Patterns of venous insufficiency in patients with varicose veins. Arch Surg 126: 687–691

Hobbs JT (1986) Errors in the differential diagnosis of incompetence of the popliteal vein and short saphenous vein by Doppler ultrasound. J Cardiovasc Surg 27:169–174

Kistner RL, Kamida CB (1995) 1994 update on phlebography and varicography. Dermatol Surg 21:71–76

Koyano K, Sakaguchi S (1987) Selective stripping operation based on Doppler ultrasonic findings for primary varicose veins of the lower extremities. Surgery 103:615–619

Large J (1985) Surgical treatment of saphenous varices with preservation of the great saphenous trunk. J Vasc Surg 2: 886–891

Masuda EM, Kistner RL (1992) Prospective comparison of duplex scanning and descending venography in the assessment of venous insufficiency. Am J Surg 164:254–259

Masuda EM, Kistner RL, Eklof B (1994) Prospective study of duplex scanning for venous reflux: comparison of Valsalva and pneumatic cuff techniques in the reverse Trendelenburg and standing positions. J Vasc Surg 20:711–720

Munn SR, Morton JB, Macbeth WAAG Mcleish AR (1981) To strip or not to strip the long saphenous vein? A varicose vein trial. Br J Surg 68:426–428

Neglen P, Raju S (1992) A comparison between descending phlebology and duplex Doppler investigation in the evaluation of reflux in chronic venous insufficiency: a challenge to phlebography as the "gold standard". J Vasc Surg 16: 687–693

Negus D (1986) Should incompetent saphenous vein be stripped to the ankle? Phlebologie 1:33–36

Papadakis K, Christodoulou C, Christodoulou D, Hobbs J, Malouf GM, Grigg M, Irvine A, Nicolaides A (1989) Number and anatomical distribution of incompetent thigh perforating veins. Br J Surg 76:581–584

Phillips GWL, Paige J, Molan MP (1995) A comparison of colour duplex ultrasound with venography and varicography in the assessment of varicose veins. Clin Radiol 50: 20–25

Rollins DL, Semrow CM, Friedell ML, Buchbinder D (1987) Use of ultrasonic venography in the evaluation of venous valve function. Am J Surg 154:189–191

Sarin S, Scurr JH, Colderidge Smith PD (1992) Assessment of stripping the long saphenous vein in the treatment of primary varicose veins. Br J Surg 79:889–893

Schanzer H, Skladany M (1994) Varicose vein surgery with preservation of the saphenous vein: a comparison between high ligation-avulsion versus saphenofemoral banding valvuloplasty-avulsion. J Vasc Surg 20:684–687

Sullivan ED, David JP, Cranley JJ (1984) Real-time B-mode venous ultrasound. J Vasc Surg 1:465–469

Thomas LM (1990) Techniques of phlebography: a review. Eur J Radiol 11:125–130

Tung KT, Chan O, Thomas ML (1990) The incidence and sites of medial thigh communicating veins: a phlebographic study. Clin Radiol 41:339–340

Valentin LI, Valentin WH, Mercado S, Rosado CJ (1993) Venous reflux localization: comparative study of venography and duplex scanning. Phlebology 8:124–127

Van Bemmelen PS, Bedford G, Beach KW, Strandness DE (1989) Quantitative segmental evaluation of venous valvular reflux with duplex ultrasound scanning. J Vasc Surg 10:425–431

Van Bemmelen PS, Beach KW, Bedford G, Stradness DE (1990) The mechanism of venous valve closure. Arch Surg 125: 617–619

Van der Heijden FHWM, Bruyninckx CMA (1993) Preoperative colour-coded duplex scanning in varicose veins of the lower extremity. Eur J Surg 159:329–333

Weber J, May R (1990) Funktionelle Phlebologie. Thieme, Stuttgart

Weiss RA (1994) Vascular studies of the legs for venous or arterial disease. Dermatol Clin 12:175–190

Widmer LK (1978) Venenerkrankungen, Häufigkeit und sozialmedizinische Bedeutung: Baslerstudie III. Huber, Bern

Wuppermann T (1986) Varizen, Ulcus cruris und Thrombose. Springer, Berlin Heidelberg New York

Zwiebel WJ, Priest DL (1990) Color duplex sonography of extremity veins. Semin Ultrasound CT MR 11:136–167

11 Venous Color Duplex Sonography of the Scrotum

F. Fobbe

CONTENTS

11.1 Preliminary Remarks

For the diagnosis of most scrotal diseases, gray-scale US is a reliable method in combination with palpation and the case history. However, two important scrotal diseases can only be diagnosed based on knowledge about the perfusion of the scrotal content: varicocele and an 'acute scrotum'. Information important for this differential diagnosis can be acquired by color duplex Doppler sonography (CDDS). This method enables not only morphological visualization but also qualitative detection of perfusion in the individual structures.

11.2 Instrumentation, Examination Technique, Normal Findings

The scrotum should be examined with a high-frequency transducer with excellent spatial resolution. If the scrotum is considerably enlarged, as for example in marked hydrocele or epididymo-orchitis, the organ may only be sufficiently insonated with a transducer working at a lower frequency (5 MHz). The US unit must be capable of color-coded visualization of slow testicular perfusion, seen especially in small children. The healthy testis should also always be examined for comparison and to adjust the correct setting of the US equipment. The frame rate in the color-coded mode should be higher than 10 images/s for the reliable differentiation of perfusion signals and artifacts. The use of amplitude-encoded CDDS is not very helpful in scrotal examinations. Although the detection of slow blood flow is better with this method, the disadvantage is that motion artifacts may be difficult to differentiate from real flow signals. As the testis and epididymis are only fixed via the spermatic cord cranially and can otherwise move freely in the serous cavity, complete absence of motion artifacts during the examination is difficult to accomplish.

If spatial resolution of the available US unit in the direct near-field is limited or hampered by artifacts, then use of a water path bridging the so-called near-field may be indicated. This might be necessary especially in neonates and small children, where the scrotal content is small and close to the surface. The CDDS examination is performed in the supine position with legs adducted. The patient holds his penis in the cranial direction against his abdominal wall. In this position, the scrotum is easily accessible from anterior, and the closed thighs serve as support. Infants and small children should be examined on the lap of a familiar person. To avoid color artifacts, the transducer must be steadily guided, and the patient must lie still. This may require sedation in infants and smaller children. As an alternative, the (hungry) child can be fed by the accompanying person. To displace air cavities from the wrinkled and hairy scrotal skin, large amounts of ultrasound jelly must be applied for the examination. In patients with suspicion of a varicocele, visualization of the pampiniform plexus in the standing position is sometimes required in addition to the examination in the supine position.

After optimal adjustment of the US unit, longitudinal and cross-sectional scans of both testes are acquired using real-time US. The normal testis in a sexually mature man is oval and has a homoge-

F. Fobbe, MD
Professor of Radiology, Auguste-Viktoria-Krankenhaus, Abteilung für Röntgendiagnostik, Rubensstrasse 125, 12157 Berlin, Germany

neously moderate to hyperechoic tissue pattern, similar to that of the normal thyroid. Occasionally, there is a band-shaped, eccentrically located, hyperreflexive structure in the testis corresponding to the mediastinum testis. In childhood, the testis is of lower echogenicity; the characteristic high echogenicity develops with maturity (Hamm and Fobbe 1995). The testis and epididymis are supplied by the testicular artery. After branching off to the epididymis and deferent duct, the vessel enters the testis at the hilum. It courses on the surface of the testis and gives off several lateral branches, which enter the inner testis together with the lobular septa (Williams 1995). Venous drainage flows from the inside to the outside: The veins concentrate in the mediastinum testis and form the pampiniform plexus with the afferent vessels from the epididymis, which leads into the testicular vein (internal spermatic vein) (Gösfay 1953; Williams 1995). There are usually several veins with different lumina accompanying the testicular vein. All of these veins are interconnected at the level of the deep inguinal ring (Gösfay 1953; Williams 1995). The spermatic cord is basically formed by the veins of the pampiniform plexus. Other components include the deferent duct, the testicular artery, the cremaster muscle, and fatty tissue. The individual components course together through the inguinal canal and separate again before the testicular hilum (Gösfay 1953; Williams 1995).

Perfusion of the normal testis can be seen easily with CDDS: In most cases, individual arterial or venous vessel segments with corresponding color-coded signals are diffusely distributed throughout the testis. However, perfusion can only be qualitatively determined. Thus, color-encoded perfusion must always be compared to the other testis. In healthy individuals, only the epididymal head is visible, which sits on the cranial testis like a hood and appears homogeneously isoreflexive or slightly hyperechoic in comparison with testicular tissue. The other parts of the epididymis are very small and not displayed in every patient. Even if the US unit is adjusted for the detection of very slow blood flow, no or only very few color-coded flow signals can be detected in the epididymis of healthy subjects. Testicular and epididymal appendages are small and cannot usually be visualized. On the gray-scale image, the spermatic cord appears as an inhomogeneous hyperechoic structure. Visualization is best carried out somewhat cranial and lateral to the epididymal head. The individual anatomic contents cannot be reliably differentiated from the surrounding fatty tissue. However, blood flow in the vessels can be visualized with CDDS. There are pulse-synchronous flow signals in the arteries, while only single, weak, color-coded, blood flow signals are detected from the veins. During the Valsalva maneuver, there is an initial, slight, longitudinal shift of the structures in the inguinal canal. Temporary (lasting less than a second) retrograde blood flow may occur in the veins of the normal pampiniform plexus.

11.3 Varicocele

Idiopathic varicocele is the most common treatable cause of sterility in men. It involves dilation of the veins in the pampiniform plexus, usually occurring on the left side (Fig. 11.1). The increased blood volume in the pampiniform plexus leads to a temperature increase in the testis and thus to disturbed spermiogenesis (Hornstein 1973; Kurgan et al. 1994). The cause of idiopathic varicocele is unclear. The following factors have been discussed as possible causes: Absent or insufficient valves in the testicular vein, impaired blood flow at the connection of the left testicular vein to the left renal vein (hemodynamically unfavorable angle of about 90°), as well as a possible compression of the left renal vein between the SMA and the aorta, causing reflux into the testicular vein (Hornstein 1973). Disturbed spermiogenesis may also occur in a mild form of so-called subclinical or functional varicocele (Hornstein 1973; Marsman 1985). It is generally understood that these varicoceles are not palpable and can only be detected with imaging devices. Varicoceles on the right side are very rare. The reason for this is probably anatomic: The right testicular vein connects at a sharp angle directly into the IVC. The inflow of blood from the right testicular vein into the IVC is thus less impeded than on the left side. However, idiopathic varicocele must be differentiated from symptomatic varicocele. The most common causes of symptomatic varicocele are renal tumors and retroperitoneal lymphomas with compression of the left renal vein. In such cases, the testicular vein serves as the bypass vein.

In the supine position with steady breathing, the veins of the pampiniform plexus are normally nearly collapsed and not easily detectable using gray-scale US. Using CDDS, there are only a few arterial or venous flow signals. During the Valsalva maneuver, there is a brief, initial reflux of venous blood. However, if there is a varicocele other than the 'subclinical' type, the dilated vessels in the pampiniform plexus are frequently visualized on the gray-scale image

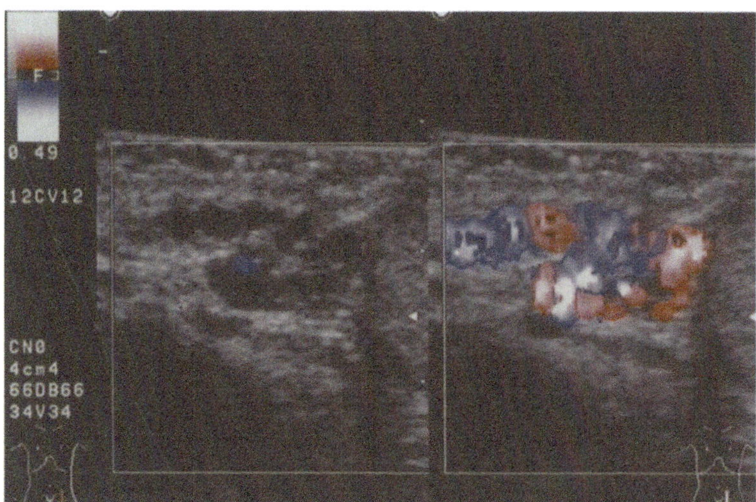

Fig. 11.1. Longitudinal scan through the upper pole of the left testis in a patient with an extensive varicocele. Dilated and tortuous veins of the pampiniform plexus are visible with almost no color coded flow signals (*left*) during normal breathing. Valsalva maneuver induces marked retrograde flow (*red* and *blue*) in the tortuous and dilated veins (*right*). This typical retrograde flow during the Valsalva maneuver is evident even in small (subclinical) varicoceles

as multiple, tortuous venous segments. Retrograde blood flow occurs during the Valsalva maneuver regardless of the extent of the varicocele and can be detected using CDDS. This retrograde blood flow continues until the end of the Valsalva maneuver. In doubtful cases, the finding should be compared to the contralateral side and/or the examination should be repeated in the standing position.

The classification of varicocele into groups by Siegmund et al. (1987) based on testicular phlebography findings cannot be paralleled with CDDS findings. However, the classification into groups has no effect on the diagnosis, and the clinical value of this classification is also unclear (Fobbe 1995).

CDDS is the only noninvasive method that can diagnose varicoceles with high sensitivity and specificity. This also applies to recurrences after vascular occlusion in the cranial region that can only be detected with great difficulty by phlebography. Following therapy, collateral veins from the retroperitoneum and the renal capsule can retain varicoceles (Chiou et al. 1997; Fobbe 1995; Fobbe et al. 1987; Kim and Lipshultz 1996; Trum et al. 1996). However, it is important to use an adequate examination technique and an appropriate device for this type of examination. The patient must be able to carry out the Valsalva maneuver. The examination has to be repeated in a standing position in doubtful cases. In my opinion, analysis of the Doppler spectrum is not required to confirm the diagnosis if a CDDS unit with 'slow-flow' capabilities is used. However, this does not agree with Lund and Nielsen's opinion (Lund and Nielsen 1994).

Large varicose veins can be detected by palpation, but not a subclinical varicocele (by definition). Even after treatment (especially after caudal sclerotherapy), recurrent or persistent varicocele cannot be reliably detected by palpation (Fobbe et al. 1987; Hamm et al. 1986). Although varicoceles can be demonstrated by thermography and CW-Doppler with high sensitivity, the low specificity of these methods requires further clarification of all positive findings by an additional method. Using gray-scale US alone, only severe varicoceles can be confirmed (Fobbe 1995; Hamm et al. 1986; Trum et al. 1996).

With phlebography, varicoceles can be detected on the left side only in patients in whom the testicular vein opens into the left renal vein. When the testicular vein connects as a variant anatomic finding, for example, to the IIV, the CIV, or veins of the renal capsule, the phlebographic diagnosis of the varicocele may be difficult (necessitating significant radiation exposure) or even impossible. Similar problems occur after surgical ligation of the testicular vein and a suspected recurrence or persistence of the varicocele. In these cases, the varicocele may be fed by lateral branches originating from the pelvic veins or the veins of the renal capsule (Fobbe et al. 1987). Testicular phlebography should only be performed in conjunction with intended transcutaneous interventional therapy (e.g., sclerotherapy).

11.4 Acute Scrotum

An acute scrotum involves a sudden and persistent strong pain in the scrotum, possibly accompanied by swelling and reddened skin. A number of diagnoses are characterized by these symptoms:

testicular torsion, epididymitis or epididymo-orchitis, hydatid torsion, acute hydrocele, strangulated inguinal hernia, abscess, vasculitis in conjunction with a Schönlein-Henoch syndrome, insect bites, or traumatic testicular rupture (Kass and Lundak 1997). With the exception of testicular torsion and epididymo-orchitis, further diagnoses can be differentiated with the aid of the case history, clinical findings, and gray-scale US. Testicular torsion and epididymo-orchitis have similar symptoms, similar findings on palpation, and identical findings on gray-scale US (Figs. 11.2 and 11.3). The usually younger patients complain of sudden and increasing unilateral pain. Occasionally, the patients are awakened by the pain. The clinical examination reveals swelling and possibly reddened skin on the affected side of the scrotum. At US, the testes and epididymis are enlarged and inhomogeneous (Hricak et al. 1996; Kass and Lundak 1997).

Acute torsion is usually characterized by a marked enlargement of the involved testis and epididymis, with an inhomogeneous and largely hyporeflexive texture (Fig. 11.3). The testis is round, and there may also be thickening of the scrotal skin and a hydrocele. No color-coded flow signals are displayed in the testis or epididymis if the blood flow is completely blocked.

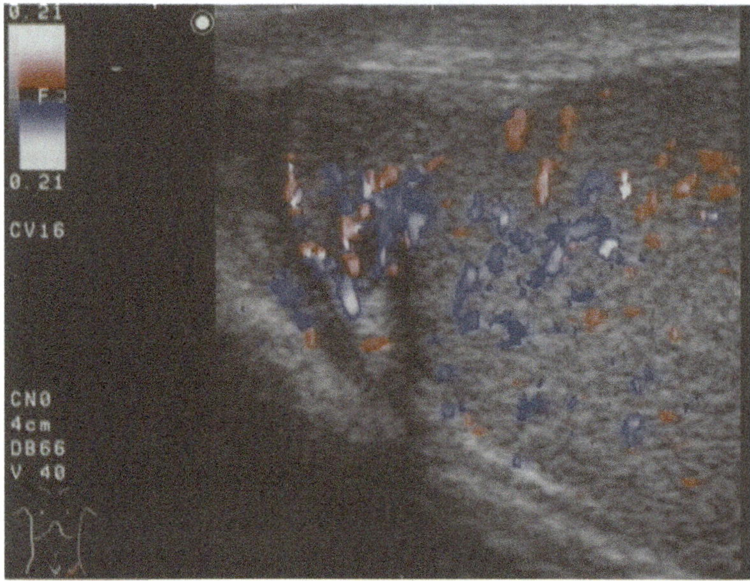

Fig. 11.2. Longitudinal scan through the upper pole of the testis and the head of the epididymis in a patient with epididymo-orchitis: enlarged testis and head of the epididymis with mixed echogenicity and markedly increased blood flow

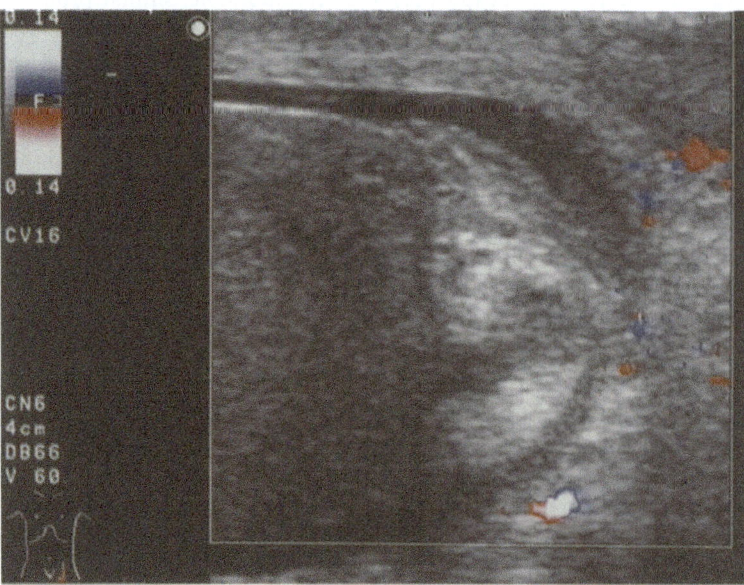

Fig. 11.3. Longitudinal scan through the lower pole of the left testis and the tail of the epididymis in a patient with an acute torsion: enlarged testis and tail of the epididymis with mixed echogenicity. Blood flow (*blue* and *red*) is only visualized in the peritesticular tissue and not in the testis or epididymis

Increased flow signals are detected in the immediate vicinity of the affected testis and epididymis as a reaction to the absence of perfusion. Epididymo-orchitis looks similar on gray-scale US and is the major differential diagnosis to torsion. In contrast to torsion, CDDS demonstrates markedly increased perfusion of the testis and epididymis.

Nevertheless, there might be diagnostic difficulty in partial torsion or torsion after spontaneous lysis. Different alterations are visualized depending on the degree of disturbed perfusion: In mildly disturbed testicular perfusion, there may be discrete diffuse swelling with a nearly homogeneous texture and slightly reduced blood flow on CDDS. These discrete differences can only be detected by comparing the morphology and blood flow to the contralateral, normal testis and epididymis. With increasingly disturbed afferent and efferent flow, the alterations become more pronounced until complete torsion is evident (Fobbe 1995). In torsion with spontaneous lysis, the morphological alterations are often discrete: Especially in cases following a short interval of disturbed perfusion, there may only be mildly pronounced, diffuse swelling of the testis and epididymis with a homogenous texture. However, in contrast to partial torsion, there may be a (reactively) increased perfusion compared with the contralateral testis. It should be emphasized that palpation and the case history always have to be taken into account in the CDDS differential diagnosis. For example, an early epididymo-orchitis (with similar morphological and blood flow changes as torsion with spontaneous lysis in CDDS imaging) is usually more painful to palpation than torsion.

Epididymo-orchitis is generally characterized by a diffuse, usually pronounced increase of perfusion in addition to the inhomogeneous, hypoechoic, enlarged testis and epididymis (Fig. 11.2). There may be thickening of the scrotal skin as well as increased perfusion. In the case of liquefaction (abscess formation), a circumscribed echo-poor area without flow signals is visualized by CDDS. A simple epididymitis (where the testis appears normal) can be adequately diagnosed by gray-scale US: The epididymis is usually circumscribed and very painful on palpation, with corresponding morphological alterations (inhomogeneous, hypoechoic enlargement, thickening of the scrotal skin). However, both testes have the same echogenicity, size, and shape (Fobbe 1995; Hricak et al. 1996).

Hydatid torsion is an exclusion diagnosis. The clinical symptoms are similar to those of testicular torsion. There is circumscribed or local pain on palpation. The gray-scale US image reveals no morphological alterations of the testes or epididymis. Sometimes there is a moderately or pronounced hydrocele. The perfusion as displayed by CDDS is identical and normal compared with the contralateral, unaffected side (Fobbe 1995; Hricak et al. 1996).

Testicular rupture, which is easily visualized by gray-scale US, may occur after severe scrotal trauma. However, torsion which can develop as a result of testicular trauma cannot be excluded. Testicular perfusion should therefore always be checked by CDDS after a severe testicular trauma (Fobbe 1995; Hricak et al. 1996).

Generally, testicular perfusion cannot by quantified by CDDS. The only possibility is a 'semiquantitative' assessment of perfusion by comparing the color signals between both testes at CDDS. This side-to-side comparison makes it possible to check simultaneously whether the US unit is properly adjusted or even suitable for displaying the slow testicular blood flow. Detecting the blood movement in the testes of small children is especially difficult and can only be done with an appropriate device. In theory, a slow blood flow is more easily recorded by amplitude-encoded color Doppler. However, all hemodynamic information (flow direction, artery versus vein) is lost with this technique, and it might be difficult to differentiate between real flow signals and artifacts. This method is therefore not suitable for examining the scrotal content (Dubinsky et al. 1998; Lee et al. 1996).

As an alternative to CDDS, scintigraphy can be performed to prove suspected testicular torsion. This method is supposed to exclude a torsion with comparable reliability to CDDS (Melloul et al. 1995; Paltiel et al. 1998). However, this examination is more time-consuming than CDDS, and though low, there is radiation exposure. Even in cases where CDDS findings are equivocal between torsion and inflammation, scintigraphy should not be used as a trouble-shooting examination, because this would lead to another temporal delay. In view of the warm ischemia time of probably just a few hours, surgical exposure should be performed immediately if the CDDS findings are unclear or equivocal (Fobbe 1995). In the same setting, hand-held CW-Doppler is likewise no alternative to CDDS: Because of the lack of morphologic information, the source of any received Doppler signal cannot be defined. Increased perfusion in the peritesticular tissue after torsion may simulate undisturbed perfusion.

The value of CDDS in the diagnosis of an acute scrotum has been evaluated in a number of publications. In the majority of these publications, CDDS is regarded as the method of choice for diagnostic imaging of patients presenting with an acute scrotum (Cartwright et al. 1995; Hendrikx 1997; Schwaibold et al. 1996; Süzer et al. 1997). However, there is a belief that CDDS does not reliably differentiate between testicular torsion and an inflammation in all cases (Allen and Elder 1995). It has to be emphasized again that all unclear CDDS findings have to be immediately clarified by surgical exposure. The diagnosis is particularly problematic for partial torsion and torsion after spontaneous lysis. Use of appropriate US equipment is mandatory. The examiner has to be well trained and experienced in the differential diagnosis of scrotal diseases. In addition to the CDDS findings, the case history, clinical symptoms, and palpation findings must definitely be included in the diagnostic process. When these prerequisites are fulfilled, CDDS is a reliable method for the diagnostic work-up of an acute scrotum.

References

Allen TD, Elder JS (1995) Shortcomings of color Doppler sonography in the diagnosis of testicular torsion. J Urol 154:1508–1510

Cartwright PC, Snow NW, Reid BS, Shultz PK (1995) Color Doppler ultrasound in newborn testis torsion. Urology 45:667–670

Chiou RK, Anderson JC, Wobig RK, Rosinsky DE, Matamoros AM, Chen WS, Taylor RJ (1997) Color Doppler ultrasound criteria to diagnose varicocels: correlation of a new scoring system with physical examination. Urology 50:953–956

Dubinsky TJ, Chen P, Maklad N (1998) Color-flow and power Doppler imaging of the testes. World J Urol 16:35–40

Fobbe F (1995) Scrotum. In: Wolf K-J, Fobbe F (eds) Color duplex sonography. Thieme, Stuttgart

Fobbe F, Hamm B, Sörensen R, Felsenberg D (1987) Percutaneous transluminal treatment of varicoceles: where to occlude the internal spermatic vein. Am J Roentgenol 149:983–987

Gösfay S (1959) Untersuchungen der V. spermatica interna durch retrograde Phlebographie bei Kranken mit Varikozele. Z Urol 2:105–115

Hamm B, Fobbe F (1995) Maturation of the testis: ultrasound evaluation. Ultrasound Med Biol 21:143–147

Hamm B, Fobbe F, Sörensen R, Felsenberg D (1986) Varicocele: combined sonography and thermography and post-therapeutic evaluation. Radiology 160:419–424

Hendrikx AJM, Dang CL, Vroegindeweij D, Korte JH (1997) B-mode and color-flow ultrasonography: a useful adjunct in diagnosing scrotal diseases? Br J Urol 79:58–65

Hornstein OP (1973) Kreislaufstörungen im Hoden-Nebenhodensystem und ihre Bedeutung für die männliche Fertilität. Andrologie 5:119–125

Hricak H, Hamm B, Kimm B (1996) Imaging of the scrotum. Raven Press, New York

Kass EJ, Lundak B (1997) The acute scrotum. Pediatr Clin North Am 5:1251–1266

Kim, ED, Lipshultz LI (1996) Role of ultrasound in the assessment of male infertility. J Clin Ultrasound 24:437–453

Kurgan A, Nunnelee JD, Zilberman M (1994) The importance of early detection of varicocele in adolescent males. Nurse Pract 19:36–37

Lee FT, Winter DB, Madsen FA, Zagzebski JA, Pozniak MA, Chosy SG, Scanlan KA (1996) Conventional color Doppler velocity sonography versus color Doppler energy sonography for the diagnosis of acute experimental torsion of the spermatic cord. Am J Roentgenol 167:785–790

Lund L, Nielsen AH (1994) Color Doppler sonography in the assessment of varicocele testis. Scand J Urol Nephrol 28: 281–285

Marsman JW (1985) Clinical versus subclinical varicocele: venographic findings and improvement of fertility after embolisaton. Radiology 155:635–638

Melloul M, Lask PD, Mukamel E (1995) The value of radionuclide scrotal imaging in the diagnosis of acute testicular torsion. Br J Urol 76:628–631

Paltiel HJ, Connolly LP, Atala A, Paltiel AD, Zurakowski D, Treves ST (1998) Acute scrotal symptoms in boys with an indeterminate clinical presentation: comparison of color Doppler sonography and szintigraphy. Radiology 207:223–232

Schwaibold H, Fobbe F, Klän R, Dieckmann KP (1996) Evaluation of acute scrotal pain by color-coded duplex sonography. Urol Int 56:96–99

Siegmund G, Gall H, Bähren W (1987) Stop-type and shunt-type varicoceles: venographic findings. Radiology 163:105–110

Süzer O, Özcan H, Küpeli S, Gheiler EL (1997) Color Doppler imaging in the diagnosis of acute scrotum. Eur Urol 32: 457–461

Trum LW, Gubler FM, Laan R, van der Veen F (1996) The value of palpation, varicoscreen contact thermography and colour Doppler ultrasound in the diagnosis of varikozele. Hum Reprod 11:1232–1235

Williams PL (ed) (1995) Gray's anatomy: the anatomical basis of medicine and surgery, 38th edn. Churchill Livingstone, London

12 Influences of Cardiac Pathology on Doppler Findings in the Venous System

C. B. Henk, S. Grampp, G. H. Mostbeck

CONTENTS

12.1 Introduction

Since the supracardiac and infracardiac venous system is connected to the right atrium and right ventricle in order to propel venous blood into the lungs, it can be expected that changes in cardiac dynamics frequently have secondary effects on the venous blood flow. These venous hemodynamic changes observed in cardiac disease are mostly apparent when the origin of the pathologic condition is located in the right portion of the heart or the pulmonary circulation. Nevertheless, many other types of heart diseases, including congenital, ischemic, pericardial, and rhythmologic disorders may also affect the hemodynamics of the venous circulation. Changes in venous flow dynamics have been reported to be a sensitive indicator of right heart diastolic function because they directly reflect right atrial pressure contours (Fig. 12.1) (Sivaciyan and Ranganathan 1978). It is evident that these changes are best observed in veins located near the right atrium because they might fade in a peripheral, more downstream position. For the radiologist performing Doppler imaging, knowledge of altered venous flow dynamics caused by cardiac disease is mandatory not only to avoid confusing it with other disorders, but also to give diagnostic support to the referring physician, since not all patients examined for venous abnormalities, ascites, or elevated liver enzymes are known to suffer from heart disease (Table 12.1).

C. B. Henk, MD
Associate Professor of Radiology, Department of Radiology, University Hospital Vienna, School of Medicine, Währinger Gürtel 18–20, 1090 Vienna, Austria
S. Grampp, MD
Associate Professor of Radiology, Department of Radiology, University Hospital Vienna, School of Medicine, Währinger Gürtel 18–20, 1090 Vienna, Austria
G. H. Mostbeck, MD
Professor of Radiology, Sozialmedizinisches Zentrum, Baumgartner Höhe mit Pflegezentrum, Otto Wagner Spital, Sanatoriumstrasse 2, 1140 Vienna, Austria

12.2 Tricuspid Regurgitation and Its Causes

This chapter discusses various pathophysiologic conditions that have one symptom in common, namely the development of tricuspid regurgitation. It leads to specific venous flow changes which can be diagnosed by Doppler imaging. First, lung disorders associated with an elevation in pulmonary arterial pressure and thus an increase in right ventricular as well as atrial pressure and volume, leading to distinct changes in the Doppler spectra of the venous circulation, are reviewed. This chapter deals further with the importance of valvular disease in the development of detectable hemodynamic alterations in the systemic veins. It reviews the various pathologic conditions where the right portion of the heart is functionally affected. This mechanism works not directly via the pulmonary circulation but secondarily due to ischemic or metabolic myocardial damage.

12.2.1 Pulmonary Heart Disease

The right ventricle has only a limited power of response to an increase in afterload (which, in that respect, is defined as pulmonary vascular resistance) compared

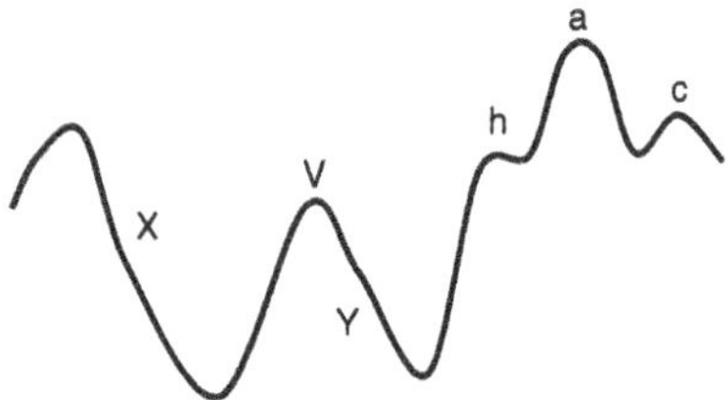

Fig. 12.1. Scheme of right atrial pressure contours

with the left ventricle. A drastic sudden increase in pulmonary resistance, as may happen with pulmonary embolism, leads to an increase in the right ventricular volume accompanied by only a mild or no elevation of ventricular and atrial pressure. If the rise of pulmonary arterial pressure develops gradually over a longer period of time, the right ventricle compensates with myocardial hypertrophy and a rise in ventricular pressure. Lung diseases that lead to a rise in pulmonary artery pressure are listed in Table 12.2. This compensation mechanism is, however, limited and finally leads to ventricular dilatation. As a functional result, the tricuspid valve becomes insufficient due to an enlargement of the orifice and annulus. Regurgitation of blood into the right atrium during ventricular systole with an elevation of right atrial pressure becomes evident. The regurgitant jet can be graded according to its length by means of Doppler echocardiography (grades I–IV) and represents the main feature for alterations in juxtacardiac vein flow (best detectable in hepatic and jugular veins as well as the superior and inferior vena cava). In severe cases, these disturbances can be propagated to the veins of the splenoportal axis and the peripheral veins of the lower extremities (see later).

Table 12.1. Changes in systemic venous waveforms and their differential diagnosis

S>D	Normal
	Atrial septal defect (mild)
S=D	Post-cardiotomy
	Severe mitral regurgitation (LV-volume overload)
S<D	Tricuspid regurgitation (mild to moderate)
	Post-cardiotomy
	Severe mitral regurgitation (LV-volume overload)
	Atrial fibrillation and flutter
	Constrictive pericarditis
Single Df	Tricuspid regurgitation (moderate to severe)
	Atrial fibrillation and flutter
Retrograde Sf	Tricuspid regurgitation (severe)
Retrograde Df (large a-wave)	AV dissociation
	Heart block
	Junctional Cannon wave
	Tricuspid stenosis
	Pulmonary hypertension
	Pulmonic stenosis
Absent Df	Tamponade
Absent a-wave	Atrial fibrillation and flutter
Prominent v-wave	Normal variant
	Tricuspid regurgitation
Atrial relaxation flow	Normal ('S-notch')
	AV dissociation

S, S-wave velocity; *D*, D-wave velocity; *Sf*, systolic flow; *Df*, diastolic flow

12.2.2 Valve and Myocardial Disease

The tricuspid valve (TV) may not only be affected secondarily due to right heart dilatation but may itself be impaired in its competence, e.g., because of

Table 12.2. Etiology of pulmonary hypertension

Disease	Mechanism
Primary pulmonary hypertension (PPH)	Principally unknown
Secondary pulmonary hypertension (SPH)	
Vascular lung disease	
Chronic pulmonary embolism	Vascular and/or microvascular obstruction
Vasculitis	Alveolar hypoxia → Vasoconstriction
Venoocclusive disease	
Parenchymal lung disease	
Restrictive	
Fibrosis	Alveolar hypoxia → Vasoconstriction
Pneumonectomy	Vascular distortion and/or loss of vessels
Obesity	
High altitudes	
Obstructive	
COPD	Alveolar hypoxia → Vasoconstriction
Emphysema	Vascular stretching, lung hyper-inflation → impeded heartbeat

infectious endocarditis or intravenous drug abuse, which are the most common causes of isolated TV disease. Compared with relative (functional) tricuspid insufficiency, primary valve disease in the right heart is rare and mostly accompanies left heart valvular disorders. Decompensated mitral stenosis, for example, leads frequently to right ventricular and thus TV dilatation via a rise in pulmonary vascular resistance originating from chronic congestion. Other causes of tricuspid regurgitation are carcinoid involvement of the leaflets, myocardial infarction with rupture of the right papillary muscle (Collins and Daly 1977), and external blunt trauma, with rupture of one or more elements of the tensor apparatus and disruption of the papillary muscle or less frequently rupture of the chordae. In several cases, laceration of the leaflet tissue itself is evident (Jahnke et al. 1967).

Very commonly, tricuspid regurgitation is a consequence of ischemic heart disease or cardiomyopathies where the global dilatation of the heart also involves the right ventricle in later stages. Tricuspid regurgitation may diminish when the heart failure is treated successfully but can be permanent with longstanding dilatation of the right ventricle.

Another rare cause of mild tricuspid incompetence that should not be overlooked is the pacing wire passing through the valve in patients carrying pacemakers. The presence of the wire may cause incomplete closure of the leaflets.

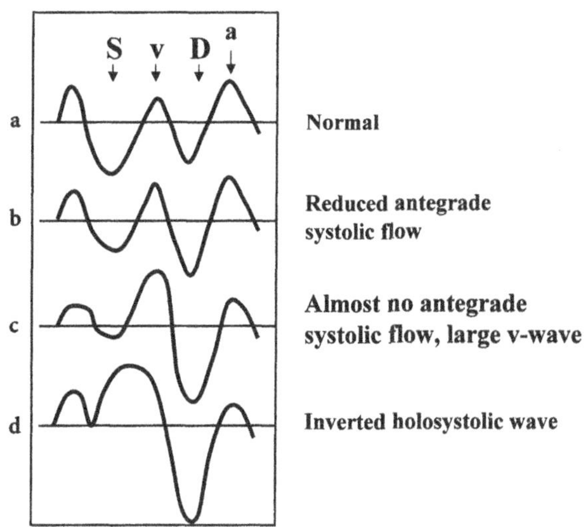

Fig. 12.2. Normal hepatic vein flow profile (**a**). Gradual development of flow changes observed in tricuspid regurgitation (**b–d**)

12.2.3 Venous Doppler Findings

As mentioned above, the propagation of the tricuspid regurgitant jet can best be noticed in the hepatic veins, the inferior vena cava (IVC), and the jugular veins. In cases of severer TV insufficiency, flow changes in the veins of the splenoportal axis and pelvic as well as leg veins can become apparent.

Hepatic Veins and IVC. The normal hepatic vein Doppler waveform consists of four major waves (Sharpiro et al. 1993; Abu-Yousef 1992) in the following sequence (Figs. 12.2a, 12.3, 12.4):

1. The first component is a large antegrade systolic wave (S) that is caused by the movement of the tricuspid annulus towards the cardiac apex. On right atrial pressure tracings, it corresponds to the x‘ descent and trough and occurs approximately 0.15 s after the QRS complex. Usually, the velocity ranges from 20 to 40 cm/s.
2. The second wave is a small retrograde v-wave caused by right atrial overfilling, corresponding to the similar v-wave on right atrial pressure tracings. It can be on or slightly above the baseline with negative velocities usually not exceeding 5–8 cm/s. On ECG tracings, it immediately follows the T-wave.
3. A third component, an antegrade diastolic wave (D), can be observed originating from the opening of the TV and the blood flowing from the right atrium into the right ventricle. It corresponds to the y‘ descent and trough and appears within 0.1 s after the T-wave on ECG tracings. Velocities vary between 15 and 35 cm/s. S/D ratios therefore also range between 1 and 2.5.
4. The fourth part is a retrograde a-wave that is caused by right atrial contraction and is similar to the a-wave on pressure tracings. It occurs soon after the p-wave on the ECG and is above the baseline, with retrograde velocities commonly lying between 0 and 35 cm/s. Frequently, a c-wave (also corresponding to the pressure-curve c-wave) can be appreciated which is due to the closure of the TV at the beginning of systole (Fig. 12.4).

The main feature that occurs in tricuspid regurgitation is a decrease in systolic antegrade flow caused by the high right ventricular pressure that is transmitted into the right atrium (Abu-Yousef 1990). Systolic flow may even reverse in severe TV disease. Several studies have shown that dampening or reversal of systolic flow correlates with the presence and the various degrees of tricuspid regurgitation as

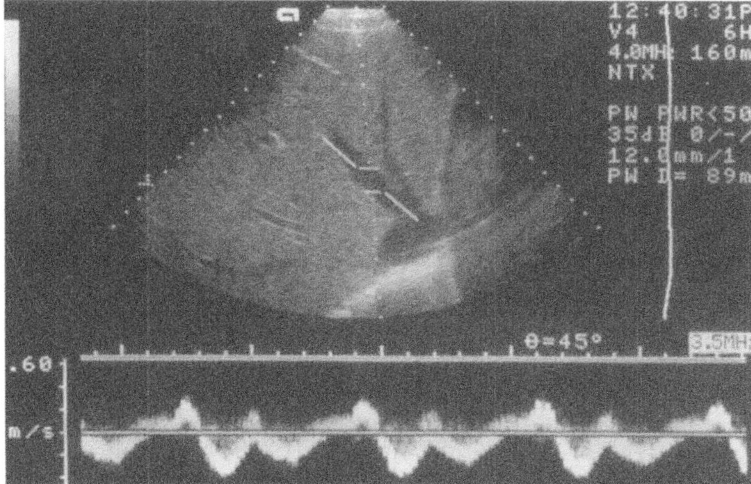

Fig. 12.3. Normal hepatic vein flow profile

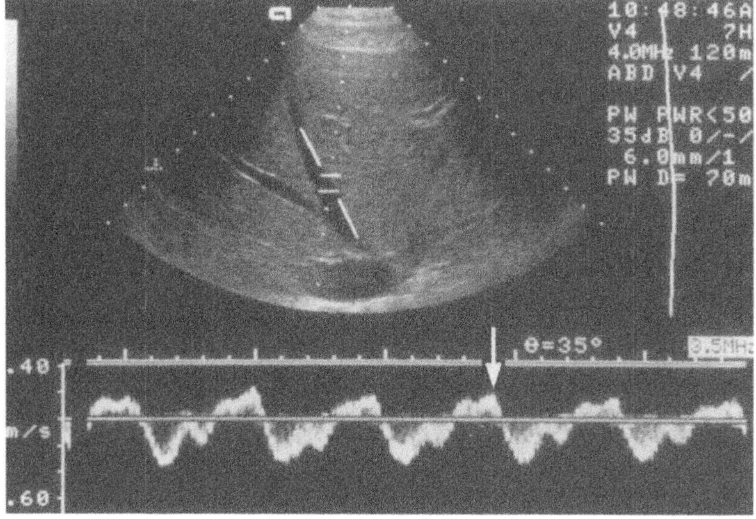

Fig. 12.4. Normal hepatic vein flow profile; note the c-wave, displayed immediately after the a-wave (*arrow*)

assessed by radionuclide ventriculography or Doppler echocardiography (Sakai et al. 1984; Pennestri et al. 1984). The hepatic vein Doppler waveform can be divided into three groups (according to Sakai et al. 1984) based on S-wave changes (Fig. 12.2b–d):

1. In the first group, S-wave flow velocities are decreased relative to the D-wave velocities (S/D 0.6, Fig. 12.5).
2. In group two, there is no systolic flow.
3. Group three shows reversed systolic blood flow.

Besides these distinct changes in the shape of the S-wave, other (minor) criteria apply in the presence of TV disease. An increase in D-wave velocities can be observed as well as a large retrograde v-wave. Moreover, retrograde a-wave velocities can also rise. However, these findings can also be seen in healthy subjects or other types of cardiac disorders, so that without S-wave abnormalities, the diagnosis of tricuspid regurgitation cannot be established. In that respect, a classic but rare pitfall is the Doppler waveform observed in left-to-right intracardiac shunts at the atrium level. Patients may show high retrograde v-wave and/or a-wave velocities together with a rise in diastolic flow velocities, but no dampening of the S-wave. Another pitfall is the evidence of atrial fibrillation or flutter. Figure 12.2 shows the gradual development of hepatic vein Doppler waveform changes typically observed in tricuspid regurgitation; Fig. 12.6 demonstrates the various forms of Doppler curves associated with TV disease.

Veins of the Splenoportal Axis. Normal subjects typically demonstrate minimal variation in portal vein

a
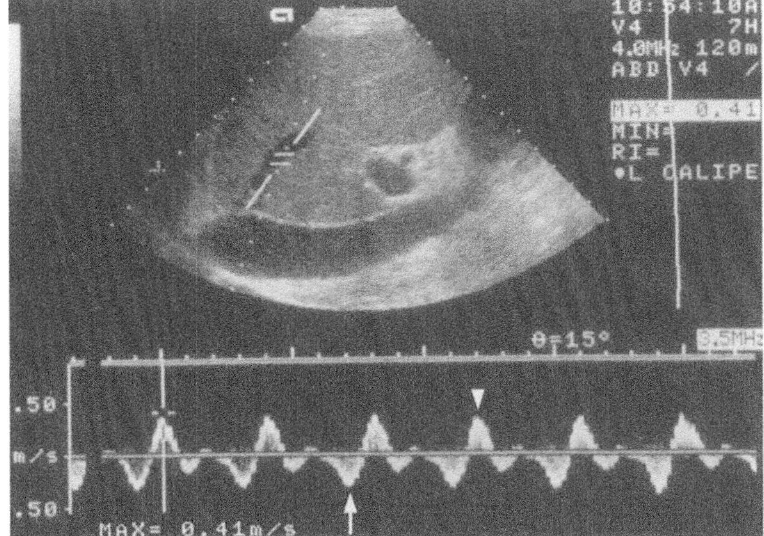

b
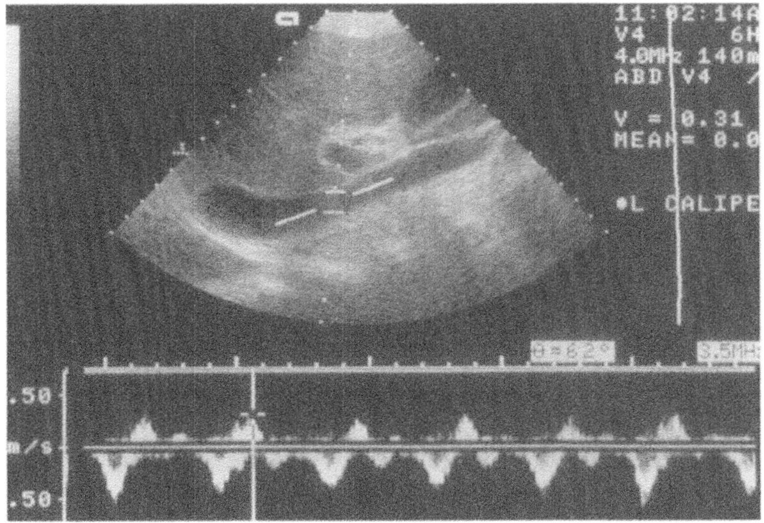

Fig. 12.5a, b. Patient with pulmonary hypertension and moderate tricuspid regurgitation. **a** Middle hepatic vein Doppler curve displays reduced S-wave velocity (S<D, *arrow*) and a large a-wave (*arrowhead*), indicating strong atrial contraction as a sign of compensated right heart disease. **b** IVC Doppler curve resembles findings in the hepatic vein

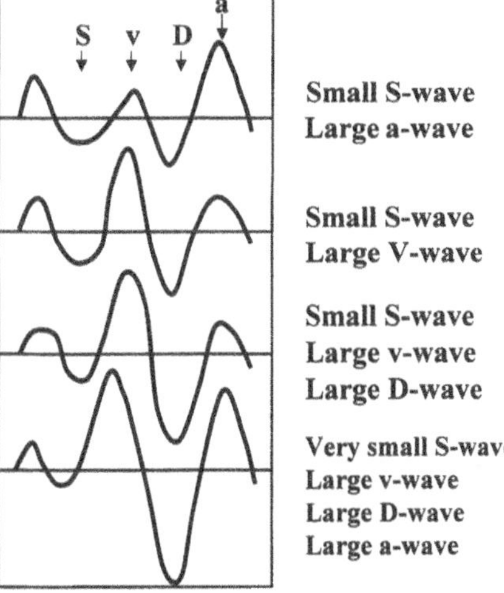

Fig. 12.6. Various flow patterns associated with tricuspid regurgitation

velocities on spectral Doppler analysis during breath-holding (Abu-Yousef 1992). In most instances, these changes cannot be observed in the splenic and the superior mesenteric veins, and blood flow in these veins shows a continuous pattern. The mildly phasic character in portal blood flow is most likely a reflection of changes in transmitted right atrial pressure, with significant dampening by resistance in venules, sinusoids, and small portal branches. In patients with tricuspid regurgitation, the exaggerated right atrial pressure changes are also reflected in the flow pattern in the portal vein. Here flow velocity during systole may be decreased or reversed as a result of the regurgitant blood flow from the right ventricle to the right atrium. The dilatation of sinusoids and the small branches of the portal and the hepatic veins, which probably occurs in tricuspid regurgitation, may also decrease their dampening effect on portal flow changes (Abu-Yousef 1990; Duerinckx et al. 1990; Hosoki et al. 1990). In severe regurgitation, pulsations are also transmitted in a hepatofugal direction to the splenic and superior mesenteric veins. However, such portal vein pulsatility is not peculiar to tricuspid regurgitation. The lack of sensitivity can be explained as a consequence of two reasons. First, portal vein flow pulsatility is in most cases a result of systolic flow inversion in the hepatic veins that may not be evident in mild or moderate TV disease, as discussed previously. The second factor is that portal vein flow may be continuous in patients with severe tricuspid regurgitation in the presence of advanced liver fibrosis. The only specific sign regarding pulsatile portal blood flow that accounts for tricuspid regurgitation is the presence of inverted flow following systole. However, this symptom can only be observed in about one-third of the patients (Loperfido et al. 1993). Furthermore, blood flow in the portal vein has been shown to be pulsatile in healthy subjects, especially in those with a low body weight (Gallix et al. 1997). Such flow modulations might be due to a lower intraabdominal pressure in lean rather than in overweight persons, a transmission of the pulsatility from the nearby inferior vena cava, or a splanchnic/hepatic artery wave transmission. For all these reasons, the finding of a pulsatile portal vein needs to be interpreted in a clinical context and does not necessarily imply dysfunction of the right side of the heart (Figs. 12.7, 12.8).

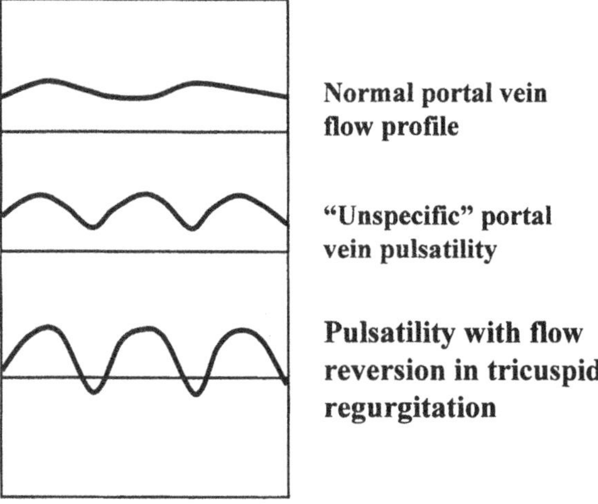

Fig. 12.7. Various portal vein flow patterns

Jugular Veins. Pulse and Doppler tracings obtained from the jugular veins are an established extracardiac diagnostic tool in the work-up of heart disease (Sivaciyan et al. 1978). The flow patterns observed in the jugular veins are very similar to the hepatic vein flow curves and directly reflect right atrial pressure changes. The main and most important waves obtained from jugular Doppler tracings are again a systolic (S) and a diastolic (D) wave (also see above, Fig. 12.2a). Tricuspid regurgitation is characterized by an S/D ratio <1, as also observed in the hepatic veins (Fig. 12.9). In severer cases, single diastolic flow (single Df) and finally retrograde systolic flow (ret. Sf) become evident. In contrast, retrograde diastolic flow (ret. Df) is not itself a feature of advanced tricuspid regurgitation; it is related to a high right atrial a-wave, indicating a vigorous atrial contraction in the presence of a decreased right ventricular compliance. Retrograde Df can be present in normal subjects during end-expiration but also in patients with right heart disorders, characterizing a compensated stage of the disease. If retrograde Df disappears in longitudinal follow-up exams, it can be considered an early sign of decompensation. Therefore, loss of retrograde flow during atrial systole plus abnormal forward flow indicates advanced right ventricular failure (Sivaciyan et al. 1978).

Generally, variations from the normal dominant systolic flow (namely S/D ratio ≤ 1) are associated with abnormal right heart hemodynamics with elevation of right atrial and end-diastolic ventricular pressures. There are only two exceptions that should be considered when establishing the differential diagnosis: post-cardiac surgery states and severe left ventricular overload.

In postcardiotomy patients, the abnormality in flow patterns in the presence of normal right ventricular pressures is best explained by a decrease in the compliance of the right atrium induced iatrogenically. Both its contractility and relaxation may be affected, contributing to a decrease in systolic blood flow. The stiffness of the atrium can further help build up 'v-wave' pressures during systole and therefore add to the diastolic flow velocity.

In patients with severe left ventricular volume overload, the reason for the change in flow pattern is perhaps explainable on the basis of a Bernheim effect on the atrial septum: The septum may bulge into the right atrium due to the high regurgitant volume and pressure build-up in the left atrium during ventricular systole, causing restriction of flow into the right side. This can be observed in severe mitral regurgitation.

Peripheral Lower Extremity Veins. The normal peripheral Doppler tracing typically shows spontaneous anterograde phasic flow. The explanation of the flow

a

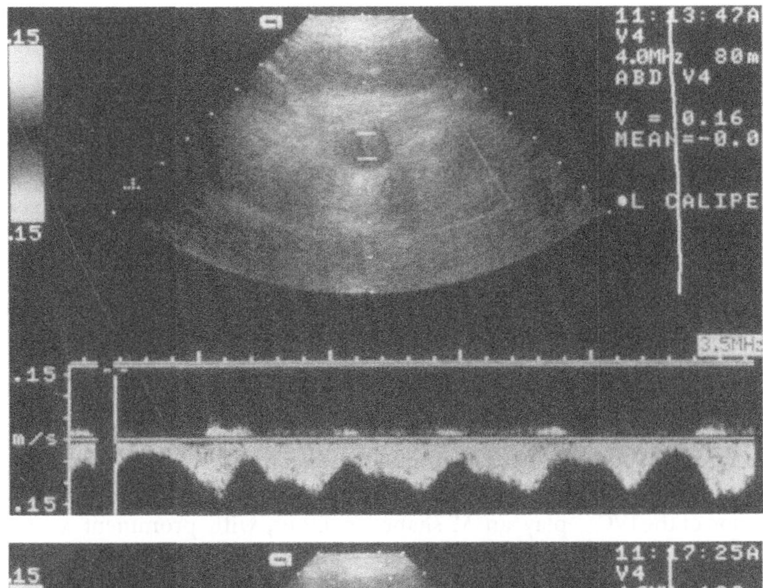

b

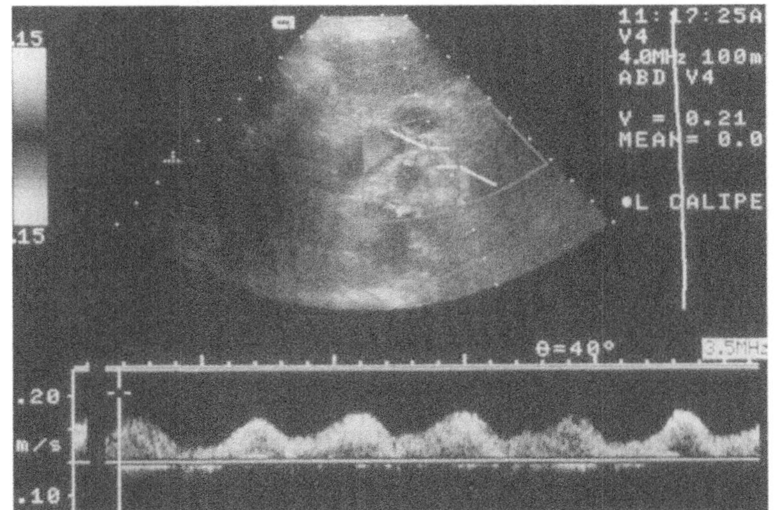

Fig. 12.8a, b. Patient with moderate tricuspid regurgitation. **a** Pulsatile portal vein flow curve with a slight amount of retrograde blood flow. **b** Propagation of pulsatility into the splenic vein

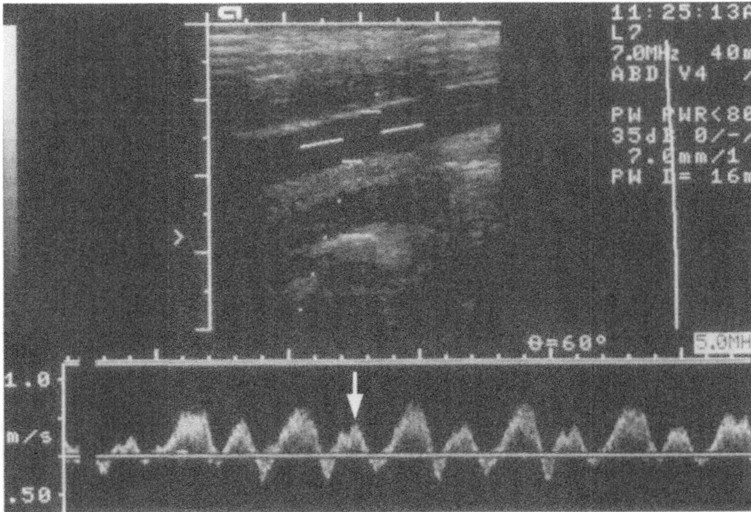

Fig. 12.9. Patient with tricuspid regurgitation: Jugular vein flow curve displays a low S-wave velocity with an S/D ratio <1. Moreover, there is retrograde diastolic flow (a-wave) and a 'notch' on top of the S-wave (x descent), corresponding to atrial relaxation (*arrow*)

phasicity is still controversial. Some authors believe it is cardiac in nature (Abu-Yousef 1992), reflecting changes in the right atrial pressure during the cardiac cycle, while others think it is respiratory in origin (Janssen et al. 1993). The most reasonable interpretation is that both factors contribute to the shaping of phasic pelvic or leg vein (LV) flow patterns. The cardiac nature of LV waveforms is indicated by their similarity to that of the hepatic veins and by correlation with simultaneous ECG tracings (see section on hepatic veins). The presence of cyclic retrograde LV flow is due to a large a-wave resulting from a large amount of stagnant blood because of right heart failure, or a combination of a large a-wave, a dampened or retrograde systolic wave (resulting from the reversal of flow that occurs in systole due to tricuspid valve incompetence), and sometimes a large retrograde v-wave (Fig. 12.10). The dilatation of the IVC and the peripheral veins that accompanies tricuspid regurgitation and congestive heart failure facilitates and speeds up the transmission of such right atrial pressure changes that make their waveforms pulsatile (Kakish et al. 1996). Especially when examining the lower extremity veins for venous thrombosis, the detection of a pulsatile waveform should alert the examiner to the possibility of underlying cardiac disease.

12.3 Pericardial Disease: Tamponade and Constrictive Pericarditis

The fundamental physiologic abnormality in patients with chronic constrictive pericarditis, as in those with cardiac tamponade, is the inability of the ventricles to fill sufficiently during diastole because of the limitations caused by the rigid pericardium or the tense pericardial fluid. In constrictive pericarditis, ventricular filling is unimpeded during early diastole but is reduced abruptly when the elastic limit of the pericardium is reached. In contrast, cardiac tamponade is characterized by impaired ventricular filling throughout diastole. In chronic constrictive pericarditis, the stroke volume is reduced. The end-diastolic pressures in both ventricles and the mean pressures in the atria, pulmonary veins, and systemic veins are all elevated to about the same levels. Despite these hemodynamic changes, the myocardial function is not affected and may actually be normal (Sivaciyan et al. 1978).

In constrictive pericarditis, the juxtacardiac venous, right and left atrial pressure pulses display an M-shaped contour, with prominent x and y descents (S-waves and especially D-waves, where D-wave velocities often exceed those of the S-waves); the y descent is the most prominent deflection and is interrupted by a rapid rise in pressure during early diastole, when ventricular filling is impeded by the constricting pericardium (Fig. 12.11). In contrast, the y descent (D-wave) is completely absent or diminished in cardiac tamponade. These characteristic changes are transmitted to the jugular and hepatic veins, where they may be recognized by Doppler flow imaging. For constrictive pericarditis, such changes in hemodynamics, although typical, are not pathognomonic but may also be observed in restrictive cardiomyopathies. In cardiac tamponade, however, complete absence of the D-wave combined with high S-wave velocities is more specific and should not be mistaken for another disorder (Fig. 12.12) (Lorrell and Braunwald 1992).

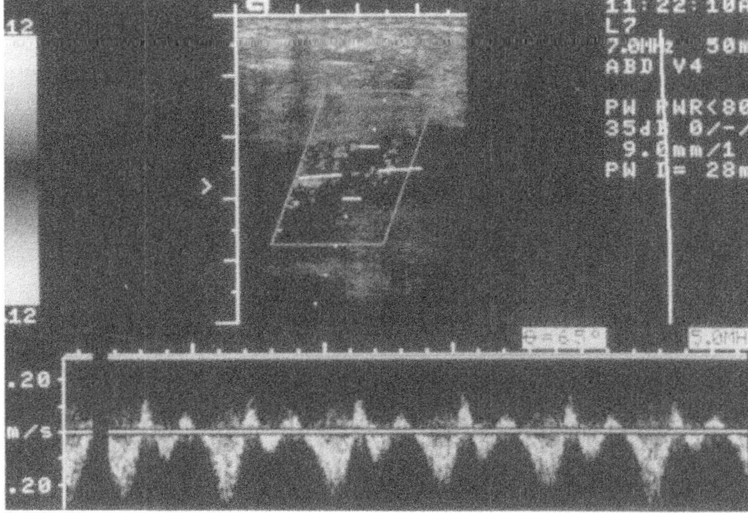

Fig. 12.10. Patient with congestive heart failure: Common femoral vein flow shows marked pulsatility similar to a waveform detectable in hepatic veins

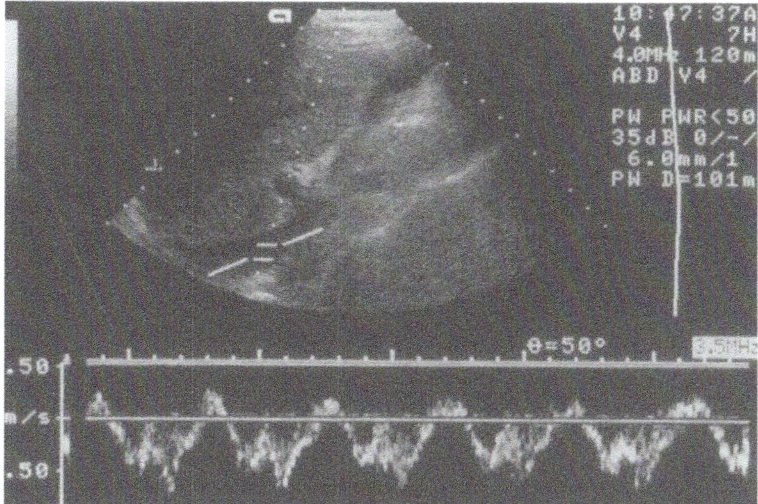

Fig. 12.11. Patient with constrictive pericarditis: IVC flow curve displays an M-shaped contour with a D-wave velocity exceeding 50 cm/s. The S-wave velocity is slightly reduced, with a S/D ratio <1

a

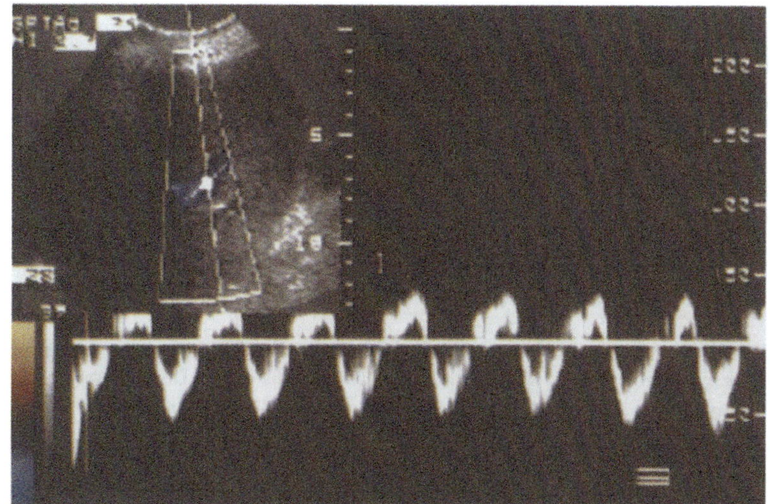

b

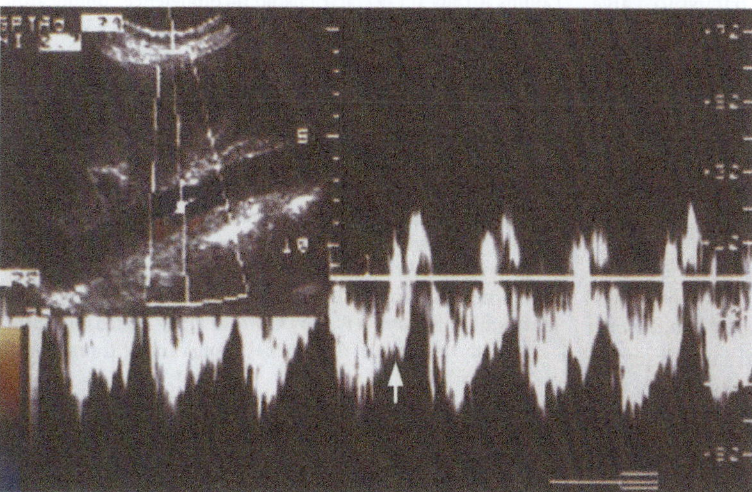

Fig. 12.12a, b. Patient with cardiac tamponade. **a** Hepatic vein flow curve demonstrates the absence of the D-wave and large a-waves (Cannon waves). **b** On the IVC flow curve, a very short D-wave can be seen (*arrow*). Note the high S-wave velocities (up to 50 cm/s)

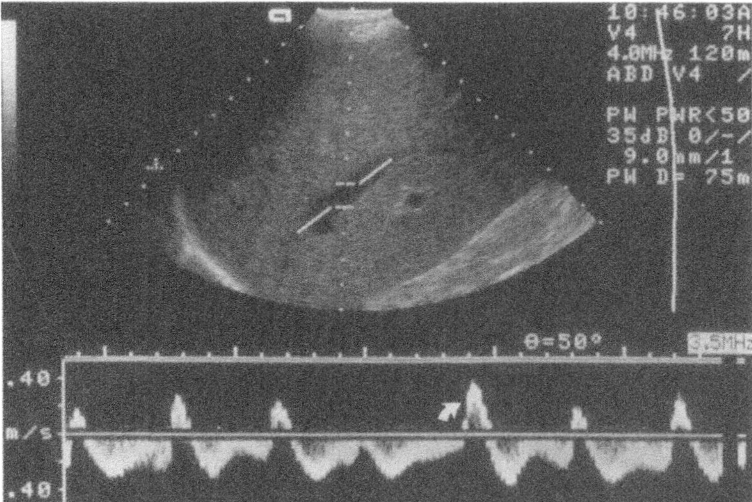

Fig. 12.13. Patient with junctional rhythm: Note the large a-waves (*arrow*) found in the middle hepatic vein as a sign of atrial contraction against a closed tricuspid valve

12.4 Rhythmologic Disorders of the Heart

Systolic flow is caused by two factors, namely atrial relaxation (x) and the descent of the ventricle base during active ventricular systole (x'), the latter being the dominant factor. Atrial relaxation flows have been shown to occur during atrioventricular dissociation or in patients with long P-R intervals. However, in healthy persons, atrial relaxation flows are depicted occasionally on Doppler imaging as a 'notch' on the upstroke of the systolic wave (Fig. 12.9) (Sivaciyan et al. 1978).

Large a-waves indicate that the right atrium is contracting against an increased resistance which occurs with tricuspid stenosis or more commonly with increased resistance to right ventricular filling (pulmonary hypertension or pulmonic stenosis). Large a-waves also occur during arrhythmias whenever the right atrium contracts while the tricuspid valve is closed by right ventricular systole. Such 'cannon' a-waves may occur regularly (as during junctional rhythm, Figs. 12.12, 12.13) or irregularly (as in atrioventricular dissociation with ventricular tachycardia or complete heart block).

In patients with atrial fibrillation, the a-wave is absent, based on the inability of the atrium to contract sufficiently. These patients show a lack of dominant systolic flow which some authors find is caused by the lack of atrial relaxation (Brawley et al. 1966). In other studies, a relationship to a decreased Starling effect on the ventricle is held responsible, due to loss of atrial systole, in turn leading to decreased ventricular contractility and diminished descent of the base (Kalamanson et al. 1971).

However, diminished systolic flow in atrial fibrillation should not be mistaken for tricuspid regurgitation (although often coexisting). The absence of an a-wave, as described above, may be helpful in the differential diagnosis.

References

Abu-Yousef MM (1990) Duplex Doppler sonography of the hepatic vein in tricuspid regurgitation. Am J Roentgenol 156:79–83

Abu-Yousef MM (1992) Normal and respiratory variations of the hepatic and portal venous duplex Doppler waveforms with simultaneous electrocardiographic correlation. J Ultrasound Med 11:263–268

Brawley RK, Oldham NH, Vasko JS et al (1966) Influence of right atrial pressure pulse on instantaneous vena cava blood flow. Am J Physiol 211:347

Collins R Daly JJ (1977) Tricuspid incompetence complicating acute myocardial infarction. Postgrad Med J 53:51

Duerinckx AJ, Grant EG, Perrella RR et al (1990) The pulsatile portal vein in cases of congestive heart failure: correlation of duplex Doppler findings with right atrial pressures. Radiology 176:655–658

Gallix BP, Taoural P, Dauzat M et al (1997) Flow pulsatility in the portal venous system: a study of Doppler sonography in healthy adults. Am J Roentgenol 169:141–144

Hosoki T, Arisawa J, Marukawa T et al (1990) Portal blood flow in congestive heart failure: pulsed duplex sonographic findings. Radiology 174:733–736

Jahnke EJ Jr, Nelson WP, Aaby GV et al (1967) Tricuspid insufficiency: the result of nonpenetrating cardiac trauma. Arch Surg 95:880

Janssen H, Trivino C, Williams D et al (1993) Hemodynamic alteration in venous blood flow produced by external pneumatic compression. J Cardiovasc Surg 34:441

Kakish ME, Abu-Yousef MM, Brown BP et al. (1996) Pulsatile

lower limb venous Doppler flow: revalence and value in cardiac disease diagnosis. J Ultrasound Med 15:747–753

Kalamanson D, Veyrat C, Chiche P (1971) Atrial versus ventricular contribution in determining systolic venous return. A new approach to an old riddle. Cardiovasc Res 5:293

Loperfido F, Lombardo A, Amico CM et al (1993) Doppler analysis of portal vein flow in tricuspid regurgitation. J Heart Valve Dis 2:174–182

Lorell B, Braunwald E (1992) Pericardial disease. In: Braunwald E (ed) Heart disease, 4th edn. Saunders, Philadelphia, pp 1465–1516

Pennestri F, Loperfido F, Salvatori M et al (1984) Assessment of tricuspid regurgitation by pulsed Doppler ultrasonography of the hepatic veins. Am J Cardiol 54:363–368

Sakai K, Nakamura K Satomi G et al (1984) Evaluation of tricuspid regurgitation by blood flow pattern in the hepatic vein using pulsed Doppler technique. Am Heart J 108: 516–523

Sharpiro RS, Winsberg F, Maldjian C et al (1993) Variability of hepatic vein Doppler tracings in normal subjects. J Ultrasound Med 12:701–703

Sivaciyan V, Ranganathan N (1978) Transcutaneous Doppler jugular venous flow velocity recording. Circulation 57: 930–938

13 Pediatric Aspects of Doppler Imaging of the Venous System

K. Vergesslich

CONTENTS

13.1 Introduction

Since the introduction of CDDS and pulsed Doppler imaging, the application of this technique for the assessment of the vascular status has been widely extended (Babcock et al. 1996). This is particularly important in the pediatric age group, where invasive catheterization can be partially avoided. Malformations of the venous system play an important role in children. Thus, some typical examples should be emphasized in this chapter. The special features of portal venous hemodynamics in portal hypertension represent another important aspect of the Doppler technique in the pediatric age group. In addition, the diagnosis of renal vein thrombosis is considerably facilitated by the application of CDDS.

K. Vergesslich, MD
Professor of Pediatric Radiology, Universitäts-Kinderklinik, Röntgen- und Ultraschalldiagnostik, Römergasse 8, 4005 Basel, Switzerland

13.2 Technique

Venous blood flow in the peripheral vessels is characterized by a laminar, continuous unidirectional flow profile with low velocity. Depending on the location of the vessel, the flow profile is influenced by respiration and cardiac activity. The wall filter should be low (50 Hz) to avoid motion artifacts of the vessel wall or adjacent organs. The sample volume has to extend over the entire vessel diameter. Lack of cooperation of the child may prolong the duration of the exam, but sedation is rarely necessary.

13.2.1 Blood Flow in Cerebral Veins and Sinuses

In the cerebral veins, a laminar, low velocity flow pattern is observed (Fig. 13.1). The blood flow can be slightly modulated by respiration within the big sinuses (Taylor et al. 1992).

13.2.2 Portal Venous Blood Flow

Portal venous blood flow is characterized by a continuous flow curve with respiratory and cardiac modulation (Fig. 13.2). The blood flow velocity is low. The flow signals of the portal vein, the splenic vein, and the SMV can only be distinguished by their anatomic location.

13.2.3 Blood Flow in the Inferior Vena Cava and Hepatic Veins

Abdominal veins adjacent to the heart show a characteristic flow profile due to cardiac modulation (Fig. 13.3) (Teichgräber et al. 1997). This applies primarily to the IVC and the hepatic veins. A triphasic blood flow curve is found:

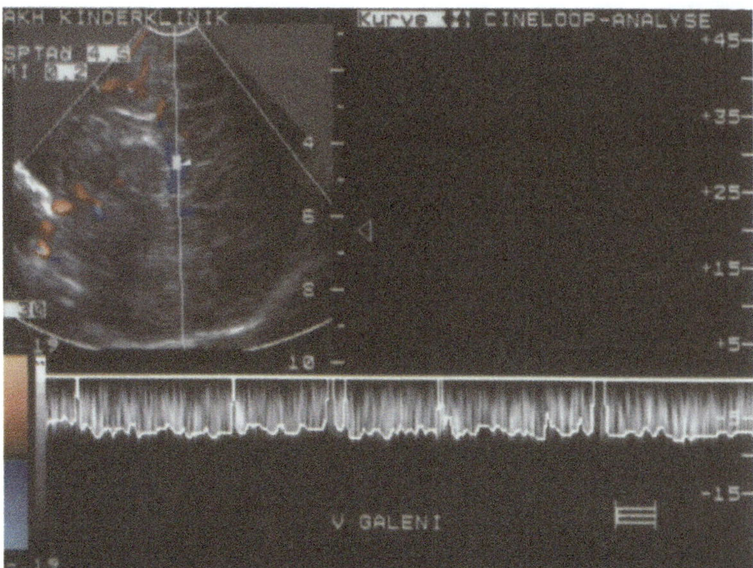

Fig. 13.1. Hemodynamics of cerebral veins. Sample volume (*arrowhead*) in vein of Galen: continuous, low velocity flow profile

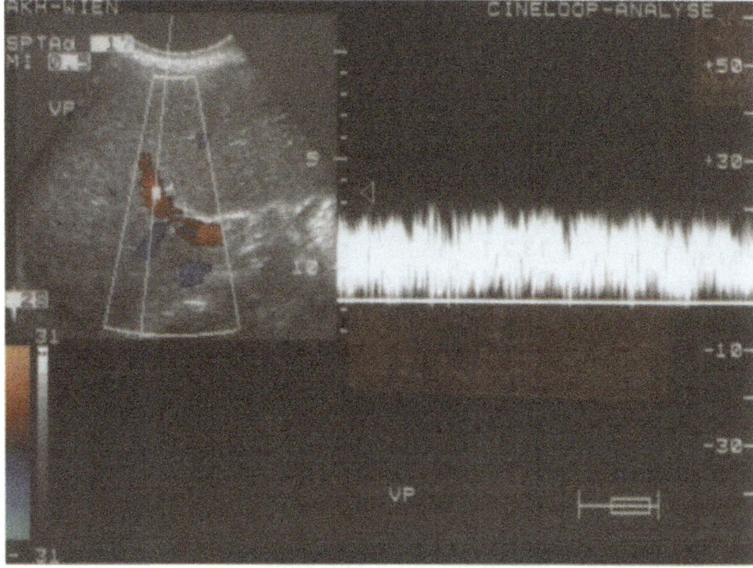

Fig. 13.2. Portal venous flow profile. Sample volume (*arrowhead*) in left portal vein: Laminar blood flow with minimal variation of flow amplitude

1. peak: early ventricular systole, atrial diastole: increased blood flow to the heart;
2. peak: early ventricular diastole: increased blood flow into the right ventricle;
3. peak: blood flow above the zero line, late diastole: flow reversal by atrial contraction.

13.3 Clinical Application

13.3.1 Arteriovenous Malformation of the Vein of Galen

Arteriovenous malformation of the vein of Galen represents the most common vascular malformation of the brain in children (Deeg and Scharf 1989). The characteristic clinical feature is cardiac decompensation in the neonatal period, caused by an extensive left to right shunt through the vascular malformation. Auscultation of a systolic–diastolic flow murmur over the anterior fontanel is characteristic, if not pathognomonic for this entity.

On real-time ultrasound, a round or oval, mostly echo-free mass is visualized behind the third ventricle and superior to the quadrigeminal plate. CDDS easily documents the vascular nature of the cystic mass. The flow within the mass is characterized by a 'mosaic pattern' caused by turbulence. In addition, the afferent and efferent vessels can also be shown.

The afferent vessel usually represents branches of the anterior cerebral artery, middle cerebral artery, posterior cerebral artery, or anterior or posterior

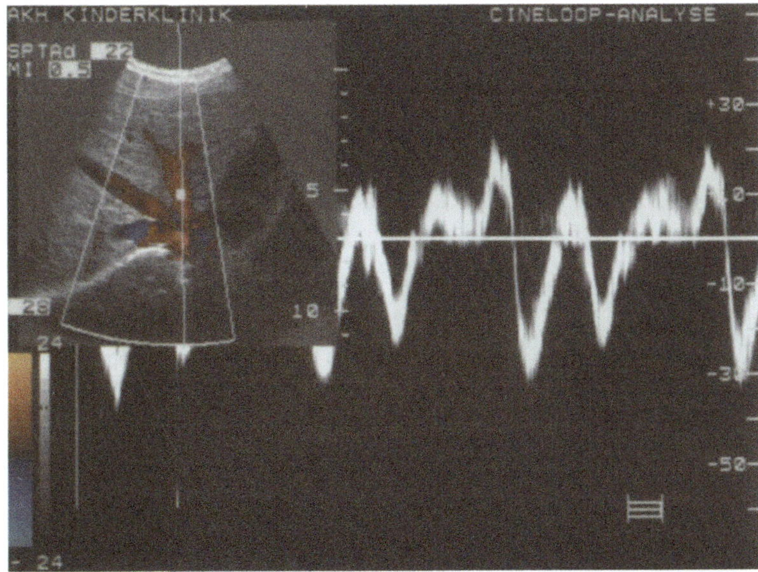

a

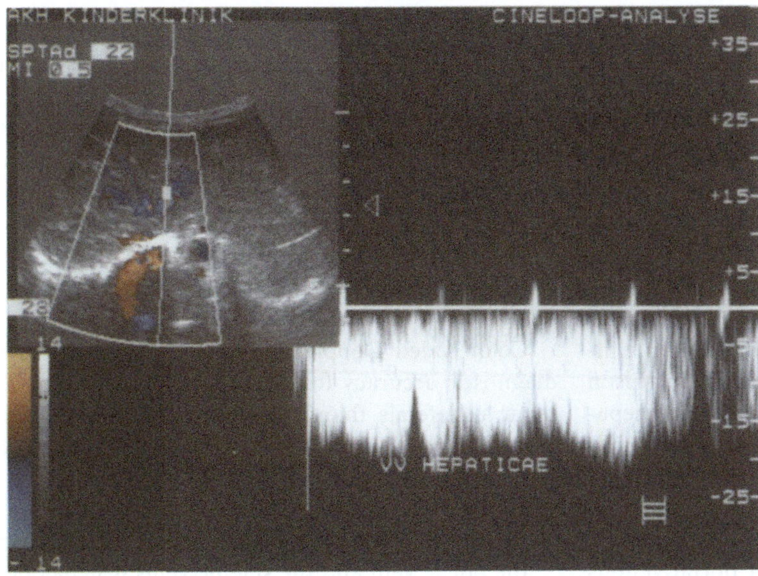

b

Fig. 13.3a,b. Hemodynamics of hepatic veins. a Regular, triphasic blood flow (cardiac modulation). b Band-like flow curve without cardiac modulation in a newborn infant with right heart decompensation

choroid artery. Often, the afferent vessel takes a serpiginous course. The flow pattern in these vessels is characterized by a high diastolic flow amplitude, caused by the low peripheral vascular resistance in the arteriovenous malformation ('vascular steal').

The blood flow volume within the draining straight sinus is elevated, estimated at about 1200 ml/min in comparison with 400 ml/min in healthy children. The basal veins, however, show normal blood flow velocities.

CDDS is considered to be the method of choice for the noninvasive diagnosis of arteriovenous malformation of the vein of Galen (Deeg and Scharf 1989). By application of a 3D reconstruction, the anatomy can be clearly differentiated (Fig. 13.4).

Therapy consists of embolization of the arteriovenous malformation. This is performed angiographically by inserting coils into the mass to make it hemodynamically ineffective. CDDS documents the efficacy of this procedure (Westra et al. 1993). Usually, blood flow in the center of the lesion is barely present, whereas the afferent vessels in the periphery of the malformation still exhibit increased flow velocities over a period of time.

13.3.2 Portal Hypertension

Portal hypertension in childhood is usually the result of chronic liver disease. The main cause

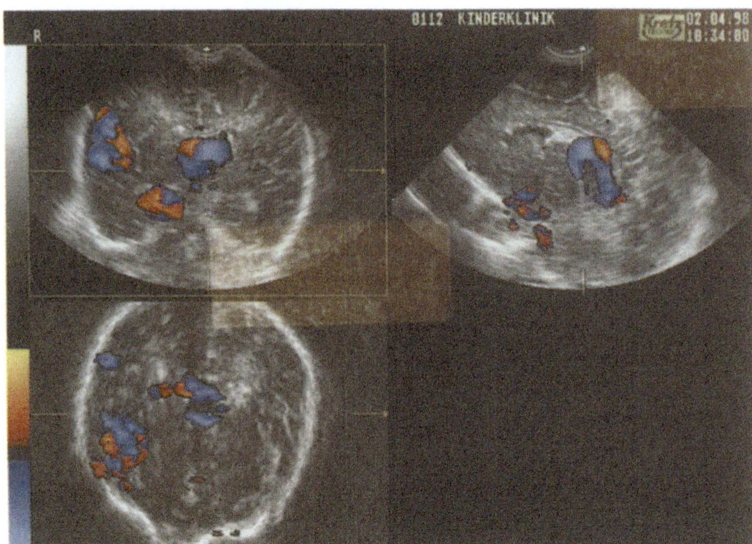

Fig. 13.4. Color-coded Doppler sonography of arteriovenous malformation of the vein of Galen, 3D reconstruction. Three malformations are clearly shown, one in the midline, one in the right temporal lobe, and one in the right hippocampal area. *Mixed red/blue color* as a sign of turbulent flow

(50–70%) is extrahepatic obstruction of the portal vein. In the majority of the patients, the pathogenesis remains unidentified. Often the symptomatology develops progressively after birth. Major causes in this age group are catheterization of the umbilical vein, omphalitis, and dehydration. In older children, abdominal trauma, pancreatitis, inflammatory or neoplastic disease adjacent to the portal vein are the major causes. In addition, storage diseases (e.g., Gaucher disease) or liver cirrhosis can ultimately lead to portal hypertension. Liver cirrhosis in children develops in α1-antitrypsin deficiency, Wilson disease, cystic fibrosis, or chronic aggressive hepatitis. The evaluation of portal hypertension in children represents a great challenge for the pediatric radiologist. Real-time sonography has become the screening procedure of choice to detect the anatomy of the porta hepatis. The increase of portal venous diameter and its reduced respiratory variability are indirect signs of the development of portal hypertension. Another sign is an absent increase of the portal venous diameter after a meal. The most important sign of portal hypertension is the documentation of portosystemic collaterals (Vergesslich et al. 1989; Subramanyam et al. 1983).

Hemodynamically, two types of portosystemic collaterals may be differentiated:

1. Closed or partially closed channels of the fetal period that are reopened (Farrant et al. 1996). They provide a linkage between the portal venous system and the venous system: Parumbilical veins in the falciform ligament (Fig. 13.5).
2. Flow reversal in vessels: Collaterals present themselves as echo-free, tubular or serpiginous structures on real-time sonography. Subramanyam et al. (1983) described 60 different collateral pathways in portal hypertension. The most important ones are: coronary vein, gastroesophageal veins, pancreaticoduodenal veins, gastrorenal and splenorenal veins, and rectal plexus (Fig. 13.6) (Subramanyam et al. 1983; Kainberger et al. 1990; Riehl et al. 1997; Besnard et al. 1994).

Color-coded Doppler sonography shows higher diagnostic accuracy for the evaluation of portosystemic collaterals than pulsed Doppler sonography. The following Doppler sonographic parameters are important for the diagnosis of portal hypertension:

- Blood flow direction. The normal flow direction in the portal vein and the splenic veins is hepatopetal. In severe portal hypertension, flow reversal may occur, leading to hepatofugal blood flow.
- Spontaneous shunting. Hemodynamically open portosystemic shunts cause flow reversal in the portal vein (Fig. 13.7).
- Quantitative assessment of portal venous hemodynamics. A significant reduction of blood flow velocity was observed in patients with liver cirrhosis, chronic aggressive hepatitis, or idiopathic portal hypertension. The concomitant increase of portal venous diameter keeps the blood flow volume constant. Sometimes a tendency to increased blood flow volume was observed. This is apparently the result of adaptation of the pressure-volume curve of the portal venous system. In severe portal hypertension, this adaptive mecha-

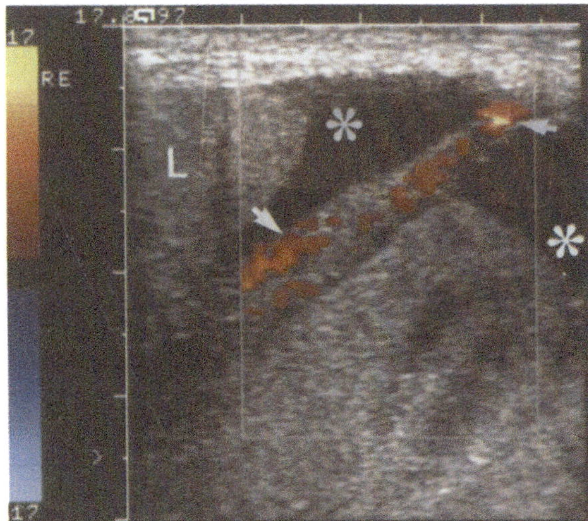

Fig. 13.5. Recanalization of paraumbilical veins. Multiple colored impulses coded in *red* (*arrows*) in the falciform ligament: hepatofugal blood flow (*L*, liver). Newborn infant with hepatic failure (*stars*, ascites) due to connatal hemochromatosis

nism cannot prevent the reduction of the portal venous blood flow volume.

The higher life expectancy of patients with cystic fibrosis makes involvement of the liver in this entity more common. The frequency of chronic liver disease in portal hypertension varies between 20% and 50%. With increasing age, the clinical presentation of liver disease becomes more common. VERGESSLICH et al. (1989) described a significant increase of the diameter and a significant reduction of blood flow velocity of the portal vein in comparison to age-matched healthy children. The concomitant rise of the portal venous blood flow volume could be partly due to the above-mentioned adaptive mechanism of the pressure-volume curve of the portal vein, in part other hemodynamic alterations in cystic fibrosis may be responsible (e.g., cardiac!). Liver function tests often become pathologic late in the course of the disease; even in the presence of portal hypertension, they do

a

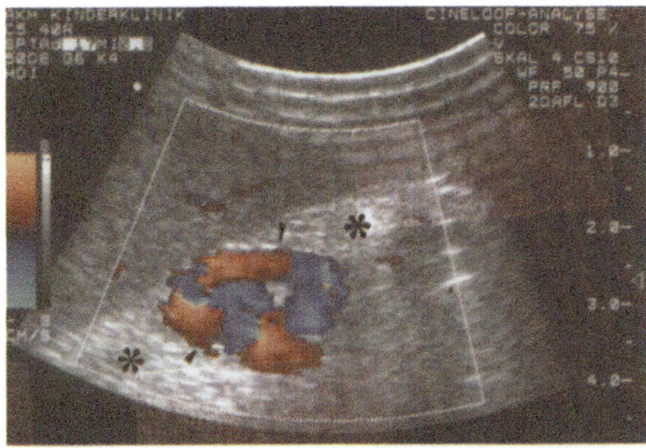

b

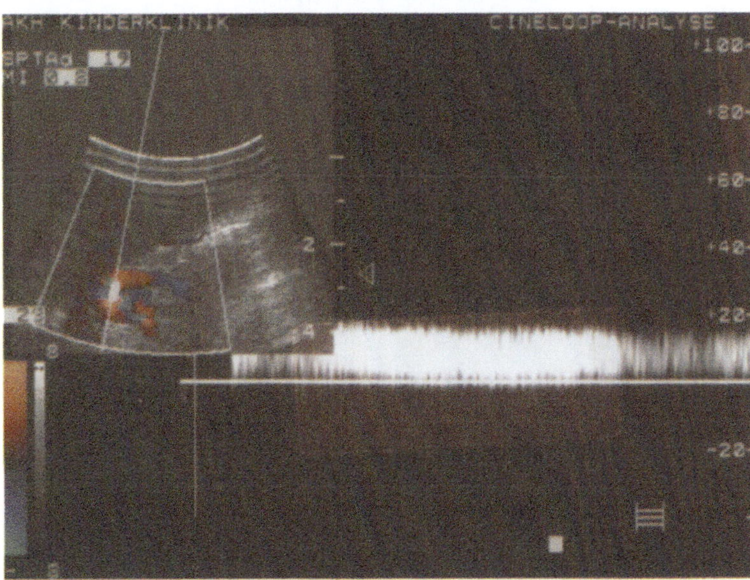

Fig. 13.6a,b. Gastroesophageal varices. **a** Tubular, vascular structures (*arrowheads*) in echogenic omentum minus (*stars*). **b** Pulsed Doppler flow curve shows typical portal venous blood flow pattern with low velocity, band-like flow curve. Two-month-old infant with biliary atresia, status after Kasai operation

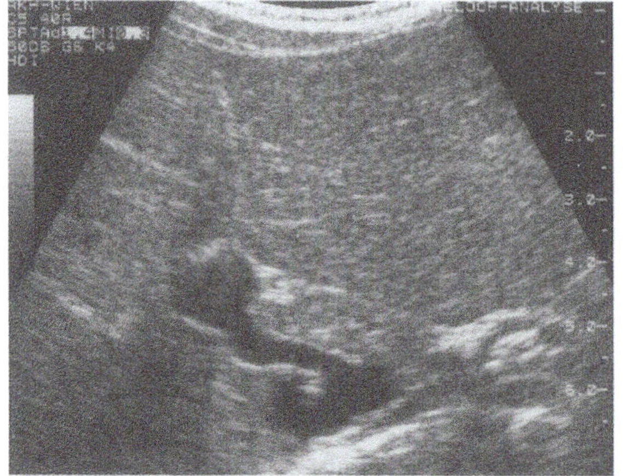

a

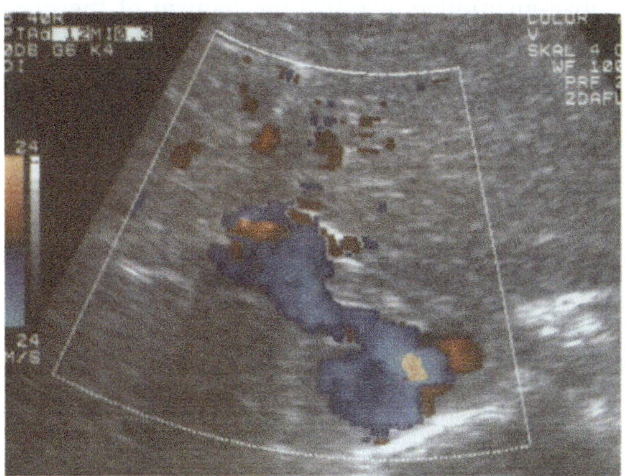

b

Fig 13.7a,b. Portocaval shunt. **a** Serpiginous communication between the portal vein and the inferior hepatic vein adjacent to the confluens. **b** Blood flow in the vascular malformation is coded in *blue*: hepatofugal blood flow. Three-year-old infant with cardiomegaly, pulmonary hypertension, and an incidentally found portocaval shunt

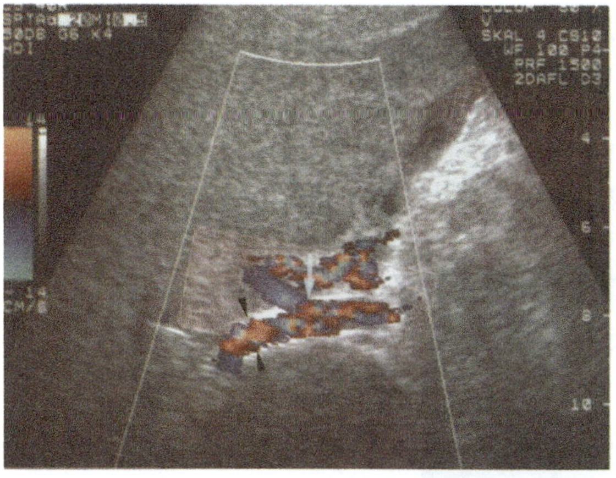

Fig. 13.8. Transjugular portosystemic shunt (TIPS). TIPS (*arrowheads*) shows regular perfusion with turbulent flow (mosaic pattern). Anastomosis (*arrow*) with portal vein. Seven-year-old boy with hepatic failure due to congenital disorder of glycosylation syndrome

not necessarily differ markedly from normal. Under these circumstances, early assessment of hemodynamic changes of the portal venous system provides important information about liver involvement in the course of the disease.

In severe portal hypertension with portosystemic collaterals, therapy consists of either a surgical portosystemic shunt or a transjugular portosystemic shunt (TIPS). This alternative to the surgical procedure is becoming more widely used in specialized centers (Fig. 13.8). Hepatofugal or splenofugal blood flow within the shunt, high mean blood flow velocity, and high volume flow are direct Doppler sonographic signs of shunt patency.

13.3.3 Abdominal Situs

Normal abdominal situs is characterized by the fact that the abdominal aorta is situated on the left side of the spine and the inferior vena cava on the right–situs solitus. In situs inversus, there is a mirror image arrangement: The aorta is on the right and the inferior vena cava on the left. In situs ambiguus, the classification of the abdominal vessels is more complicated.

13.3.3.1 Situs Ambiguus with Left Isomerism

The hepatic veins drain into an azygos continuation, the inferior vena cava is absent. This anomaly is associated with polysplenia, two left-sided lungs (lingula), and a left atrium (no septum).

13.3.3.2 Situs Ambiguus with Right Isomerism

In this anomaly, no spleen is present (asplenia), there are two right lungs (middle lobe), anomalous drainage of the pulmonary veins, and a right atrium (absent septum). Often there is an association with congenital heart disease with right heart obstruction (pulmonary atresia).

13.3.4 Renal Vein Thrombosis

Renal vein thrombosis occurs either in the neonatal period (e.g., after dehydration) or secondarily in the course of nephrotic syndrome, coagulopathies, or

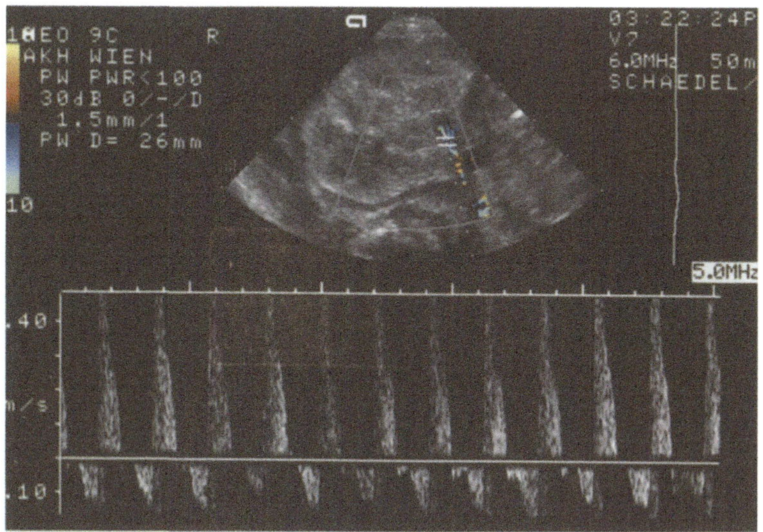

Fig. 13.9. Renal vein thrombosis. Diastolic flow reversal in the renal artery as a result of increased peripheral vascular resistance. Aliasing due to high systolic flow velocities. Newborn infant with oliguria and hematuria

tumors. On real-time sonography, the affected kidney is enlarged in size, and the echogenicity is inhomogeneously increased. Eventually, thrombosis of the IVC or a tumor can be demonstrated. On pulsed Doppler sonogram, the following characteristic features can be noted:

- Flow in the renal vein is absent or markedly reduced;
- Diastolic blood flow in the arteries is decreased, absent, or reversed;
- The resistive index increases to 1 or even above 1 (Fig. 13.9).

13.4 Conclusion

CDDS is a valuable diagnostic tool in the evaluation of normal and pathologic hemodynamic states of the venous system in children. The constant technologic development continuously produces new diagnostic possibilities, making other invasive procedures partly unnecessary.

References

Babcock AS et al (1996) Power Doppler sonography: basic principles and clinical application in children. Pediatr Radiol 26:109–115

Besnard M et al (1994) Portal cavernoma in congenital hepatic fibrosis. Pediatr Radiol 24:61–65

Deeg KH, Scharf J (1989) Colour Doppler imaging of arteriovenous malformation of the vein of Galen in a newborn. Neuroradiology 32:60–63

Farrant P et al (1996) Ultrasound diagnosis of portocaval anastomosis in infants–a report of eight cases. Br J Radiol 69:389–393

Kainberger FM et al (1990) Color-coded Doppler evaluation of cholecystic varices in portal hypertension. Pediatr Radiol 21:71–72

Riehl JD et al (1997) Spontaneous portosystemic shunts in liver cirrhosis: demonstration by color coded duplex ultrasonography. Ultraschall Med 6:272–276

Subramanyam BR et al (1983) Sonographic evaluation of patients with portal hypertension. Am J Gastroenterol 78: 369–373

Taylor GA et al (1992) Intracranial venous system in the newborn: evaluation of normal anatomy and flow characteristics with color Doppler US. Radiology 183:449–452

Teichgräber JD et al (1997) Characterization of hepatic venous flow via duplex doppler sonography. Ultraschall Med 6: 267–272

Vergesslich KA et al (1989) Portal venous blood flow in cystic fibrosis: assessment by duplex Doppler sonography. Pediatr Radiol 19:371–374

Westra SJ et al (1993) Pediatric intracranial vascular malformations: evaluation of treatment results with color-coded Doppler ultrasound. Radiology 186:775–783

Abbrevaitions

ACD	Amplitude Coded Color Doppler
A/D	Analog/Digital
A-mode	Amplitude mode
ATV	Anterior Tibial Vein
AV	Axillary Vein
BCV	Brachiocephalic Vein
B-mode	Brightness (gray-scale) mode
BV	Brachial Vein
CDDS	Color Duplex Doppler Imaging
CDI	Color Doppler Imaging
CFV	Common Femoral Vein
CIV	Common Iliac Vein
CT	Computed Tomography
CV	Contrast Venography
CVI	Color Velocity Imaging
CW	Continuous-wave
DFT	Discrete Fourier Tranformation
DFV	Deep Femoral Vein
DS	Duplex Scanning
DVT	Deep Venous Thrombosis
EIV	External Iliac Vein
FR	Frame Rate
FV	Fibular Vein
GSV	Great (Long) Saphenous Vein
HV	Hepatic Vein
IIV	Internal Iliac Vein
IJV	Internal Jugular Vein
IMV	Inferior Mesenteric Vein
IVC	Inferior Vena Cava
MHz	Megahertz
MI	Mechanical Index
MR	Magnetic Resonance
MRI	Magnetic Resonance Imaging
MTI	Moving Target Indicator
PE	Pulmonary Embolism
PI	Pulsatility Indice
POPV	Popliteal Vein
POV	Portal Vein
PRF	Pulse Repetition Frequency
PTV	Posterior Tibial Vein
PV	Perforating Veins
PW	Pulsed-wave
QA	Quality Assurance
RBC	Red Blood Cell
RI	Resistence Index
RV	Renal Vein
SFV	Superficial Femoral Vein
SMV	Superior Mesenteric Vein
SPV	Splenic Vein
SSV	Small (Short) Saphenous Vein
SV	Subclavian Vein
SVC	Superior Vena Cava
TDA	Time-Domain analysis
TI	Thermal Index
TIB	Thermal Indexmodel for bone at focus
TIC	Thermal Index model for transcranial application
TIPS	Transjugular Intrahepatic Portosystemic Shunt
TIS	Thermal Index model for soft tissue
VTE	Venous Thromboembolism

Subject Index

List of Contributors

MANFRED BALDT, MD
Associate Professor of Radiology
Bilddiagnostik Wolfsberg
Roßmarkt 14
9400 Wolfsberg
Austria

ROLAND DORFFNER, MD
Associate Professor of Radiology
Department of Radiology
Hospital of the Brothers of St. John
Esterhazystr. 26
7000 Eisenstadt
Austria

FRANZ FOBBE, MD
Professor of Radiology
Auguste-Viktoria-Krankenhaus
Abteilung für Röntgendiagnostik
Rubensstr. 125
12157 Berlin
Germany

STEPHAN GRAMPP, MD
Associate Professor of Radiology
Department of Radiology
Univ. Hosp. Vienna, School of Medicine
Währinger Gürtel 18–20
1090 Vienna
Austria

NORBERT GRITZMANN, MD
Professor of Radiology
Department of Radiology
Hospital of the Brothers of St. John
Kajetanerplatz 1
6020 Salzburg
Austria

CHRISTINE B. HENK, MD
Associate Professor of Radiology
Department of Radiology
Univ. Hosp. Vienna, School of Medicine
Währinger Gürtel 18–20
1090 Vienna
Austria

ALOIS HOLLERWEGER, MD
Department of Radiology
Hospital of the Brothers of St. John
Kajetanerplatz 1
6020 Salzburg
Austria

FRANZ KARNEL, MD
Röntgeninstitut
Kaiser-Franz-Josef-Spital
Kundratstraße 3
A-1100 Vienna
Austria

CHRISTIAN KOLLMANN, PhD
Institut für Biomedizinische Technik und Physik
AKH Vienna
Währinger Gürtel 18–20
1090 Vienna
Austria

REINHARD KUBALE, MD
Associate Professor of Radiology
Institut für Radiologie, Sonographie
und Nuklearmedizin Pirmasens
Ringstr. 60-64
66953 Pirmasens
Germany

JASMIN LISKUTIN, MD
CT und MR Institut Hernalser Spitz
Jörgerstr. 52
1170 Vienna
Austria

Peter Macheiner, MD
Department of Radiology
Hospital of the Brothers of St. John
Kajetanerplatz 1
6020 Salzburg
Austria

M. Merz, MD
Innere Abteilung
Kreiskrankenhaus Sigmaringen
Hohenzollernstr. 40
72488 Sigmaringen
Germany

Gerhard H. Mostbeck, MD
Professor of Radiology
Department of Radiology
Sozialmedizinisches Zentrum
Baumgartner Höhe mit Pflegezentrum
Otto Wagner Spital
Sanatoriumstr. 2
1140 Vienna
Austria

Günther Nics, MD
Röntgeninstitut
Kaiser-Franz-Josef-Spital
and Röntgenordination Hollabrunn
Kundratstraße 3
1100 Vienna
Austria

Thomas Rettenbacher, MD
Department of Radiology
Hospital of the Brothers of St. John
Kajetanerplatz 1
6020 Salzburg
Austria

Karl-Heinz Seitz, MD
Associate Professor of Internal Medicine
Innere Abteilung
Kreiskrankenhaus Sigmaringen
Hohenzollernstr. 40
72488 Sigmaringen
Germany

Gertraud Strasser, MD
Department of Radiology
Sozialmedizinisches Zentrum
Baumgartner Höhe mit Pflegezentrum
Otto Wagner Spital
Sanatoriumstr. 2
1140 Vienna
Austria

Klara Vergesslich, MD
Professor of Pediatric Radiology
Universitäts-Kinderklinik
Röntgen und Ultraschalldiagnostik
Römergasse 8
4005 Basel
Switzerland

Hans Peter Weskott, MD
Klinikum Hannover
Siloah KH, Med. Klinik II
Roesebeckstr. 15
30449 Hannover
Germany

Thomas Zontsich, MD
Ambulatorium für Computertomographie,
Ultraschall und moderne Schnittbilddiagnostik
Ferdinand Porsche Ring 10
2700 Wiener Neustadt
Austria

Medical Radiology Diagnostic Imaging and Radiation Oncology

Titles in the series already published

Diagnostic Imaging

Innovations in Diagnostic Imaging
Edited by J. H. Anderson

Radiology of the Upper Urinary Tract
Edited by E. K. Lang

The Thymus - Diagnostic Imaging, Functions, and Pathologic Anatomy
Edited by E. Walter, E. Willich, and W. R. Webb

Interventional Neuroradiology Edited by A. Valavanis

Radiology of the Pancreas
Edited by A. L. Baert, co-edited by G. Delorme

Radiology of the Lower Urinary Tract
Edited by E. K. Lang

Magnetic Resonance Angiography
Edited by I. P. Arlart, G. M. Bongartz, and G. Marchal

Contrast-Enhanced MRI of the Breast
S. Heywang-Köbrunner and R. Beck

Spiral CT of the Chest
Edited by M. Rémy-Jardin and J. Rémy

Radiological Diagnosis of Breast Diseases
Edited by M. Friedrich and E.A. Sickles

Radiology of the Trauma
Edited by M. Heller and A. Fink

Biliary Tract Radiology
Edited by P. Rossi

Radiological Imaging of Sports Injuries
Edited by C. Masciocchi

Modern Imaging of the Alimentary Tube
Edited by A. R. Margulis

Diagnosis and Therapy of Spinal Tumors
Edited by P. R. Algra, J. Valk, and J. J. Heimans

Interventional Magnetic Resonance Imaging
Edited by J. F. Debatin and G. Adam

Abdominal and Pelvic MRI
Edited by A. Heuck and M. Reiser

Orthopedic Imaging
Techniques and Applications
Edited by A. M. Davies and H. Pettersson

Radiology of the Female Pelvic Organs
Edited by E. K.Lang

Magnetic Resonance of the Heart and Great Vessels
Clinical Applications
Edited by J. Bogaert, A.J. Duerinckx, and F. E. Rademakers

Modern Head and Neck Imaging
Edited by S. K. Mukherji and J. A. Castelijns

Radiological Imaging of Endocrine Diseases
Edited by J. N. Bruneton in collaboration with B. Padovani and M.-Y. Mourou

Trends in Contrast Media
Edited by H. S. Thomsen, R. N. Muller, and R. F. Mattrey

Functional MRI
Edited by C. T. W. Moonen and P. A. Bandettini

Radiology of the Pancreas
2nd Revised Edition
Edited by A. L. Baert
Co-edited by G. Delorme and L. Van Hoe

Emergency Pediatric Radiology
Edited by H. Carty

Spiral CT of the Abdomen
Edited by F. Terrier, M. Grossholz,and C. D. Becker

Liver Malignancies
Diagnostic and Interventional Radiology
Edited by C. Bartolozzi and R. Lencioni

Medical Imaging of the Spleen
Edited by A. M. De Schepper and F. Vanhoenacker

Radiology of Peripheral Vascular Diseases
Edited by E. Zeitler

Diagnostic Nuclear Medicine
Edited by C. Schiepers

Radiology of Blunt Trauma of the Chest
P. Schnyder and M. Wintermark

Portal Hypertension
Diagnostic Imaging-Guided Therapy
Edited by P. Rossi
Co-edited by P. Ricci and L. Broglia

Recent Advances in Diagnostic Neuroradiology
Edited by Ph. Demaerel

Virtual Endoscopy and Related 3D Techniques
Edited by P. Rogalla, J. Terwisscha Van Scheltinga, and B. Hamm

Multislice CT
Edited by M. F. Reiser, M. Takahashi, M. Modic, and R. Bruening

Pediatric Uroradiology
Edited by R. Fotter

Transfontanellar Doppler Imaging in Neonates
A. Couture and C. Veyrac

Radiology of AIDS
A Practical Approach
Edited by J.W.A.J. Reeders and P.C. Goodman

CT of the Peritoneum
Armando Rossi and Giorgio Rossi

Magnetic Resonance Angiography
2nd Revised Edition
Edited by I. P. Arlart, G. M. Bongratz,and G. Marchal

Pediatric Chest Imaging
Edited by Javier Lucaya and Janet L. Strife

Applications of Sonography in Head and Neck Pathology
Edited by J. N. Bruneton in collaboration with C. Raffaelli and O. Dassonville

Imaging of the Larynx
Edited by R. Hermans

3D Image Processing
Techniques and Clinical Applications
Edited by D. Caramella and C. Bartolozzi

Imaging of Orbital and Visual Pathway Pathology
Edited by W. S. Müller-Forell

Pediatric ENT Radiology
Edited by S. J. King and A. E. Boothroyd

Radiological Imaging of the Small Intestine
Edited by N. C. Gourtsoyiannis

Imaging of the Knee
Techniques and Applications
Edited by A. M. Davies and V. N. Cassar-Pullicino

Perinatal Imaging
From Ultrasound to MR Imaging
Edited by Fred E. Avni

Radiological Imaging of the Neonatal Chest
Edited by V. Donoghue

Diagnostic and Interventional Radiology in Liver Transplantation
Edited by E. Bücheler, V. Nicolas, C. E. Broelsch, X. Rogiers, and G. Krupski

Radiology of Osteoporosis
Edited by S. Grampp

Imaging Pelvic Floor Disorders
Edited by C. I. Bartram and J. O. L. DeLancey
Associate Editors: S. Halligan, F. M. Kelvin, and J. Stoker

Imaging of the Pancreas
Cystic and Rare Tumors
Edited by C. Procassi and A. J. Megibow

High Resolution Sonography of the Peripheral Nervous System
Edited by S. Peer and G. Bodner

Imaging of the Foot and Ankle
Techniques and Applications
Edited by A. M. Davies, R. W. Whitehouse, and J. P. R. Jenkins

Radiology Imaging of the Ureter
Edited by F. Joffre, Ph. Otal, and M. Soulie

Imaging of the Shoulder
Techniques and Applications
Edited by A. M. Davies and J. Hodler

Radiology of the Petrous Bone
Edited by M. Lemmerling and S. S. Kollias

Interventional Radiology in Cancer
Edited by A. Adam, R. F. Dondelinger, and P. R. Mueller

Duplex and Color Doppler Imaging of the Venous System
Edited by G. H. Mostbeck

Multidetector-Row CT of the Thorax
Edited by U. J. Schoepf

Intracranial Vascular Malformations and Aneurysms
From Diagnostic Work-Up to Endovascular Therapy
Edited by M. Forsting

Functional Imaging of the Chest
Edited by H.-U. Kauczor

Radiology of the Pharynx and the Esophagus
Edited by O. Ekberg

Radiological Imaging in Hematological Malignancies
Edited by A. Guermazi

Imaging and Intervention in Abdominal Trauma
Edited by R. F. Dondelinger

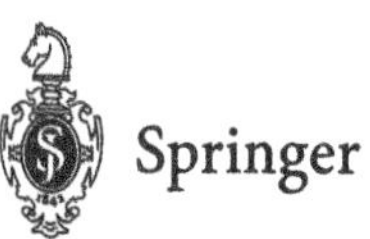

Springer

MEDICAL RADIOLOGY Diagnostic Imaging and Radiation Oncology

Titles in the series already published

RADIATION ONCOLOGY

Lung Cancer
Edited by C.W. Scarantino

Innovations in Radiation Oncology
Edited by H. R. Withers and L. J. Peters

Radiation Therapy of Head and Neck Cancer
Edited by G. E. Laramore

Gastrointestinal Cancer – Radiation Therapy
Edited by R.R. Dobelbower, Jr.

Radiation Exposure and Occupational Risks
Edited by E. Scherer, C. Streffer, and K.-R. Trott

Radiation Therapy of Benign Diseases
A Clinical Guide
S. E. Order and S. S. Donaldson

Interventional Radiation Therapy Techniques – Brachytherapy
Edited by R. Sauer

Radiopathology of Organs and Tissues
Edited by E. Scherer, C. Streffer, and K.-R. Trott

Concomitant Continuous Infusion Chemotherapy and Radiation
Edited by M. Rotman and C. J. Rosenthal

Intraoperative Radiotherapy – Clinical Experiences and Results
Edited by F. A. Calvo, M. Santos, and L.W. Brady

Radiotherapy of Intraocular and Orbital Tumors
Edited by W. E. Alberti and R. H. Sagerman

Interstitial and Intracavitary Thermoradiotherapy
Edited by M. H. Seegenschmiedt and R. Sauer

Non-Disseminated Breast Cancer
Controversial Issues in Management
Edited by G. H. Fletcher and S.H. Levitt

Current Topics in Clinical Radiobiology of Tumors
Edited by H.-P. Beck-Bornholdt

Practical Approaches to Cancer Invasion and Metastases
A Compendium of Radiation Oncologists' Responses to 40 Histories
Edited by A. R. Kagan with the Assistance of R. J. Steckel

Radiation Therapy in Pediatric Oncology
Edited by J. R. Cassady

Radiation Therapy Physics
Edited by A. R. Smith

Late Sequelae in Oncology
Edited by J. Dunst and R. Sauer

Mediastinal Tumors. Update 1995
Edited by D. E. Wood and C. R. Thomas, Jr.

Thermoradiotherapy and Thermochemotherapy
Volume 1:
Biology, Physiology, and Physics
Volume 2:
Clinical Applications
Edited by M.H. Seegenschmiedt, P. Fessenden, and C.C. Vernon

Carcinoma of the Prostate
Innovations in Management
Edited by Z. Petrovich, L. Baert, and L.W. Brady

Radiation Oncology of Gynecological Cancers
Edited by H.W. Vahrson

Carcinoma of the Bladder
Innovations in Management
Edited by Z. Petrovich, L. Baert, and L.W. Brady

Blood Perfusion and Microenvironment of Human Tumors
Implications for Clinical Radiooncology
Edited by M. Molls and P. Vaupel

Radiation Therapy of Benign Diseases
A Clinical Guide
2nd Revised Edition
S. E. Order and S. S. Donaldson

Carcinoma of the Kidney and Testis, and Rare Urologic Malignancies
Innovations in Management
Edited by Z. Petrovich, L. Baert, and L.W. Brady

Progress and Perspectives in the Treatment of Lung Cancer
Edited by P. Van Houtte, J. Klastersky, and P. Rocmans

Combined Modality Therapy of Central Nervous System Tumors
Edited by Z. Petrovich, L. W. Brady, M. L. Apuzzo, and M. Bamberg

Age-Related Macular Degeneration
Current Treatment Concepts
Edited by W. A. Alberti, G. Richard, and R. H. Sagerman

Radiotherapy of Intraocular and Orbital Tumors
2nd Revised Edition
Edited by R. H. Sagerman, and W. E. Alberti

Biological Modification of Radiation Response
Edited by C. Nieder, L. Milas, and K. K. Ang

Palliative Radiation Oncology
R. G. Parker. N. A. Janjan, and M. T. Selch

Clinical Target Volumes in Conformal and Intensity Modulated Radiation Therapy
A Clinical Guide to Cancer Treatment
Edited by V. Grégoire, P. Scalliet, and K. K. Ang

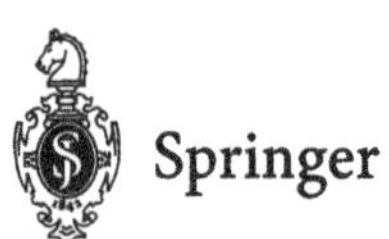

Springer

The manufacturer's authorised representative in the EU is Springer Nature Customer Service Centre GmbH, Europaplatz 3, 69115 Heidelberg, Germany. If you have any concerns regarding our products, please contact ProductSafety@springernature.com

Printed and bound by CPI Group (UK) Ltd, Croydon, CR0 4YY
28/04/2026
02098462-0010